Nursing Care in Pediatric Respiratory Disease

D1199532

618.92
N93t

Nursing Care in Pediatric Respiratory Disease

Edited by

Concettina (Tina) Tolomeo, DNP, APRN, FNP-BC, AE-C

Nurse Practitioner
Director, Program Development
Yale University School of Medicine
Department of Pediatrics
Section of Respiratory Medicine
New Haven, CT

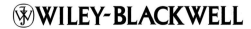
WILEY-BLACKWELL

A John Wiley & Sons, Inc., Publication

02/12

EP

64.99

This edition first published 2012 © 2012 by John Wiley & Sons, Inc.

Wiley-Blackwell is an imprint of John Wiley & Sons, formed by the merger of Wiley's global Scientific, Technical and Medical business with Blackwell Publishing.

Registered office: John Wiley & Sons Inc., The Atrium, Southern Gate, Chichester, West Sussex, PO19 8SQ, UK

Editorial offices: 2121 State Avenue, Ames, Iowa 50014-8300, USA
The Atrium, Southern Gate, Chichester, West Sussex, PO19 8SQ, UK
9600 Garsington Road, Oxford, OX4 2DQ, UK

For details of our global editorial offices, for customer services and for information about how to apply for permission to reuse the copyright material in this book please see our website at www.wiley.com/wiley-blackwell.

Authorization to photocopy items for internal or personal use, or the internal or personal use of specific clients, is granted by Blackwell Publishing, provided that the base fee is paid directly to the Copyright Clearance Center, 222 Rosewood Drive, Danvers, MA 01923. For those organizations that have been granted a photocopy license by CCC, a separate system of payments has been arranged. The fee codes for users of the Transactional Reporting Service are ISBN-13: 978-0-8138-1768-2/2012.

Designations used by companies to distinguish their products are often claimed as trademarks. All brand names and product names used in this book are trade names, service marks, trademarks or registered trademarks of their respective owners. The publisher is not associated with any product or vendor mentioned in this book. This publication is designed to provide accurate and authoritative information in regard to the subject matter covered. It is sold on the understanding that the publisher is not engaged in rendering professional services. If professional advice or other expert assistance is required, the services of a competent professional should be sought.

Library of Congress Cataloging-in-Publication Data

Nursing care in pediatric respiratory disease / edited by Concettina Tolomeo. – 1st ed.
      p. ; cm.
   Includes bibliographical references and index.
   ISBN-13: 978-0-8138-1768-2 (pbk. : alk. paper)
   ISBN-10: 0-8138-1768-4 (pbk. : alk. paper)
   1. Pediatric respiratory diseases–Nursing.   I. Tolomeo, Concettina.
   [DNLM: 1. Respiratory Tract Diseases–nursing.   2. Child.   3. Pediatric Nursing–methods. WY 163]
   RJ431.N87 2012
   618.92'2–dc23
                              2011021938

A catalogue record for this book is available from the British Library.

This book is published in the following electronic formats: ePDF 9780470962947; ePub 9780470962978; Mobi 9780470963005

Set in 9.5/12 pt Palatino by Toppan Best-set Premedia Limited
Printed and bound in Singapore by Fabulous Printers Pte Ltd

Disclaimer

The publisher and the author make no representations or warranties with respect to the accuracy or completeness of the contents of this work and specifically disclaim all warranties, including without limitation warranties of fitness for a particular purpose. No warranty may be created or extended by sales or promotional materials. The advice and strategies contained herein may not be suitable for every situation. This work is sold with the understanding that the publisher is not engaged in rendering legal, accounting, or other professional services. If professional assistance is required, the services of a competent professional person should be sought. Neither the publisher nor the author shall be liable for damages arising herefrom. The fact that an organization or Website is referred to in this work as a citation and/or a potential source of further information does not mean that the author or the publisher endorses the information the organization or Website may provide or recommendations it may make. Further, readers should be aware that Internet Websites listed in this work may have changed or disappeared between when this work was written and when it is read.

1   2011

On the cover: The Vest® Airway Clearance System is a registered trademark of Hill-Rom Services, Inc. REPRINTED WITH PERMISSION-ALL RIGHTS RESERVED.

This textbook is dedicated to my parents,
Nicolantonio and Caterina Tolomeo

Contents

Contributors

Dawn Baker, MSN, CPNP, CCRC
Nurse Practitioner
University of Florida
Gainesville, FL

Anita Bhandari, MD
Assistant Professor of Pediatrics
University of Connecticut School of Medicine
Farmington, CT;
Division of Pediatric Pulmonology
Connecticut Children's Medical Center
Hartford, CT

Kathryn Blake, PharmD, BCPS, FCCP
Senior Research Scientist
Center for Pharmacogenomics and Translational Research
Nemours Children's Clinic
Jacksonville, FL

Rosalynn Bravo, BS, MS, APRN, CPNP, AE-C
Division of Pediatric Pulmonology
Connecticut Children's Medical Center
Hartford, CT;
Adjunct Nursing Faculty
Capital Community College
Hartford, CT;
Clinical Instructor
Yale University School of Nursing
New Haven, CT

Michael Bye, MD, FAAP
Professor of Clinical Pediatrics
Attending Physician
Pediatric Pulmonary Medicine
Columbia University Medical Center
New York, NY

Melissa M. Dziedzic, MSN, CPNP, CORLN
Pediatric Nurse Practitioner
Connecticut Pediatric Otolaryngology
Madison, CT;
Lecturer in Surgery
Yale University School of Medicine;
Clinical Instructor in Pediatrics
Yale University School of Nursing
New Haven, CT

Lisa M. Gagnon, MSN, CPNP
Pediatric Nurse Practitioner
Connecticut Pediatric Otolaryngology
Madison, CT;
Lecturer in Surgery
Yale University School of Medicine;
Clinical Instructor in Pediatrics
Yale University School of Nursing
New Haven, CT

Antoinette Gardner, RN, MEd, CCRC, AE-C
Clinical and Research Nurse Coordinator
LSU Health Sciences Center
Pediatric Pulmonary
Shreveport, LA

Julie Honey, MSN, CPNP
Pediatric Nurse Practitioner
Summit Pediatric Pulmonology
Summit, NJ

Kimberly Jones, MD
Associate Professor
Chief, Pediatric Pulmonary
LSU Health Sciences Center
Shreveport, LA

Lewis J. Kass, MD
Founder
Westchester Pediatric Pulmonology and Sleep Medicine
Mount Kisco, NY;
Director
Pediatric Sleep Medicine
Pediatric Sleep Disorders Center at Norwalk Hospital
Norwalk, CT

Catherine Kier, MD
Associate Professor of Pediatrics
Stony Brook University School of Medicine;
Division Chief
Pediatric Pulmonary
Allergy and Immunology
Stony Brook Long Island Children's Hospital
Stony Brook, NY

Wendy S.L. Mackey, MSN, APRN-BC, CORLN
Pediatric Nurse Practitioner
Connecticut Pediatric Otolaryngology
Madison, CT;
Lecturer in Surgery
Yale University School of Medicine;
Clinical Instructor in Pediatrics
Yale University School of Nursing
New Haven, CT;
Adjunct Faculty
Quinnipiac University School of Nursing
Hamden, CT

Neal Nakra, MD, FAAP
Pediatric Pulmonologist
Codirector
Cystic Fibrosis Center
St. Joseph's Children's Hospital
Paterson, NJ

Linda Niemiec, MSN, RN, CPNP
Clinical Instructor of Nursing
New York University
New York, NY

Concettina Tolomeo, DNP, APRN, FNP-BC, AE-C
Nurse Practitioner
Program Development
Director
Yale University School of Medicine
Department of Pediatrics
Section of Respiratory Medicine
New Haven, CT

Pnina Weiss, MD
Assistant Professor of Pediatrics
Section of Respiratory Medicine
Director of Subspecialty Resident Education
Yale University School of Medicine
Section of Respiratory Medicine
New Haven, CT

Marcia Winston, MSN, CPNP, AE-C
Certified Pediatric Nurse Practitioner
Certified Asthma Educator
The Children's Hospital of Philadelphia
Division of Pulmonary Medicine
Philadelphia, PA

Preface

Pediatric respiratory disorders are responsible for a number of acute and chronic health conditions in the United States and worldwide. Nurses and nurse practitioners are often the first to come in contact with and recognize respiratory problems in children in either the school or a primary care setting. Therefore, the nursing profession as a whole must be knowledgeable in this area of care. The purpose of this book is to provide both nurses and nurse practitioners with the information required to safely and confidently care for children with common respiratory disorders and their families. The first three chapters of the book are intended to provide readers with a foundation for the specific conditions discussed later in the book. Chapter 1 presents an overview of the anatomy and physiology of the respiratory system; Chapter 2 provides a systematic approach to the assessment of a child with respiratory symptoms; and Chapter 3 provides information regarding common respiratory treatments and their methods of delivery. The remainder of the book details specific childhood respiratory conditions and their management in both hospital and ambulatory settings. The selection of which conditions to include was not an easy task as all conditions are important. However, the final conditions selected include a combination of common disorders encountered in both hospital and ambulatory settings and throughout the childhood years, from infancy to adolescence. Specific topic areas include apnea of prematurity, bronchopulmonary dysplasia, pneumonia, bronchiolitis, obstructive sleep apnea, foreign body aspiration, pneumothorax, respiratory failure, asthma, cystic fibrosis, ciliary dyskinesia, and bronchiectasis. Additionally, because the upper airway is so closely related to the lower airways, a chapter devoted to an overview of upper airway conditions has been included. Topics presented in this chapter include laryngotracheobronchitis, epiglottitis, vocal cord dysfunction, vocal cord paralysis, laryngomalacia, rhinitis, and sinusitis. To make the book user friendly, each chapter follows the same outline, which includes epidemiology, pathophysiology, signs and symptoms, diagnosis, complications, management, and nursing care of the child and family. Furthermore, the book is written such that the roles of both the nurse and the nurse practitioner are addressed.

Respiratory illnesses and nursing are two areas that are near and dear to my heart. As an infant, I was diagnosed and hospitalized with laryngotracheobronchitis. In addition, as a child, when everyone else wanted to be a teacher or an actress and played school or dress up, I wanted to be a nurse. Therefore, I am both honored and privileged to have played a role in making this book a reality for all nurses and nurse practitioners interested in respiratory conditions. I hope that you enjoy the practical nature of this book and find it to be a useful reference during both your educational preparation as well as your career as a nursing professional.

Concettina (Tina) Tolomeo

Acknowledgments

I would like to thank the following people for helping make this book possible:

Dr. Kathleen Conboy-Ellis for making the initial proposal.

Shelby Allen and Melissa Wahl at Wiley-Blackwell for always being there.

The nursing schools at Southern Connecticut State University and Case Western Reserve University for providing excellent educational experiences.

My colleagues for their support and willingness to contribute to this worthwhile endeavor.

My patients and their families for teaching me the practical side of pediatric respiratory medicine and what it's like to live with respiratory problems.

My family, mamma, papá, Elvira, Marisa, Giacomo, Greg, Kyle, Louie, Adriana, Antonia, Giana, and Nico, for their never-ending love and support and for being the best family a person could ask for. I love you!

C.T.

Reviewers

Alia Bazzy-Asaad, MD
Associate Professor of Pediatrics
Chief, Section of Pediatric Respiratory Medicine
Yale University School of Medicine
New Haven, CT

Aaron Chidekel, MD
Associate Professor of Pediatrics
Jefferson Medical College of Thomas Jefferson University
Philadelphia, PA
Chief, Division of Pulmonology
Nemours/duPont Hospital for Children
Wilmington DE

Melinda DeSell, MS, CRNP
Pediatric Nurse Practitioner
Division of Pediatric Otolaryngology
Johns Hopkins Hospital
Baltimore, MD

Marie E Egan, MD
Associate Professor of Pediatrics and Cellular and Molecular Physiology
Yale University School of Medicine
Section of Respiratory Medicine
New Haven, CT

Richard A. Ehrenkranz, MD
Professor of Pediatrics and of Obstetrics, Gynecology, and Reproductive Sciences
Division of Perinatal Medicine
Yale University School of Medicine
New Haven, CT

Antonina G. Evans, BPharm, RPh, AE-C
Clinical Consultant
Catalyst Rx
Las Vegas, NV

Edward Vincent S. Faustino, MD
Assistant Professor of Pediatrics
Yale University School of Medicine
Section of Pediatric Critical Care Medicine
New Haven, CT

Maureen George, PhD, RN, AE-C, FAAN
Assistant Professor
University of Pennsylvania School of Nursing
Family and Community Health Division
Center for Health Equity Research
Philadelphia, PA

Stephen Jones, MS, RN, CPNP, ET
Pediatric Clinical Nurse Specialist/Nurse Practitioner and Enterostomal
Therapist
Children's Hospital at Albany Medical Center
Albany, NY
Founder and Principal, Pediatric Concepts
Averill Park, NY

Holger Link, MD, MRCP (UK)
Clinical Associate Professor
Doernbecher Pediatric Sleep Disorders Program
Oregon Health & Science University
Portland, OR

Barbara Sabo, MSN, APRN, NNP-BC
APRN, Coordinator ECMO Program
Yale New Haven Children's Hospital
Newborn Special Care Unit
New Haven, CT

Pnina Weiss, MD
Assistant Professor of Pediatrics
Section of Respiratory Medicine
Director of Subspecialty Resident Education
Yale University School of Medicine
Section of Respiratory Medicine
New Haven, CT

Nursing Care in Pediatric Respiratory Disease

Pediatric pulmonary anatomy and physiology

Neal Nakra, MD, FAAP

INTRODUCTION

In ancient Greece, Erasistratus (304–250 BC), an anatomist and royal physician, was among the first to distinguish between veins and arteries. He described the function of the lungs was to bring air into the body to be transferred to the arteries and then into the heart (Mason, 1962). Our understanding of the anatomy and physiology of the human respiratory system has progressed significantly over the past 2,000-plus years. This chapter will explore the structure of the lung and describe the physiological properties that support ventilation and gas exchange through different stages of development of the respiratory system, from fetus to maturity.

ANATOMY OF THE RESPIRATORY SYSTEM

Embryology

To appreciate the complex physiology of breathing, one must understand the events that occur before the first breath is taken at birth. *In utero*, the lung does not participate in gas exchange. The responsibility of fetal oxygenation and elimination of carbon dioxide lies with the placenta until the

Nursing Care in Pediatric Respiratory Disease, First Edition. Edited by Concettina (Tina) Tolomeo.
© 2012 John Wiley & Sons, Inc. Published 2012 by John Wiley & Sons, Inc.

lung takes over the process immediately upon transition from prenatal to postnatal life.

Lung growth *in utero* can be divided into five overlapping stages: (1) the embryonic period during the first 5 weeks, (2) the pseudoglandular period from 6 to 16 weeks of gestation, (3) the canalicular period from 16 to 24 weeks of gestation, (4) the saccular period from 24 to 36 weeks, and (5) the alveolar phase from 36 weeks to term and continuing for at least 3 years postnatally (Jeffery, 1998). The alveoli continue to multiply and grow during the first few years of life, following the growth in height of each child.

During the embryonic period, the primitive foregut, seen in the third week of embryogenesis, forms and is the origin of the lung. Over the course of the next 3–4 weeks, branches of the right and left lung form through budding and dividing (see Figure 1.1).

During the pseudoglandular period, there is a differentiation of the primitive airway epithelium (Post & Copland, 2002). At the time of branching, the bronchi are enveloped in the mesenchyme that develops into connective tissue, smooth muscle, and cartilaginous rings, among other things. By the end of the 16th week, the bronchial tree is developed without further formation of airways.

During the canalicular stage, further branching of the bronchioles leads to respiratory bronchioles. The lobules of the lungs start to form, and there is a decrease in interstitial tissue. The differentiation of cuboidal epithelium into types I and II pneumocytes begins at this time (DiFiore & Wilson, 1994). Cartilage starts centrally and proceeds peripherally, ending around the 25th week. It is at this point that the number of bronchial generations with cartilage is the same as the adult lung.

The saccular phase is the period when there is growth of the pulmonary parenchyma, continued development of the surfactant system, and a reduction in the connective tissue between the airspaces. During the alveolar period, branching becomes more extensive. There is an exponential increase in the surface area as saccules, which will eventually form alveoli, develop (Burri, 1984). It is during this time that surface epithelium and blood vessels come into even closer contact, allowing for the future exchange of gases. This process continues for at least 3 years after birth.

The fetal lung is the main source of amniotic fluid in the uterus. Abnormal lungs secondary to poor intrauterine growth are among the many abnormalities associated with a low amount of amniotic fluid. Type II pneumocytes appear in the alveolar epithelium and begin to function around the 24th week of life. These cells go on to produce a surfactant, which is a mixture of phospholipids and proteins. The surfactant decreases the surface tension of the lung, allowing for maturation and, upon delivery, expansion of the lung with the newborn's first breaths. When expectant mothers begin premature labor, administration of glucocorticoids to the mother accelerates the maturation of type II pneumocytes and therefore the production of surfactants (Liggins & Howie, 1972). The molecular

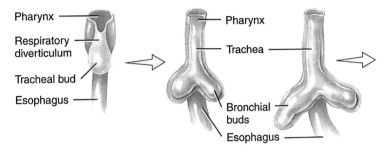

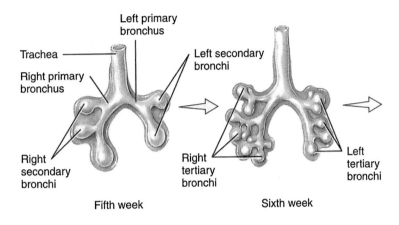

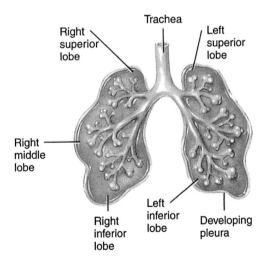

Figure 1.1 Development of the bronchial tubes and lungs. Reprinted from Tortora and Derrickson (2009), with permission from John Wiley & Sons, Inc.

properties of surfactants and the physiological role they play is discussed in the section "Surface Tension Properties of the Lung."

Just before full-term birth, there is approximately 50 mL of surfactant-rich fluid in the lung. This fluid is removed by a combination of active channel transport, lymphatic drainage, and the physics of natural childbirth. Most of the protein-rich portion of this fluid is removed by the lymphatic system. At birth, expansion of the chest cavity with high negative intrathoracic pressures pushes the fluid from the alveoli into the interstitium, then onto the lymphatic channels. By the end of the first few hours after birth, the majority of fluid that was in the lungs during the 9 months of gestation is replaced by air.

During gestation, the lungs do not function as the source of oxygen for the developing organs of the body. That task is completed by the placenta. As a result, the lungs receive poorly oxygenated blood in comparison to the more "vital" fetal organs (see Figure 1.2).

Fetal circulation receives highly oxygenated blood from the placenta through the liver to the right side of the heart. Most of the blood is shunted through the foramen ovale to the left side of the heart. It then either flows through the ascending aorta to the head or through the descending aorta to the systemic circulation. The venous blood that returns from the head flows through the right side of the heart to the pulmonary artery. However, most of this blood is shunted via the ductus arteriosus into the descending aorta to the systemic circulation and the lower part of the body. That blood which does not go through the ductus arteriosus is the blood that oxygenates the lungs. Again, it needs to be pointed out that this blood has already passed through the brain, an organ requiring large amounts of oxygen. As a result, 9 months of this poorly oxygenated circulating blood results from and contributes to the high pulmonary vascular resistance *in utero.*

Replacement of lung fluid by air upon delivery and breathing by the newborn contributes to the decrease in the pulmonary vascular resistance. The subsequent increase in the partial pressure of oxygen (PO_2) and the decrease in the partial pressure of carbon dioxide remove stimuli for vasoconstriction. All of this occurs in association with the reversal of the right-to-left shunt through the ductus arteriosus and foramen ovale present *in utero.* The ductus closes completely during the first few days after birth.

Pulmonary vascular development and the tracheobronchial tree

There are two types of airways based on structure and function: (1) cartilaginous airways (bronchi), which make up the conducting system, and (2) membranous, noncartilaginous airways (bronchioles) (see Figure 1.3). The bronchi and nonrespiratory bronchioles serve as conductors of the gas stream, while the respiratory bronchioles and alveolar ducts (terminal respiratory units) serve as sites of gas exchange. The cartilaginous rings of the trachea, except for the cricoid, are not complete and occur over the anterior two-thirds of its surface. The posterior portion is membranous and pliable (Johnson, 2008). The conducting airways' blood supply comes from branches of the bronchial arteries and the terminal respiratory units from branches of the pulmonary arteries.

From the trachea to the alveolar sacs, the airway divides 23 times. The first 16 generations form the conducting zone, while the last 7 generations form the transitional and respiratory zone (Sircar, 2008). As stated

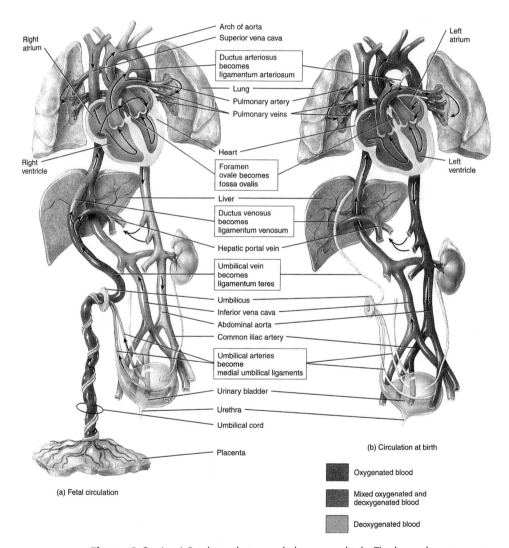

(a) Fetal circulation

(b) Circulation at birth

Oxygenated blood

Mixed oxygenated and deoxygenated blood

Deoxygenated blood

Figure 1.2 (a–c) Fetal circulation and changes at birth. The boxes between parts (a) and (b) describe the fate of certain fetal structures once postnatal circulation is established. Reprinted from Tortora and Derrickson (2009), with permission from John Wiley & Sons, Inc.

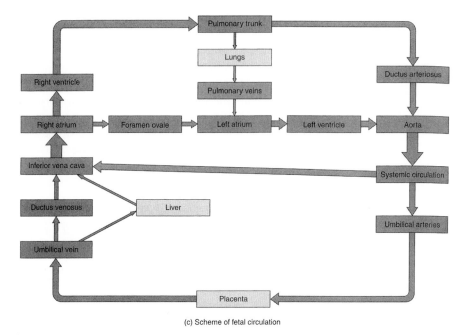

(c) Scheme of fetal circulation

Figure 1.2 (*Continued*)

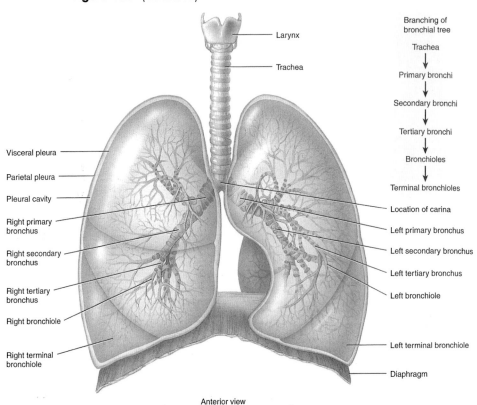

Larynx

Trachea

Branching of
bronchial tree

Trachea
↓
Primary bronchi
↓
Secondary bronchi
↓
Tertiary bronchi
↓
Bronchioles
↓
Terminal bronchioles

Visceral pleura

Parietal pleura

Pleural cavity

Right primary
bronchus

Right secondary
bronchus

Right tertiary
bronchus

Right bronchiole

Right terminal
bronchiole

Location of carina

Left primary bronchus

Left secondary bronchus

Left tertiary bronchus

Left bronchiole

Left terminal bronchiole

Diaphragm

Anterior view

Figure 1.3 Branching of airways from the trachea: the bronchial tree. Reprinted from Tortora and Derrickson (2009), with permission from John Wiley & Sons, Inc.

previously, the conducting airways are in place and are fully formed by birth. However, alveoli are just starting to develop at this point.

While the lung bud is forming, the right and left pulmonary arteries are growing as well; branches of the pulmonary arteries follow branches of the bronchi. By the end of the pseudoglandular period, the conducting airways are complete and have an adult pattern, as are all conventional and super-numerary arteries leading to the terminal respiratory units. The pattern of veins from the sites of gas exchange to the hilum, similar to the conducting airways, is complete halfway through gestation. Conversely, just as alveo-lar formation continues after birth, the arteries within the terminal unit continue to form for several years after birth.

RESPIRATORY AND NONRESPIRATORY FUNCTIONS OF THE LUNG

Nongas exchange functions

The upper airway and tracheobronchial tree do not participate in gas exchange; however, they provide other very important functions. The upper airway warms and humidifies the inspired air and filters out par-ticulate matter. By the time the air reaches the alveoli, it is near body temperature. The hairs in the nostril filter particles larger than $10\,\mu m$ in diameter. Most of the smaller particles do not travel past the pharynx and are trapped by the tonsils and adenoids. Cilia, which line the respiratory tract down to the terminal bronchioles, pick up any particles between 2–$10\,\mu m$ in size that may have passed through the conducting airways. The cilia are covered in a layer of mucus produced by mucus glands and goblet cells. The cilia move in a synchronized beat carrying these particles up to the larynx where they are swept up to the hypopharynx and swallowed. An abnormality in structure or function of the cilia results in primary ciliary dysfunction, a condition that results in buildup of secretions and a subsequent propensity of bacterial growth in this medium (Johnson, 2008). A similar picture is seen in the lungs of patients with cystic fibrosis, not because of an abnormality of the cilia but because of an abnormality of the mucus layer.

Gases and gas exchange

Transfer of gases through the airways

In humans, as the airway branches from the trachea, the branches become smaller and more numerous. Initially from the trachea, the right and left main bronchi divide to lobar (secondary) followed by segmental (tertiary) bronchi and finally to terminal (0.5 mm in diameter) bronchioles. The walls of the primary bronchi are constructed like the trachea, but as the branches

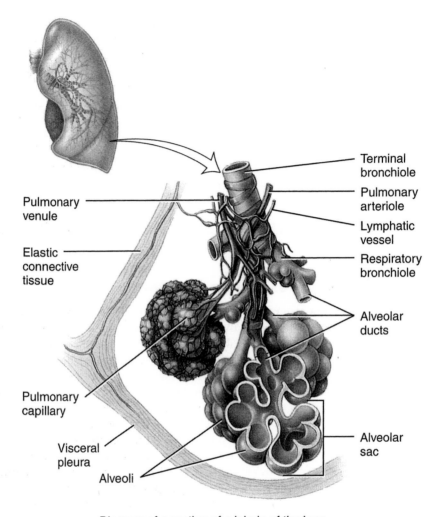

Diagram of a portion of a lobule of the lung

Figure 1.4 Microscopic anatomy of a lobule of the lungs. Reprinted from Tortora and Derrickson (2009), with permission from John Wiley & Sons, Inc.

of the tree decrease in size, the cartilaginous rings and the mucosa are replaced by smooth muscle. To this point, there are no alveoli. As a result, this portion of the lung is anatomical dead space, as there is no participation in gas exchange. These branches mark the first 16 generations of airways and, based on their main function in the lung, are referred to as the conducting airways. This would be analogous to the branches of a tree (see Figure 1.4).

The area where gas exchange occurs is known as the respiratory zone. The occasional alveoli off the walls of the respiratory bronchioles are the first site of gas exchange in the respiratory tree. Alveoli, which is Latin for little cavities, are particular to mammalian lungs. They contain collagen and elastic fibers and are lined with epithelium. The elastic fibers allow the alveoli to stretch with inhalation and retract during exhalation (this is explained in more detail in the section "Control of Ventilation"). Further distal are alveolar ducts and alveolar sacs, which are completely lined with alveoli. Harkening back to the earlier analogy, the respiratory zone would be the leaves on the tree.

Each human lung contains about 300 million alveoli. Each alveolus is wrapped in a fine mesh of capillaries. The alveoli in the respiratory zone of the lungs constitute a total surface area of about 75 m² (Pavelka & Roth, 2005). The gas exchange tissue is referred to as the pulmonary parenchyma, while the nonparenchyma consists of the conducting airways, lymphatics, noncapillary blood vessels, and the supplying structures.

Transfer of gas in the parenchyma

Diffusion

Inspired fresh air moves via bulk movement through the conducting airways. Here, different gases move together along a total pressure gradient. Because of the vast branching of the bronchi and the subsequent increase in the cross-sectional area of the respiratory zone, the velocity of the bulk flow rapidly decreases. As a result, once in the respiratory zone, further movement occurs via diffusion. Diffusion, the movement from an area of high to low pressure, is the principle by which oxygen and carbon dioxide move in different directions between the air and blood. Unicellular organisms do not require respiratory structures for diffusion. However, for more complex organisms, specialized organs have evolved, including gills in fish and lungs in humans (Rhoades & Planzer, 1996). In all these organisms, the underlying basis for the diffusion of gas is the presence of thin walls and a rich supply of blood vessels to allow for exchange and transport of gases.

Different gases move according to each of their partial pressure gradients. From the alveolar sacs, oxygen diffuses into the pulmonary capillary blood. An important concept to discuss here is Fick's law, which describes diffusion through tissues. Essentially, the rate of transfer of a gas across a surface is directly proportional to the product of the tissue surface area and the difference in gas partial pressure between the two sides of a tissue and is inversely proportional to the thickness of the tissue:

$$V_{gas} = [A \times (P_1 - P_2)]/T,$$

where V_{gas} = volume of gas diffusing through a tissue per time;
A = surface area of the tissue;
$P_1 - P_2$ = partial pressure difference of gas across the tissue; and
T = thickness of the tissue.

Based on these relationships, it becomes clear how the human lung is ideal for gas transfer: The gas exchange surface is very thin (0.2–0.5 µm) and the surface area vast.

After diffusing through the alveolar–capillary interface, that is, the air–blood barrier, the oxygen molecule enters the red blood cell in the pulmonary capillary, combining with hemoglobin (Hb). The exchange of oxygen from the alveolus into the pulmonary capillary blood occurs rapidly with the pressures equalizing in the two areas in 0.25 second. However, the blood requires 0.75 second to move through the pulmonary capillary bed under resting conditions. Approximately 85–95% of the alveolar surface is intertwined with pulmonary capillaries, with 280 billion capillaries supplying 300 million alveoli (Levitzky, 2007).

Because the PO_2 in a red blood cell entering a pulmonary capillary equals the PO_2 in the alveolus one-third of the way through the capillary, the transfer of oxygen is defined as perfusion limited. In other words, the amount of oxygen taken up by the blood is dependent on the amount of blood flow through the capillaries. The fact that under normal circumstances oxygen transfer is perfusion limited does not do justice to the enormous diffusion reserve of the human lung. The PO_2 in the red blood cell at the initial portion of the pulmonary capillary is 40 mmHg. Across the thin alveolar wall, the PO_2 is 100 mmHg. Now, applying Fick's law, consider the enormous surface area of the respiratory zone, the microscopic thickness of the blood–gas barrier, and the large pressure gradient between the barrier. It becomes obvious under normal conditions why the PO_2 in the red cell approximates the PO_2 of the alveolar gas in 0.25 second.

As with much of physiology, abnormal conditions, or pathophysiology sheds more light on normal conditions. Perfusion limitation is most often seen in disease states where there is decreased surface area and/or increased thickness of the alveolar–capillary interface. The rate of diffusion will be slowed, but the PO_2 of the end capillary red cell is still able to equal the PO_2 of alveolar gas. However, with vigorous and prolonged exercise, there is up to a threefold increase in cardiac output and pulmonary blood flow (West, 2003). With the increase in transit time through the pulmonary capillary bed, blood runs through the pulmonary capillaries in less than 0.75 second. In conditions where there is an increased thickness or a decreased surface area, the PO_2 in the capillaries is unable to equalize the partial pressure in the alveolus, leading to diffusion limitation. Disease states in which there is an increased thickness of the alveolar–capillary interface include neonatal chronic lung disease and interstitial lung disease. A decrease in the surface area is seen in emphysema (Bates, 1962). In someone without lung disease, the increase in transit time through the pulmonary circulation will not affect end-capillary PO_2. Clinically, this is part of the explanation for decreased exercise tolerance in these disease states.

Now take for example persons without lung disease, but place them in an abnormal environment. Again, according to Fick's law, one of the factors in the diffusion of a gas is the difference in partial pressures. The atmospheric PO_2, that is, the pressure that determines the pressure gradient, is assumed to be constant, which at sea level it is. However, the pressure gradient changes in a location of higher altitude. Elevations of 6,500 ft (2,000 m) are classified as high altitude because of this difference in the PO_2, but depending on the person, this effect of altitude may be experienced at lower elevations.

At sea level, oxygen has a partial pressure of 159 mmHg. In Mexico City, it is approximately 125 mmHg, while at the top of Everest, it drops to 48 mmHg (Wilmore & Costill, 2005). Therefore, at the top of Everest, the PO_2 is nearly equal to the PO_2 at the initial portion of the pulmonary capillary, markedly decreasing the pressure gradient that is the driving force for the transfer of oxygen into Hb (Peacock, 1998) (see Figure 1.5).

The human body attempts to overcome the difference in the pressure gradient of oxygen by controlling what it can, in this case, increasing the transportation capability of oxygen. Erythropoietin (EPO) is a glycoprotein released by the kidney that increases the production of red blood cells in the bone marrow. Within hours at high altitudes, EPO levels increase, and 4 days later, new red blood cells are produced (Harris, Terrio, Miser, & Yetter,

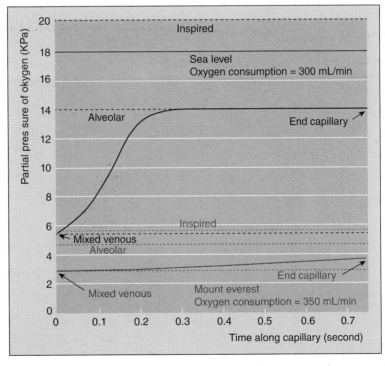

Figure 1.5 Calculated time course for change in partial pressure of oxygen in the pulmonary capillary. At sea level, oxygen pressure reaches almost alveolar levels in a third of available time. At the summit of Mount Everest, the mixed venous oxygen pressure is lower and never reaches alveolar levels. Reprinted from Peacock (1998), with permission from BMJ Publishing Group, Ltd.

1998). This leads to 75% acclimatization at 7–10 days and 100% acclimatization by 15–20 days. Synthetic EPO has been used by athletes as a performance-enhancing drug to increase Hb and, therefore, oxygen carrying capacity. This has most notably been seen in the Tour de France cycling event.

In individuals accustomed to high altitudes, the concentration of 2,3-diphosphoglycerate (2,3-DPG) in the blood is increased. 2,3-DPG allows these individuals to deliver a larger amount of oxygen to tissues under conditions of lower oxygen tension. This is further explored in the section "Oxyhemoglobin."

In 1968, the Olympics were held in Mexico City. These were the first games staged at a high altitude (7,349 ft [2,300 m]). The number of world records set and the categories in which they were set in fueled extensive research. The higher altitude led to reduced wind resistance and drag upon the competitors' bodies. This explained why records in almost every short distance track event from the 100 to 1,500 m were set. However, this was not the case with long-distance events. Athletes in events that involved prolonged aerobic activity and, subsequently, dependency upon maximal amounts of oxygen were adversely affected by the decrease in the atmospheric PO_2 (Jenkins, 2005). Because of this, the International Association of Athletic Federations specifically denotes track and field records that have been broken at altitudes greater than 1,000 m.

A significant amount of research was conducted in the wake of the Mexico City Olympics. As a result, the initial United States Olympic Training Center was built in 1978 on an Air Force base in Colorado Springs, Colorado, to take advantage of the physiological principles of high-altitude training.

As stated previously, under normal conditions, the diffusion of oxygen in the human lung is perfusion limited. In contrast, the diffusion of carbon monoxide (CO) is diffusion limited. This is because carbon monoxide bonds very strongly to Hb. This diffusion can occur with a large amount of carbon monoxide without a significant increase in the partial pressure of carbon monoxide (PCO) (Levitzky, 2007).

These gas properties were utilized in developing a pulmonary function test that measures diffusion in the lung. Because the diffusion of oxygen is not measurable, CO is used for testing. This test, the diffusing capacity of the lung for carbon monoxide (DL_{CO}), is based on the high affinity of Hb for CO and on the negligible partial pressure for CO in Hb. Again using Fick's law, the diffusing capacity of the lung is equal to the volume of carbon monoxide transferred divided by the alveolar PCO. The single-breath DL_{CO} test uses this calculation. A single inspiration of dilute CO is made, and after a 10-second breath hold, the rate of disappearance of CO is measured allowing the difference in partial pressures of inspired and expired carbon monoxide to be determined. The enormity of the surface area of the lung and the inability to measure the thickness of the blood–gas barrier precludes using these two factors in the above-mentioned calculation. However, both of these aspects impact the volume of CO transferred and the PCO. Therefore, abnormalities in these areas will lead to abnormal DL_{CO} measurements.

Conditions that *decrease* alveolar surface area and therefore *decrease* DL_{CO} include (1) uneven distribution of oxygen in the lung as seen in emphysema and (2) lung injury secondary to bleomycin administration. Conditions that *increase* the alveolar–capillary barrier and therefore decrease DL_{CO} include (1) interstitial or alveolar edema and (2) interstitial or alveolar fibrosis as seen with vasculitis, such as sarcoidosis and scleroderma. Conditions that *increase* DL_{CO} include (1) polycythemia, (2) increased pulmonary blood volume as occurs in exercise or congestive heart failure, and (3) alveolar hemorrhage. The increase in Hb available to bind CO is common to all of these conditions, explaining higher DL_{CO} measurements.

TRANSPORT OF GAS IN THE RED BLOOD CELL

Oxyhemoglobin

The movement of oxygen from the outside environment down the respiratory tract into the alveoli has been discussed. The following explains the mechanisms by which oxygen moves from the alveolus into the pulmonary capillaries and, more specifically, the physiology of the binding of oxygen to Hb.

Heme is an iron compound that is bound to globin, a protein made up of four polypeptides. The iron atom at the center of the heme group is bound to four symmetrically arranged pyrroles and one of four polypeptide chains. The combination of alpha and beta polypeptide chains and the difference in amino acid sequences determines the type of Hb, including normal adult hemoglobin (HbA), fetal hemoglobin (HbF), and hemoglobin S (HbS) (sickle), among others. Each of the four polypeptide chains can bind a molecule of oxygen, though with different affinity (Levitzky, 2007).

HbF has two alpha chains and two gamma chains and has a higher affinity for oxygen than does normal HbA, which has two alpha chains and two beta chains. This distinction is important for oxygen transportation from the placenta *in utero*, where HbF is the predominant form. Beta chains begin to be produced toward the end of the saccular phase, approximately 6 weeks before birth. HbF all but disappears from circulation by 4 months of age in the infant without hemoglobinopathies.

Oxygen combines with Hb to form oxyhemoglobin. One gram of Hb can combine with 1.39 mL of oxygen (Dominguez de Villota, Ruiz Carmona, Rubio, & de Andrés, 1981). However, some Hb exists as methemoglobin, or is combined with carbon monoxide. Therefore, the oxygen capacity, the maximum amount of oxygen that can combine with Hb, under normal conditions, is 1.34 mL O_2/g Hb. Using the example of a person with an Hb concentration of 15 g/dL, the oxygen carrying capacity would be

$$\frac{15\,\text{g Hb}}{100\,\text{mL of blood}} \times \frac{1.34\,\text{mL O}_2}{\text{g Hb}} = \frac{20.1\,\text{mL O}_2}{100\,\text{mL blood}}.$$

The oxygen saturation of Hb is the amount of oxygen attached to Hb divided by the oxygen capacity. The normal oxygen saturation for arterial blood is over 97%, while in venous blood, it is about 75%.

Oxygen in the blood is transported in two forms: bound to Hb and dissolved in the plasma. While the majority of the oxygen is bound to Hb, a small proportion is dissolved, with the amount dependent on the PO_2. For each 1 mmHg PO_2, there is 0.003 mL O_2 dissolved in 100 mL of plasma. Therefore, the total oxygen concentration of blood (mL O_2/100 mL of blood) is equal to the summation of these two forms:

$$(1.34 \times \text{Hb} \times \text{percentage saturation of Hb}) + 0.003\ PO_2.$$

These relationships explain how one can have normal saturation of Hb and PO_2 but still have a low oxygen concentration of blood if there is severe anemia.

The relationship of the PO_2 of plasma and the Hb saturation is represented graphically by the oxygen dissociation curve (see Figure 1.6).

At normal conditions (pH 7.4, PCO_2 40 mmHg, and 37°), a sigmoid curve describes the relationship between PO_2 on the x-axis and the percent

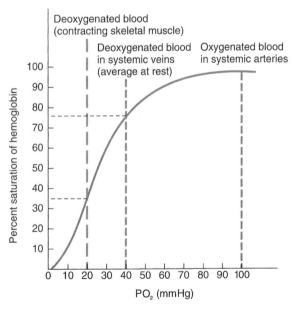

Figure 1.6 Oxygen–hemoglobin dissociation curve showing the relationship between hemoglobin saturation and PO_2 at normal body temperature. Reprinted from Tortora and Derrickson (2009), with permission from John Wiley & Sons, Inc.

saturation of Hb on the y-axis. This figure helps in understanding much of the physiology of Hb and its ability to carry oxygen to the tissues, dissociate with it, and then carry CO_2 back to the lungs.

The oxygen dissociation curve demonstrates why the Hb molecule is the ideal vehicle for combining and dissociating with oxygen. As discussed earlier, the PO_2 at the initial portion of the pulmonary capillary is 40 mmHg, while across the alveolar wall, the PO_2 is 100 mmHg. On the curve, between 40 and 60 mmHg there is steep increase in oxygen saturation. Under normal circumstances, oxygen is transferred rapidly from the alveolus to the red blood cell, and Hb is saturated with oxygen one-third of the way through the pulmonary capillary. The reason for this speed is the continued difference in PO_2 between the alveolar and the pulmonary capillary even after the oxygen has been transferred (100 mmHg vs. 60 mmHg).

Above approximately 60 mmHg, the curve flattens, indicating that the oxygen concentration and Hb saturation do not increase as much for a given increase in the PO_2. This allows for the circumstance when the alveolar PO_2 falls, without causing a significant decrease in the capillary uptake of oxygen. How then can the oxygen concentration of blood increase past this point? Looking back at the formula, it would require (1) an increase in the Hb concentration via transfusion or (2) supplemental oxygen to increase the amount of oxygen dissolved in plasma.

At the lower portion of the curve, below PO_2 of 50 mmHg, the curve is very steep, denoting a decreased affinity of Hb for oxygen. PO_2 levels in this range are found in peripheral tissues, facilitating the unloading of oxygen from Hb in this environment. The steep slope for this range of PO_2 allows for the transfer of large amounts of oxygen for small decreases in capillary PO_2. The PO_2 at which Hb is 50% saturated is known as the P50. For a healthy adult, P50 is 26.6 mmHg and can be visualized by drawing a line from 50% Hb saturation down to the x-intercept.

There are a variety of abnormal conditions that will affect the oxyhemoglobin dissociation curve. Conditions that decrease the affinity of Hb for oxygen will shift the curve to the right, indicating that it will be more difficult for Hb to bind oxygen (see Figures 1.7 and 1.8). As a corollary, a shift to the right leads to more unloading of oxygen for a given PO_2. This situation occurs with an increase in PCO_2, hydrogen ion concentration, temperature, and the concentration of 2,3-DPG (an end product of red cell metabolism). Physiologically, this occurs in exercising muscles, where the environment is acidic, hot, and hypercarbic and is most in need of oxygen. 2,3-DPG is increased in chronic hypoxia, chronic lung disease, anemia and (as stated previously) at high altitudes. These are all instances in which the unloading of oxygen would ideally be maximized.

On the other hand a decrease in the PCO_2, which is mostly secondary to a decrease in the hydrogen ion concentration (this will be discussed further in the section "Acid–Base Balance"), leads to a left shift and an increased affinity for oxygen. Naturally, this is what is seen in the lungs.

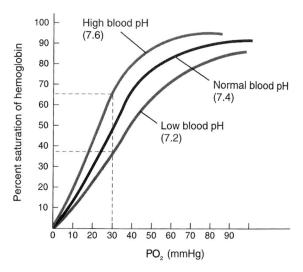

(a) Effect of pH on affinity of hemoglobin for oxygen

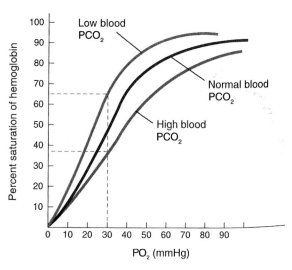

(b) Effect of PCO$_2$ on affinity of hemoglobin for oxygen

Figure 1.7 Oxygen–hemoglobin dissociation curves showing the relationship of (a) pH and (b) PCO$_2$ to hemoglobin saturation at normal body temperature. As pH increases or PCO$_2$ decreases, O$_2$ combines more tightly with hemoglobin so that less is available to tissues. The broken lines emphasize these relationships. Reprinted from Tortora and Derrickson (2009), with permission from John Wiley & Sons, Inc.

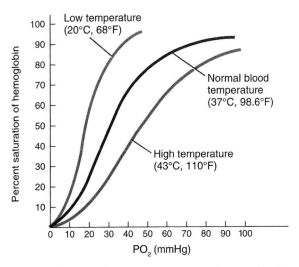

Figure 1.8 Oxygen–hemoglobin dissociation curves showing the effect of temperature changes. Reprinted from Tortora and Derrickson (2009), with permission from John Wiley & Sons, Inc.

Hb binds with carbon monoxide 240 times more readily than with oxygen. The presence of carbon monoxide on one of the four heme sites causes a stronger binding of oxygen on the other sites. Even small amounts of CO make it difficult for Hb to release oxygen to the tissues, leading to a leftward shift of the curve. A CO concentration as low as 667 ppm can cause up to 50% conversion of Hb to carboxyhemoglobin (Tikuisis, Kane, McLellan, Buick, & Fairburn, 1992). This will lead to severe hypoxemia despite a normal Hb concentration and PO_2 of blood (see Figure 1.9).

As mentioned earlier, there are different types of Hb, the most common of which are HbA, HbF, and HbS. Their properties are highlighted by their individual oxygen dissociation curve. HbA is the normal adult Hb, while HbS has a difference in the beta chain with a valine substituted for glutamic acid. HbS is the Hb chain seen in sickle cell disease. The dissociation curve for HbS is shifted to the right in comparison to HbA. HbF has a dissociation curve that is shifted to the left relative to HbA. This makes sense physiologically, as fetal arterial oxygen pressures are low and the leftward shift enhances the placental uptake of oxygen. At the placenta, there is also a higher concentration of 2,3-DPG, which causes the HbA to release more oxygen, to be taken up by the fetus.

Carboxyhemoglobin

The uptake and delivery of oxygen from the lungs to the tissues is one-half of the equation. The other half has to do with the tissues' production of carbon dioxide (CO_2) and its transport to the lungs for elimination via exhalation. Like oxygen, carbon dioxide is found dissolved in blood, but

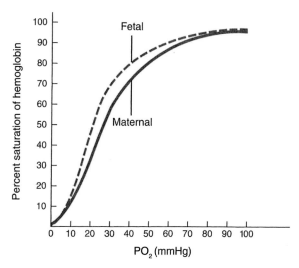

Figure 1.9 Oxygen–hemoglobin dissociation curves comparing fetal and maternal hemoglobin. Reprinted from Tortora and Derrickson (2009), with permission from John Wiley & Sons, Inc.

for carbon dioxide, this makes up a much more significant portion. CO_2 is 20 times as soluble as O_2, leading to 10% of CO_2 exhaled from the lungs coming from the dissolved form of CO_2 (see Figure 1.10).

Within the red blood cell is an enzyme, carbonic anhydrase, which catalyzes the combination of CO_2 and water (H_2O) into carbonic acid (H_2CO_3). Carbonic acid quickly dissociates into hydrogen ions (H^+) and bicarbonate (HCO_3^-):

$$CO_2 + H_2O \rightarrow H_2CO_3 \rightarrow HCO_3^- + H^+.$$

This catalyzed reaction is reversed in the lungs, where H^+ reacts with bicarbonate to form carbonic acid and then CO_2, which is exhaled into the outside environment. Approximately 80–90% of carbon dioxide in the blood is carried in the form of bicarbonate. As shown by this reaction, blood with high carbon dioxide levels will result in a higher H^+ concentration and therefore a lower pH (more acidic).

Hb that has unloaded oxygen in peripheral tissues is known as reduced Hb, or deoxyhemoglobin. Deoxyhemoglobin is a weaker acid than oxyhemoglobin and therefore combines with H^+, which is liberated during the dissociation of carbonic acid. This allows for more CO_2 to be transported as bicarbonate ion. The binding of H^+ with amino acids of Hb also lowers the affinity of Hb for oxygen. An acidic environment with more H^+ ion available will result in a shift of the oxygen dissociation curve to the right, where the affinity of Hb for oxygen is lower. Hence, we have the Haldane effect, which states that deoxygenation of blood leads to an increased

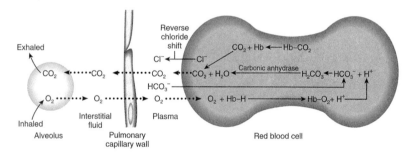

(a) Exchange of O_2 and CO_2 in pulmonary capillaries (external respiration)

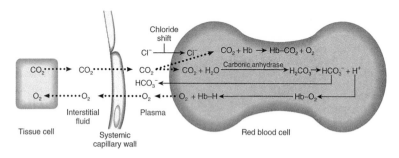

(b) Exchange of O_2 and CO_2 in systemic capillaries (internal respiration)

Figure 1.10 Summary of chemical reactions that occur during gas exchange. (a) As carbon dioxide (CO_2) is exhaled, hemoglobin (Hb) inside red blood cells (RBCs) in pulmonary capillaries unloads CO_2 and picks up O_2 from alveolar air. Binding of O_2 to Hb–H releases hydrogen ions (H^+). Bicarbonate ions (HCO_3^-) pass into the RBC and bind to released H^+, forming carbonic acid (H_2CO_3). The H_2CO_3 dissociates into water (H_2O) and CO_2, and the CO_2 diffuses from the blood into alveolar air. To maintain electrical balance, a chloride ion (Cl^-) exits the RBC for each HCO_3^- that enters (reverse chloride shift). (b) CO_2 diffuses out of tissue cells that produce it and enters RBCs, where some of it binds to Hb (Hb–O_2). Other molecules of CO_2 combine with water to produce bicarbonate ions (HCO_3^-) and hydrogen ions (H^+). As Hb buffers H^+, the Hb releases O_2 (Bohr effect). To maintain electrical balance, a chloride ion (Cl^-) enters the RBC for each HCO_3^- that exists (chloride shift). Reprinted from Tortora and Derrickson (2009), with permission from John Wiley & Sons, Inc.

ability of venous blood to carry CO_2 (seen at the tissues) and unload more CO_2 in the presence of oxyhemoglobin (seen at the lungs).

Carbon dioxide binds to Hb at the α-amino group and forms carbaminohemoglobin, the third form CO_2 is carried in the blood (Guyton & Hall, 2006). This causes a change in the protein, which facilitates the release of oxygen, shifting the oxygen dissociation curve to the left, and is known as the Bohr effect. The converse is also true, as more CO_2 can bind to carbaminohemoglobin than HbO_2. As such, the release of O_2 in the peripheral tissues leads to an increased loading of CO_2. Once in the lung capillaries, deoxyhemoglobin combines with oxygen and releases CO_2.

The carbon dioxide dissociation curve is more linear in comparison with the oxygen dissociation curve. Of particular importance is the increased slope of the curve for CO_2 versus O_2 when plotting partial pressure on the x-axis and concentration on the y-axis of the respective gases. What this demonstrates is in the physiological range of PCO_2, between 40–50 mmHg, there is a greater change in CO_2 concentration per change in PCO_2 than there is change in oxygen concentration per change in PO_2. This is why there is a significantly larger difference in the PO_2 compared to carbon dioxide in the arterial versus venous blood.

ACID–BASE BALANCE

The lungs play a significant role in the precise regulation of the acid–base balance in the human body. Understanding the acid–base balance and the role the lung plays in maintaining it requires reviewing the Henderson–Hasselbach equation. In the context of respiratory physiology where blood is a buffer solution, the equation can be derived as the following:

$$pH = pK_A + \log[(HCO_3^-)/(CO_2)].$$

pK_A is the negative logarithm of the dissociation constant of carbonic acid. It can be viewed as a constant and at physiological pH and a temperature of 37°C, it is 6.1. At the same temperature, 0.03 mmol of carbon dioxide dissolves in 1 L of plasma; therefore, the CO_2 concentration is equal to ($PCO_2 \times 0.03$). If the bicarbonate level is normal at 24 mmol/L, inserting these values in the above equation yields

$$7.4 = 6.1 + \log[(24)/0.03 \times PCO_2)],$$

a PCO_2 of 40 mmHg, consistent with what is measured by blood gas analysis.

pH is the negative log of the hydrogen ion concentration, and as such, small changes of pH are actually representative of large changes in H^+ concentration ([H^+]) in the opposite direction. For example, an increase in pH from 7.4 to 7.7 represents a 50% decrease in [H^+]. The normal pH range is 7.35–7.45. A drop leads to acidemia, while an increase renders the blood more basic, resulting in alkalemia. The respiratory system primarily regulates the PCO_2, while the kidney regulates the HCO_3^- concentration. Acidosis is the condition that causes an increase in [H^+] or a decrease in [HCO_3^-], while alkalosis is the condition that causes a decrease in [H^+] or an increase in [HCO_3^-].

The fact that in the above-mentioned Henderson–Hasselbach equation PCO_2 is in the denominator explains why an increase in PCO_2 (outside the normal range of 35–45 mmHg) leads to a fall in pH, that is, an increase in acidity. This is known as *respiratory acidosis*. Without adequate exhalation, as seen in acute respiratory failure, CO_2 accumulates quickly and respiratory acidosis develops. Short-term changes in PCO_2 (that occur prior to the onset of renal compensation) increase the ratio of CO_2 to HCO_3^-, leading to this acidosis. Causes of acute respiratory acidosis include depression of the central respiratory center by cerebral disease or drugs (including anesthetics and narcotics), or airway obstruction related to asthma or chronic obstructive pulmonary disease (COPD) exacerbation. The body's ability to sense these changes and the control centers of breathing are discussed in the section "Control of Ventilation."

There are also instances of chronic retention of CO_2 often due to neuromuscular disease, either acquired, such as myasthenia gravis, amyotrophic lateral sclerosis, and Guillain–Barré syndrome, or congenital, such as muscular dystrophy. Chronic CO_2 retention also occurs in chronic lung diseases such as neonatal chronic lung disease secondary to extreme prematurity and immaturity of the premature lung. Chronic retention of CO_2 leads to respiratory acidosis. The kidney responds by retaining HCO_3^-. When the kidney is unable to completely reverse the acidosis, a pH below 7.4 will ensue, and this is referred to as compensated respiratory acidosis.

An increase in pH will be secondary to alkalosis. As expected from the Henderson–Hasselbach equation, this can occur because of a decrease in PCO_2, and it is termed *respiratory alkalosis*. Just as respiratory acidosis is caused by hypoventilation, hyperventilation will lead to respiratory alkalosis. Essentially, alveolar ventilation is higher than required for the body's production of carbon dioxide, resulting in a PCO_2 less than 35 mmHg. Hyperventilation is seen with anxiety, fever, and overventilation via a mechanical ventilator. This is also often seen at higher altitudes with hypoxia. One of the body's adjustments to the high altitude will be an increase in the renal excretion of HCO_3^- in an attempt to normalize pH.

In *metabolic acidosis*, the primary problem can be the loss of HCO_3^-, an increase in the production of acid, or a decrease in excretion of H^+ ions all leading to a decrease in the $[(HCO_3^-)/CO_2)]$ ratio. A review of the Henderson–Hasselbach equation demonstrates why a decrease in this ratio will lead to a decrease in the pH. Metabolic acidosis is a common occurrence in the intensive care unit and is present with a variety of disease processes including diabetic ketoacidosis and sepsis leading to tissue hypoxia and lactic acid production. A significant amount of diarrhea leads to loss of bicarbonate. Type I renal tubular acidosis is secondary to a defect in the secretion of H^+ ions in the distal renal tubular and subsequent decrease in reabsorption of bicarbonate.

An increase in HCO_3^- or an excessive loss of acid will lead to an increase in pH and *metabolic alkalosis*. Examples of conditions that result in loss of H+ ions include persistent vomiting with loss of hydrochloric acid and renal loss of hydrogen secondary to high aldosterone levels. Contraction alkalosis is secondary most often to diuretic use, leading to water loss but retention of HCO_3^-, which will bind H^+ ions, increasing blood pH. Excessive ingestion of bicarbonate, as seen with antacids, also leads to an increase in bicarbonate.

Primary acid–base disturbances are often partially balanced by compensation. When the disturbance is respiratory in nature, be it acidosis or alkalosis, renal compensatory mechanisms take effect. When the disturbances are metabolic, respiratory compensation occurs.

Changes in ventilation that result in changes in PCO_2 and respiratory compensation are controlled via the central and peripheral receptors (see the section "Control of Ventilation"). In metabolic acidosis, with the increase in hydrogen ion concentration, the respiratory system will hyperventilate to increase the exhalation of CO_2 in an attempt to normalize blood pH. Winter's formula allows us to determine if this respiratory compensation for metabolic acidosis is adequate:

$$PCO_2 = [(1.5 \times HCO_3^-) + 8] \pm 2.$$

For a given HCO_3^-, the formula will give the range expected of PCO_2 for adequate respiratory compensation, allowing comparison with the actual PCO_2 measured in the child's blood (Lewis, 2008). In the case of metabolic alkalosis, the respiratory system attempts to compensate by hypoventilating and retaining CO_2, thereby lowering the pH closer to 7.4.

Renal tubular cells actively secrete H^+ ions into the renal tubular fluid, and the proximal tubule of the kidney accounts for the resorption of 80% of all filtered HCO_3^-. Overall, the kidney secretes 70 mEq of H^+ ions and 70 mEq of HCO_3^- ions on a daily basis. However, during respiratory acidosis, the kidney compensates by retaining HCO_3^-, mostly in the proximal tubule of the kidney, and by excreting H^+ ions. The summation of this process allows the pH of the urine to go as low as 4.0, while attempting to increase the blood pH closer to 7.4. In cases of respiratory alkalosis, the renal secretion of H^+ ions is decreased. The reabsorption of HCO_3^- is also decreased, leading to an increase in the secretion of HCO_3^-. The net result is the attempt to decrease the blood pH closer to 7.4.

Whether the respiratory compensation is an attempt to increase or decrease PCO_2 based on the metabolic derangement, compensation occurs rapidly, on the order of minutes. This is in comparison to renal compensatory methods for respiratory derangements. The kidneys compensate for respiratory acid–base derangement by increasing or decreasing the excretion of acids and the retention of bicarbonate. Renal compensation is typically on the order of 3–6 days (Levitzky, 2007).

RESPIRATORY MECHANICS

Oxygen enters the body from the outside environment, through the conducting airways, into the respiratory zone, diffusing into the pulmonary capillaries and combining with Hb. Entry of oxygen requires an expansion of the lungs to accommodate a volume of air from which oxygen is derived.

To understand the process of normal breathing, one needs to understand the inherent properties of the lung and the chest wall. Functionally, the chest wall is made up of the rib cage, diaphragm, and abdominal contents. At baseline, the lung's tendency is to recoil inward, while the chest wall tends to recoil outward. The pleural pressure combines them into a functioning unit. The opposing forces generate a negative intrapleural pressure of −3- to −5-cm H_2O. The lung volume at which the lung and chest wall recoil are balanced is known as functional residual capacity (FRC). At the end of expiration, the muscles of respiration are relaxed and the lung volume is at FRC (see Figure 1.11).

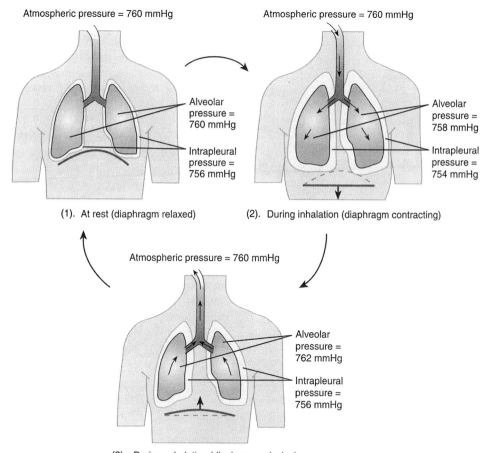

Atmospheric pressure = 760 mmHg

Atmospheric pressure = 760 mmHg

Alveolar pressure = 760 mmHg

Intrapleural pressure = 756 mmHg

Alveolar pressure = 758 mmHg

Intrapleural pressure = 754 mmHg

(1). At rest (diaphragm relaxed)

(2). During inhalation (diaphragm contracting)

Atmospheric pressure = 760 mmHg

Alveolar pressure = 762 mmHg

Intrapleural pressure = 756 mmHg

(3). During exhalation (diaphragm relaxing)

Figure 1.11 Pressure changes in pulmonary ventilation. During inhalation, the diaphragm contracts, the chest expands, the lungs are pulled outward, and the alveolar pressure decreases. During exhalation, the diaphragm relaxes, the lungs recoil inward, and alveolar pressure increases, forcing air out of the lungs. Reprinted from Tortora and Derrickson (2009), with permission from John Wiley & Sons, Inc.

An appreciation of the terminology of the various lung volumes is required prior to understanding the dynamics of ventilation. Chest wall and lung recoil properties determine pressure and volume changes during the breathing cycle. One inhalation produces a tidal volume (V_t), which, when exhaled, leaves a volume (FRC) in the lungs. Performing a maximal inhalation generates the vital capacity (VC), which is the maximal volume of air one can inhale during one breathing maneuver. The volume of air left in the lungs after a forceful exhalation from VC is the residual volume (RV). The summation of RV and VC equals the total lung capacity (TLC) (see Figure 1.12).

During forced inhalation, inspiratory muscles contract, leading to an increase in the thoracic volume. However, these muscles must overcome the inward recoil of the chest wall back to its resting position. TLC is the volume at which inspiration ceases because the muscles of inhalation cannot overcome the inward recoil of the chest wall. In forced exhalation, the contraction of expiratory muscles leads to a decrease in thoracic volume. The pressure needed to empty the lungs must overcome the outward recoil of the chest wall to its resting position. The volume left in the lungs at which the muscles of exhalation cannot overcome this outward recoil is the RV (see Figure 1.13).

The outward recoil out of the chest wall leads to a negative pressure; this negative pressure facilitates inhalation. Inhalation normally occurs via negative pressure; when alveolar pressure falls below atmospheric pressure to the point that it overcomes airway resistance, air flows into the lungs. This is in comparison to positive pressure ventilation, which is commonly utilized in intensive care units as the mode of breathing for children on ventilators.

Static properties: Compliance and elasticity

Compliance is the relationship between changes in volume and changes in pressure. In other words, compliance reflects the "ease" with which an object can be stretched. This contrasts with elasticity, which is a measure of the opposition to stretch. On a volume–pressure curve, the slope of the line is the measure of compliance and is measured as

$$\text{Compliance} = \frac{\text{Change in volume}}{\text{Change in pressure}}.$$

The classic clinical conditions that illustrate this are emphysema and fibrosis. Adult patients with emphysema have lungs that are more distensible and are therefore more compliant with elastic fibers that are easily stretched (Tortora & Derrickson, 2009). The patient with interstitial fibrosis has stiffer, less compliant lungs. The volume–pressure curve for the more compliant lung will be steeper than a normal individual, while the curve for the less compliant lung will be less steep. Conversely, the elastic recoil

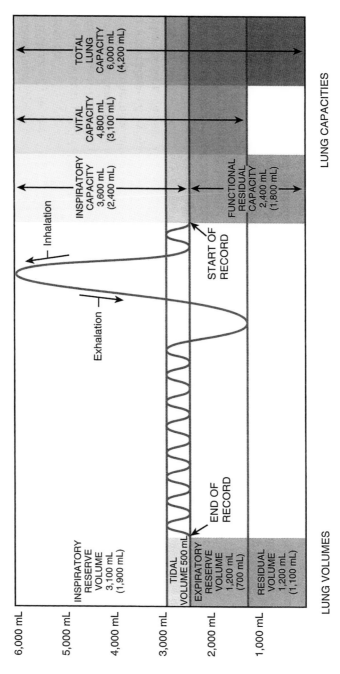

LUNG VOLUMES

LUNG CAPACITIES

Figure 1.12 Spirogram of lung volumes and capacities. The average values for a healthy adult male and female are indicated, with the values for a female in parentheses. Note that the spirogram is read from right (start of record) to left (end of record). Reprinted from Tortora and Derrickson (2009), with permission from John Wiley & Sons, Inc.

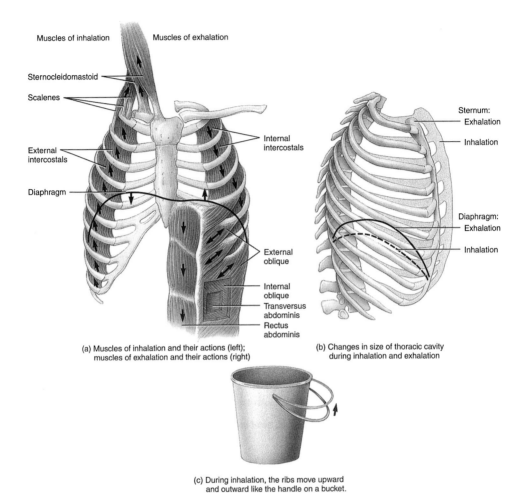

Muscles of inhalation   Muscles of exhalation

Sternocleidomastoid

Scalenes

External intercostals

Diaphragm

Internal intercostals

External oblique

Internal oblique

Transversus abdominis

Rectus abdominis

Sternum:
Exhalation
Inhalation

Diaphragm:
Exhalation
Inhalation

(a) Muscles of inhalation and their actions (left); muscles of exhalation and their actions (right)

(b) Changes in size of thoracic cavity during inhalation and exhalation

(c) During inhalation, the ribs move upward and outward like the handle on a bucket.

Figure 1.13 Muscles of inhalation and exhalation and their actions. Reprinted from Tortora and Derrickson (2009), with permission from John Wiley & Sons, Inc.

for the more compliant lung will be less, while the less compliant lung will have higher elastic recoil.

Muscles of breathing

Inspiration

As stated previously, breathing normally takes places via negative pressure; the decrease in pleural and hence alveolar pressure to below atmospheric pressure is secondary to contraction of the muscles of inspiration. The most important muscle of inspiration is the diaphragm. The diaphragm is a thin muscle that delineates the thorax from the abdomen, attaching to the lower ribs on each side. The diaphragm contracts during inspiration, forcing abdominal contents down and thereby increasing the cephalad/ caudal dimensions of the thorax. This lifts the ribs up and out, increasing the transverse dimension of the thorax. Also involved in inspiration are the external intercostal muscles that connect adjacent ribs. When they contract, the ribs are pulled upward and forward, increasing anterior– posterior and lateral diameters of the thorax, commonly referred to as the "bucket-handle" movement of the ribs (see Figure 1.13).

Paralysis of the diaphragm leads to paradoxical movement, with the diaphragm moving up on inspiration with the fall in intrathoracic pressure. Paralysis of the intercostal muscle has little effect on breathing. Other muscles that play more of a role during exercise include the scalene muscles, which elevate the first two ribs, and the sternocleidomastoid muscles, which raise the sternum. Neuronal inputs and brainstem control of inspiration are discussed in the section "Control of Ventilation."

As previously stated, prior to the initiation of inspiration, the intrapleural pressure is between -3- and -5-cm H_2O. The transmural pressure is equal to the alveolar pressure minus the intrapleural pressure. The muscles of inspiration increase thoracic cavity volume, thereby decreasing the alveolar pressure (making more negative) and the transmural pressure. An increase in the transmural pressure gradient distends the alveolar walls, increasing the alveolar volume and allowing for the inspiration of air until, once again, alveolar pressure is not less than atmospheric pressure.

Expiration

Expiration during regular tidal breathing is passive. At the end of inspiration, the elastic properties of the distended alveoli are such that the alveolar pressure is greater than atmospheric pressure, allowing for the flow of air out of the lung (see Figure 1.11). During hyperventilation, whether done voluntarily or with exercise, expiration becomes active, as the lungs attempt to overcome the outward recoil of the chest. The muscles that make up the abdominal wall are key to this movement. They contract, leading to an increase in intra-abdominal pressure as the diaphragm is pushed up. The Valsalva maneuver is a variation on this theme, where expiration is forced against a closed glottis, increasing abdominal pressure. This occurs in coughing, sneezing, and defecation (Levitzky, 2007).

Surface tension properties of the lung

In addition to the physical and mechanical properties that allow lung expansion and ventilation, the lung has specific properties that facilitate the ease with which it can be inflated and deflated. These are related to the alveolar cell types and alveolar surface tension. There are two types of alveolar epithelial cells, conveniently named type I and type II cells. Type I cells are squamous epithelial alveolar cells that have long cytoplasmic extensions that spread out over the alveolar walls and help form the structure of the wall. Type II cells are compact with microvilli that extend into the alveoli.

Type II cells produce a surfactant, a phospholipid made in the lung from fatty acids. It coats the surface of the alveolus and decreases its surface tension. Eighty-five to ninety percent of a surfactant consists of lipids of which 85% is phospholipids. Along with the phospholipids, a surfactant has four different types of surfactant proteins: The hydrophilic proteins SP-A and SP-D and the hydrophobic proteins SP-B and SP-C. Seventy-five percent of the phospholipids are dipalmitoyl phosphatidylcholine (DPCC), or lecithin. DPCC's molecular properties allow surfactants to reduce elastic recoil secondary to surface tension, thereby increasing compliance. DPCC has one hydrophobic molecular end, while the other end is hydrophilic. Normally, liquid surface molecules are attracted to each other leading to surface tension. However, the repulsive forces of the two ends of DPCC oppose this attractive force, decreasing the surface tension. A surfactant's surface tension decreases to a higher degree as the surface area layer is reduced because the molecules of DPCC are brought closer together, leading to an increase in the repulsive force.

As a result of the properties of surfactants, smaller alveoli have lower surface tensions, normalizing the alveolar pressure throughout the lung. Overall, the reduction in elastic recoil and the increase in compliance lead to a decrease in the work of breathing of inspiration. By allowing the surface tension to decrease as lung volume decreases, surfactants stabilize the lung and prevent atelectasis. Surface tension forces lead to transudation of fluid from the capillaries into the alveolar spaces, but by decreasing surface tension, surfactants also keep the alveoli dry. Furthermore, surfactants protect the lung against epithelial injury and provides a barrier against infection (Anandarajan, Paulraj, & Tubman, 2009).

Surfactant production begins in the fourth month of gestation but is not fully functional until after the seventh month (Levitzky, 2007). Infants born during this gestational period develop classic respiratory distress syndrome (RDS). Problems include difficulty inflating alveoli because the lungs are stiff, secondary to the decrease in pulmonary compliance. In those alveoli that are inflated, there are areas of collapse secondary to instability associated with lack of surfactant. This leads to the classic heterogenous picture of RDS: areas of hyperinflation and pockets of atelectasis. Current strategies to prevent RDS include antenatal maternal treatment with steroids to enhance fetal lung maturation or postnatal treatment with synthetic surfactant to the newborn.

Antenatal glucocorticoid therapy administered to women at risk for preterm delivery has reduced the incidence of RDS and overall mortality in the offspring (Liggins & Howie, 1972). Antenatal glucocorticoid therapy causes maturation of the lung architecture (Ballard & Ballard, 1995; Smolders-de Haas et al., 1990). In essence, the maternal treatment with glucocorticoids allows for a swift pulmonary maturation through the saccular phase into the alveolar stage. The decreased severity and incidence of RDS lead to a decrease in the need for surfactant therapy, supplemental oxygen, and mechanical ventilation (National Institute of Child Health and Human Development, 1994).

A similar clinical picture is seen in term infants who have inherited surfactant deficiencies secondary to mutations of the surfactant proteins SP-B and SP-C. This leads to intracellular accumulation of proteins and extracellular deficiency of surfactant proteins. These mutations are a cause of both familial and sporadic interstitial lung disease. Mutations in the adenosine triphosphate (ATP)-binding cassette gene (ABCA3) in newborns result in fatal surfactant deficiency. ABCA3 is critical for proper surfactant function.

Airway resistance

In addition to the properties of the muscles of breathing and the lung parenchyma, properties of the conducting airways are important determinants of airflow into the lungs. In straight tubes, flow is described as laminar, which is flow that occurs at a low rate in parallel streams through a tube. With laminar flow, the resistance is inversely proportional to the radius of the tube to the fourth power. As a result, a decrease in the radius by half will increase the resistance 16-fold.

In the human lung, laminar flow occurs in the smallest airways; hence, one would expect that a decrease in radius in these airways, as might occur with an infection, would result in a large increase in airway resistance to airflow. However, the main areas of resistance are not in these smallest airways. This is because despite the remarkably narrow radius of the small airways, the exponential number of these airways greatly reduces the overall effect of the radius in terms of resistance. It is the medium-sized bronchi (up to the seventh generation) that are the site of 80% of the resistance in the human lung (West, 2003).

At low lung volumes, the small airways can collapse, especially at the base of the lung. Though this area ventilates more efficiently, it is not well expanded. It is thought that children who have increased airway resistance, a hallmark of poorly controlled asthma, breathe at higher lung volumes to decrease airway resistance. Understanding this pathophysiology helps to understand the mainstays of asthma treatment.

Bronchial airway smooth muscles have receptors that, when stimulated, lead to contraction or relaxation of the muscles. In some children, airway smooth muscle contraction can be stimulated by certain triggers, including environmental (pollen, grass, etc.), viral, or exercise. Beta adrenergic receptors, found in the airway smooth muscle, lead to relaxation of the smooth muscle when stimulated by a beta adrenergic agonist. This is the means by which albuterol sulfate, a beta adrenergic agonist, acts as a rescue medicine during an asthma exacerbation and provides relief by increasing airway radius and decreasing resistance.

Regional differences of the lung

Alveoli at the top of the lung are more fully expanded at FRC than those at the bottom of the lung. This is secondary to higher transpulmonary pressure at the top of the lung. Factors that lead to this gradient in trans-pulmonary pressure include the effect of gravity on the chest wall and the effect of the weight of the lung. These downward acting forces on the lung require higher pressure at the lower rather than the higher areas to balance the forces. Therefore, the pressure near the base is less negative than at the apex. Because the transpulmonary pressure at the base is small, the resting volume of the lung in this region is also small; in essence, the basal lung is more compressed.

However, this gradient decreases during inspiration, and at full inspira-tion, that is, at TLC, the alveoli are virtually uniform in size from the apices to the bases in the lung. As the lung volume increases above FRC, alveoli at the bottom expand more than those at the top of the lung. As a result, during normal breathing at rest, the base of the lungs ventilates more than the uppermost regions of the lung. The lower portion of the lung is on the steeper part of the pressure–volume curve, leading to more expansion on inspiration in comparison to the apex. Lungs with higher volumes (apex vs. basal segments) are more difficult to inflate as they require larger expanding pressure; in essence, they are stiffer.

This regional difference in ventilation coincides with a higher blood flow at the base in comparison to the top of the lungs. The higher rate of ventilation and perfusion leads to a more efficient exchange of gases. This apex/base difference dissipates when in the supine position, but the pos-terior portion of the lung (now the lower part) is higher than the anterior portion (now the upper part).

CONTROL OF VENTILATION

This section presents the triad of components involved in ventilation: the central and peripheral receptors that sense changes in pH, PCO_2, and PO_2 in the blood and cerebrospinal fluid (CSF); the brainstem neurons that receive the inputs from these receptors; and the muscles of respiration that receive the signals sent out by the neurons.

Breathing is a tightly regulated process that is controlled by the central nervous system. In order to adjust tidal volume and respiratory rate to meet the demands of maintaining normal gas exchange and pH, feedback is needed from the lungs, the respiratory muscles, and the blood. The sensors that detect PO_2 and PCO_2 levels in the blood and CSF are located centrally and peripherally in the body.

The central chemoreceptors are bathed in brain extracellular fluid (ECF) on the ventral surface of the medulla, near cranial nerves 9 and 10. The ventral respiratory group controls voluntary forced expiration and acts to increase the force of inspiration. An increase in H^+ ion concentration will increase ventilation, as well as the converse; a decrease in H^+ ion concentration will decrease ventilation (Coates, Li, & Nattie, 1984). This is consistent with the Henderson–Hasselbach equation, which shows that a decrease in pH (an increase H^+ ion concentration) is seen with an increase in PCO_2, as might occur in hypoventilation. The result will be an increase in respiratory drive to lower PCO_2 and increase pH. Under normal conditions, the most important factor in the control of ventilation is the arterial PCO_2.

The ECF is composed of and affected by CSF and local blood flow and metabolism. The interactions of these components are dictated by the environment of the brain. The CSF is separated from the blood by the blood–brain barrier (BBB). Unlike H^+ ions, CO_2 is able to diffuse through the BBB. When blood PCO_2 rises, this difference in permeability allows CO_2 to move from the cerebral blood vessels, through the BBB, into the CSF. Once in the CSF, the pH will decrease with an increase in H^+ ions, stimulating chemoreceptors. An increase in PCO_2 increases diffusion because CO_2 causes vasodilation of cerebral blood vessels. Vasodilation is an important effect of CO_2 that allows the close control of ventilation and enables the quick resolution of changes in blood CO_2. How this stimulation leads to an increase in respiration and therefore a decrease in PCO_2 is presented later in this section.

The peripheral chemoreceptors are found in the carotid bodies at the bifurcation of the common carotid arteries and above and below the aortic arch in the aortic bodies (see Figure 1.14). Peripheral chemoreceptors act most importantly to detect arterial decreases in PO_2 and pH and increases in PCO_2. They are the sole means to an increase in ventilation secondary to a decrease in arterial PO_2. In fact, those with bilateral absence of carotid bodies have an absolute loss of hypoxic ventilatory drive. In comparison to central chemoreceptors, carotid bodies play a much smaller role in controlling ventilation secondary to PCO_2. At sea level, carbon dioxide is the main stimulus to ventilation, but at a higher altitude (above 3,000 m), hypoxia plays more of a role in increasing ventilation (Peacock, 1998). There is also a distinction in regard to the peripheral chemoreceptors themselves, as the carotid, but not aortic, bodies respond to a decrease in arterial pH.

The CSF has a lower buffering capacity in comparison with blood due to a lower protein concentration. This allows for a more rapid return of pH in the CSF versus blood when there is an alteration in the concentration of CO_2. This is an important factor when comparing central to peripheral chemoreceptors and their collective import on the control of ventilation.

Various other receptors are present, all with significantly less effect on ventilation. Among these are pulmonary stretch receptors within the airway smooth muscle. These receptors signal distention of the lung, leading to a slowing of the respiratory rate via prolongation of the expiratory phase. Irritant receptors are found in airway epithelial cells and are stimulated by irritants, such as dust, cigarette smoke, and odors, leading to bronchoconstriction (Harries, Parkes, Lessof, & Orr, 1981). As such, they

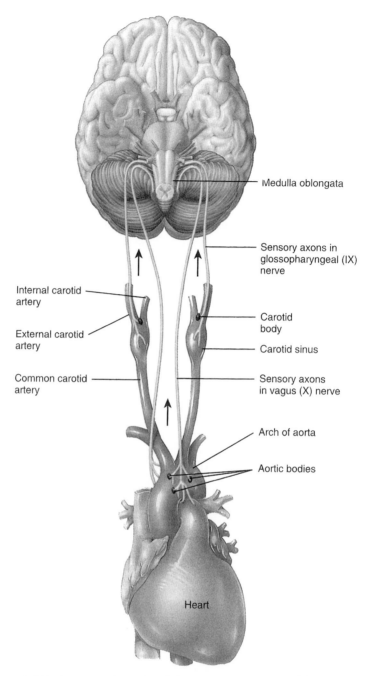

Medulla oblongata

Sensory axons in glossopharyngeal (IX) nerve

Internal carotid artery

External carotid artery

Common carotid artery

Carotid body

Carotid sinus

Sensory axons in vagus (X) nerve

Arch of aorta

Aortic bodies

Heart

Figure 1.14 Locations of peripheral chemoreceptors. Reprinted from Tortora and Derrickson (2009), with permission from John Wiley & Sons, Inc.

play a role in the bronchospasm seen with asthma exacerbations upon exposure to environmental triggers. J-receptors are believed to be in the alveolar walls, in close proximity to the capillaries. They respond to the accumulation of interstitial fluid in the lung parenchyma, seen in pulmonary edema, and to pulmonary capillary engorgement.

All of these receptors, whether central or peripheral, send signals to the central controller of respiration found in the brain. The brain stem houses groups of neurons known as the respiratory centers. Coordination of the muscles of respiration is orchestrated by the groups of neurons. During studies conducted in the 1960s, the medulla was isolated as the location of respiratory control (Batsel, 1964). This was based on experiments that showed that despite transection of the brain above the pontomedullary junction (pons and medulla in the brain stem), rhythmic respiration continued, but transaction of the medulla and below led to termination of respiration (Levitzky, 2007) (see Figure 1.15).

The region of each collection of neurons has a distinct function. In the medulla, the nuclei in the ventral region control voluntary forced exhalation and can increase the force of inspiration. In the dorsal region of the medulla, the group of neurons controls inspiration.

During normal breathing, the ventral medulla area is quiet, as inspiration is signaled by the dorsal region leading to contraction of inspiratory

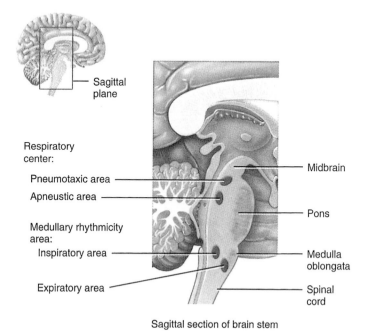

Sagittal section of brain stem

Figure 1.15 Locations of areas of the respiratory center. Reprinted from Tortora and Derrickson (2009), with permission from John Wiley & Sons, Inc.

muscles, and expiration is brought on by the natural chest wall recoil, discussed in the previous section on ventilation. However, as stated in that section, exhalation can become active (e.g., in exercise), during which the ventral medulla fires.

The apneustic center is located in the lower pons and is involved in the transition between inspiration and expiration. Its name is derived from the fact that when it sends stimulatory impulses to the dorsal medulla, it leads to prolongation of inspiration, causing long, deep breaths. This is seen in animal experiments when transection above this area leads to a prolonged inspiratory gasp followed by transient expiratory effort (apnea).

The pneumotaxic center is located in the upper pons and sends inhibitory impulses to the dorsal medulla, shortening inspiration and, as a result, leading to an increase in the respiratory rate. Sometimes it is viewed as an area that allows for small adjustments to respiration as normal rhythmic breathing still occurs with transaction of this area.

The cerebral cortex also has some, though limited, effect on ventilation. This is seen most notably with voluntary hyperventilation. Voluntary hypoventilation cannot be achieved to the same degree as hyperventilation because of the tight regulation of PCO_2 and PO_2.

REFERENCES

Anandarajan, M., Paulraj, S., & Tubman, R. (2009). ABCA3 deficiency: An unusual cause of respiratory distress in the newborn. *The Ulster Medical Journal*, 78(1), 51–52.

Ballard, P. L., & Ballard, R. A. (1995). Scientific basis and therapeutic regimens for use of antenatal glucocorticoids. *American Journal of Obstetrics and Gynecology*, 173, 254.

Bates, D. V. (1962). Respiratory disorders associated with impairment of gas diffusion (alveolo-capillary block syndrome). *Annual Review of Medicine*, 13, 301–318.

Batsel, H. L. (1964). Localization of bulbar respiratory center by microelectrode sounding. *Experimental Neurology*, 9, 410–426.

Burri, P. H. (1984). Fetal and postnatal development of the lung. *Annual Review of Physiology*, 46, 617–628.

Coates, E. L., Li, A., & Nattie, E. E. (1984). Widespread sites of brain stem ventilatory chemoreceptors. *Journal of Applied Physiology*, 75(1), 5–14.

DiFiore, J. W., & Wilson, J. M. (1994). Lung development. *Seminars in Pediatric Surgery*, 3, 221–232.

Dominguez de Villota, E. D., Ruiz Carmona, M. T., Rubio, J. J., & de Andrés, S. (1981). Equality of the in vivo and in vitro oxygen-binding capacity of haemoglobin in patients with severe respiratory disease. *British Journal of Anaesthesia*, 53(12), 1325–1328.

Guyton, A. C., & Hall, J. E. (2006). *Textbook of medical physiology* (11th ed.). Philadelphia: Elsevier Saunders.

Harries, M. G., Parkes, P. E. G., Lessof, M. H., & Orr, T. S. C. (1981). Role of bronchial irritant receptors in asthma. *Lancet, 317*(8210), 5–7.

Harris, M. D., Terrio, J., Miser, W. F., & Yetter, J. F., 3rd (1998). High altitude medicine. *American Family Physician, 57*(8), 1907–1914, 1924–1926.

Jeffery, P. (1998). The development of large and small airways. *American Journal of Respiratory Cell and Molecular Biology, 179*, 1632–1639.

Jenkins, S. (2005). *Sports science handbook: Volume 1: The essential guide to kinesiology, sport & exercise science* (p. 26). Essex, UK: Multi-Science Publishing.

Johnson, S. B. (2008). Tracheobronchial injury. *Seminars in Thoracic and Cardiovascular Surgery, 20*(1), 52–57.

Levitzky, M. G. (2007). *Pulmonary physiology* (7th ed., pp. 87, 139). New York: McGraw Hill.

Lewis, J. L. (2008). *Acid-base disorders: Acid-base regulation and disorders.* Whitehouse Station, NJ: Merck Manual Professional.

Liggins, G. C., & Howie, R. N. (1972). A controlled trial of antepartum glucocorticoid treatment for prevention of the respiratory distress syndrome in premature infants. *Pediatrics, 50*, 515.

Mason, S. F. (1962). *A history of the sciences* (p. 57). New York: Collier Books.

National Institute of Child Health and Human Development (1994). National Institutes of Health consensus statement. Effect of corticosteroids for fetal maturation on perinatal outcomes. Report on the Consensus Development Conference on the Effect of Corticosteroids for Fetal Maturation on Perinatal Outcomes. U.S. Department of Health and Human Services, Public Health Service, NIH. Pub No. 95-3784.

Pavelka, M., & Roth, J. (2005). *Alveoli: Gas exchange and host defense. Functional ultrastructure: An atlas of tissue biology and pathology* (pp. 224–225). Vienna: Springer.

Peacock, A. J. (1998). Oxygen at high altitude. *British Medical Journal, 317*(7165), 1063–1066.

Post, M., & Copland, I. (2002). Overview of lung development. *Acta Pharmacologica Sinica, (23,* Suppl.), 4–7.

Rhoades, R., & Planzer, R. (1996). *Human physiology* (3rd ed., p. 618). Fort Worth: Saunders College Publishing/Harcourt Brace College Publishers.

Sircar, S. (2008). *Principles of medical physiology* (pp. 309–310). New York: Thieme.

Smolders-de Haas, H., Neuvel, J., Schmand, B., Treffers, P. E., Koppe, J. G., & Hoeks, J. (1990). Physical development and medical history of children who were treated antenatally with corticosteroids to prevent respiratory distress syndrome: A 10- to 12-year follow-up. *Pediatrics, 86*(1), 65–70.

Tikuisis, P., Kane, D. M., McLellan, T. M., Buick, F., & Fairburn, S. M. (1992). Rate of formation of carboxyhemoglobin in exercising humans exposed to carbon monoxide. *Journal of Applied Physiology, 72*(4), 1311–1319.

Tortora, G. J., & Derrickson, B. (2009). *Principles of anatomy and physiology* (12th ed., p. 894). Hoboken, NJ: John Wiley & Sons.

West, J. B. (2003). *Respiratory physiology, the essentials* (6th ed., p. 24). Baltimore, MD: Lippincott Williams & Wilkins.

Wilmore, J. H., & Costill, D. L. (2005). *Physiology of sport and exercise* (3rd ed.). Champaign, IL: Human Kinetics.

Pediatric respiratory health history and physical assessment

Concettina Tolomeo, DNP, APRN, FNP-BC, AE-C

RESPIRATORY HEALTH HISTORY AND PHYSICAL EXAMINATION

The significance of a thorough health history and physical examination in the diagnosis of pediatric respiratory disorders should not be underestimated. Gaining an understanding of the child's symptoms from his/her perspective, as well as the perspective of the family, is invaluable. Determining the impact of the symptoms on the family unit is also important in the subsequent care and management of the problem.

Often, information elicited from both the health history and physical examination leads the health-care provider not only to the correct diagnosis but also to the identification of underlying causative factors. Once this initial assessment is complete, further testing may be employed to confirm the suspected diagnosis.

When conducting the health history and physical examination, the nurse should always consider the child's developmental level. Children less than 2 years of age fall in the sensorimotor stage of cognitive developmental. During this stage, physical handling of objects and events dictate the thought process. In addition, imitation dominates during this period (Edelman & Mandle, 2010). Therefore, the nurse should allow children of this age to hold items like a stethoscope; this provides them with the opportunity to become comfortable with the equipment as well as with the

Nursing Care in Pediatric Respiratory Disease, First Edition. Edited by Concettina (Tina) Tolomeo.
© 2012 John Wiley & Sons, Inc. Published 2012 by John Wiley & Sons, Inc.

nurse. During the preoperational stage (2–7 years of age), thought is governed by what is seen, heard, or experienced (Edelman & Mandle, 2010). Thus, for children of this age, the nurse should explain what she will be doing and should show the child how she will do it. This is also a good age to start to ask children to describe their own symptoms. Concrete operation is the stage from 7 to 11 years of age. During this stage, language is refined and mental reasoning processes take on logical approaches to solving concrete problems (Edelman & Mandle, 2010). Therefore, during this stage, the nurse should provide a clear explanation of what will take place and why. The nurse should also direct questions to the child a well as the parent. Finally, formal operation is the stage between 11 and 15 years of age. During this time, actual logical thought and manipulation of abstract concepts materialize (Edelman & Mandle, 2010). For this age group, the nurse should again explain what will happen during the examination and should allow children to verbalize their symptoms. Pictures are also helpful for this age group.

Respiratory health history

Obtaining an accurate and complete history is essential in the overall assessment and diagnosis of pediatric respiratory disorders. Before beginning the history portion of the visit, it is important that the nurse properly introduce himself/herself to the child and family. Building rapport with the child and family will allow the nurse to glean quality, pertinent information regarding the reason for the visit. Health history questions should be organized so that all components are addressed. Additionally, questions should be age specific and open-ended, thereby allowing the child and the family the ability to share their concerns and to explain completely the reason for the visit.

In addition to a list of current allergies and medications, the respiratory health history includes the chief complaint, history of the present illness, past medical history (including birth history), review of systems, family history, social history, and environmental history. The chief complaint should be in the child's/parents' own words. The history of the present illness is an investigation of the current symptoms. It should include when the symptoms first appeared, the frequency of the symptoms, duration of symptoms, the quality of the symptoms (i.e., sharp or stabbing), onset of symptoms (sudden or gradual), when symptoms occur (i.e., at rest or with activity), where symptoms occur (i.e., at home or in school), aggravating and alleviating factors, therapies attempted (including alternative therapies), and response to therapies (Lippincott, 2007). Common respiratory symptoms include coughing, wheezing, shortness of breath, chest pain, chest tightness, sputum production, and hemoptysis (coughing up blood). A thorough evaluation of the symptoms is necessary. The following presents a list of questions that can be utilized to characterize common respiratory symptoms.

Cough

- When does the cough occur? Does the cough occur both day and night?
- Does the cough occur with activity? What type of activity does it occur with? Does the cough stop with rest?
- Does the cough limit his/her activity? If yes, in what way?
- Does the cough keep the child up at night/wake the child? How often does this occur?
- Does the cough sound wet or dry?
- Describe the cough. What does it sound like? Is it hacking, barking, or whooping?
- Is there a recent history of choking?
- Is the cough productive of mucus? If yes, does it occur daily? How much mucus is produced? What color is it?
- Do any other symptoms occur with the cough? If yes, what symptoms occur?

Wheeze

- When does the wheeze occur? Does the wheeze occur both day and night?
- Describe the wheeze. What does it sound like?
- Does the wheeze occur when the child breathes in or breathes out?
- Does the child wheeze after meals? If yes, does he/she gag or choke during meals?
- Does the child wheeze with activity? What type of activity does it occur with? Does the wheeze stop with rest?
- Does the wheeze limit his/her activity? If yes, in what way?
- Does the child wake up wheezing? How often?
- (If the child is old enough) Point to where you hear/feel the wheezing.
- Do any other symptoms occur with the wheeze? If yes, what symptoms occur?

Shortness of breath

- When does the shortness of breath occur? Does the shortness of breath occur both day and night?
- Does the shortness of breath occur at rest?
- Does the shortness of breath occur with activity? What type of activity does it occur with? Does the shortness of breath stop with rest? Is the shortness of breath out of proportion with the other children he/she is playing with?
- Does the shortness of breath limit his/her activity? If yes, in what way?
- (If the child is old enough) Is it difficult to get the air in, out, or both?

- Do any other symptoms occur with the shortness of breath? If yes, what symptoms occur?

Chest pain

- When does the chest pain occur?
- Does it occur when the child takes a breath in, at rest, or with activity? What type of activity does it occur with? Does the chest pain stop with rest?
- Describe the pain.
- Did the child sustain any injuries to the chest?
- Has the child had a fever?
- Do any other symptoms occur with the chest pain? If yes, what symptoms occur?

Chest tightness

- When does the chest tightness occur?
- Does it occur at rest or with activity? What type of activity does it occur with? Does the chest tightness stop with rest?
- Point to where you (the child) feel the tightness.
- Do any other symptoms occur with the tightness? If yes, what symptoms occur?

Sputum production

- How often is mucus produced?
- How much mucus is produced (use measurements child/parents can understand, such as teaspoon, tablespoon, or cup)?
- What color is the mucus?

Hemoptysis

- What color was it (i.e., pink, red, or brown)?
- How much bleeding occurred (use measurements child/parents can understand, such as teaspoon, tablespoon, or cup)?
- Is this the first time it happened? If no, how often has it occurred?
- Has the child traveled outside of the country or been exposed to foreign travelers?

The child's birth history can be useful in determining the reason for the current symptoms. It is important to ascertain whether the child was born full term or preterm and if there were any respiratory complications after birth. If born preterm, ask what the child's gestational age was at birth.

Airway hyperresponsiveness has been demonstrated in both children who were born premature and those who had been diagnosed with broncho-pulmonary dysplasia (Bhandari & Panitch, 2006).

The nurse must establish if the child required supplemental oxygen or mechanical ventilation during the newborn period. If supplemental oxygen and mechanical ventilation were utilized, the nurse must determine the duration of therapy and whether the child was discharged home on these therapies or medications. A history of airway problems, stridor, or difficulty tolerating extubation is also helpful.

When obtaining a past medical history, the nurse must ask about any previous respiratory-related illnesses, such as bronchopulmonary dysplasia, foreign body aspiration, respiratory syncytial virus, chronic sinusitis, or asthma. Non-respiratory-related illnesses should also be uncovered as they may have an impact on the respiratory system (e.g., gastroesphageal reflux may present with coughing, and frequent episodes of otitis media may be due to immotile cilia). Any previous emergency department visits or hospitalizations should be documented. Finally, it is important to note the child's immunization history to determine if immunizations are up-to-date.

A head-to-toe review of systems should also be conducted. The nurse should ask about headaches, nasal congestion, rhinorrhea, postnasal drip, snoring, reflux, and eczema. Positive pertinent findings can have an impact on the current diagnosis.

It is often difficult to obtain an accurate environmental, social, or family history because of the sensitive nature of certain questions. However, these areas are vital components of the respiratory health history and should be investigated.

Important environmental factors include age of dwelling, location of dwelling, type of heating and cooling used, as well as the presence of carpets, pets, smokers, cockroaches, mice, or mold. Social history should include the number of occupants in the home, whether the child attends day care or school, the number of missed daycare/school days due to respiratory symptoms, whether the child smokes, and the type of activities the child participates in. When obtaining a family history, the nurse should go back two generations and determine if there is a family history of any respiratory-related illnesses such as asthma, bronchiectasis, cystic fibrosis, or chronic obstructive lung disease. The nurse should also ask about allergies, eczema, heart disease, and obstructive sleep apnea.

In addition to obtaining information from the child and parents, the health history component of the assessment is a prime opportunity to offer age-appropriate anticipatory guidance. During the infant and toddler years, it is important to remind parents to keep children away from sick contacts, large crowds, and small objects. The nurse should also discuss the dangers associated with smoking with school-age and adolescent children. Furthermore, parents should be reminded of the importance of annual influenza vaccinations.

Physical examination

The respiratory physical examination should include all aspects of health assessment, including inspection, palpation, percussion, and auscultation. All techniques should be performed systematically. In order to assure that each respiratory examination is comprehensive, the nurse should follow the same sequence each time she performs an examination, keeping in mind there may be times when the sequence will need to be adjusted to accommodate the anxious child. Furthermore, as noted previously, for the pediatric population, it is important to perform each aspect of the physical examination, keeping the child's developmental level in mind.

Prior to performing a physical examination, it is imperative that the nurse is aware of thoracic landmarks. Knowledge of common landmarks will assist with both examination and documentation. Proper documentation of findings ultimately leads to improved communication with other members of the health-care team.

The midsternal line runs down the midline of the sternum. Similarly, the vertebral line runs down the spinal process posteriorly. The midclavicular line, which is present on both the right and left, runs parallel to the midsternal line. The line starts at the midclavicle position. Anterior axillary lines are also present on both sides and also run parallel to the midsternal line. The anterior axillary lines start at the anterior axillary folds. The midaxillary lines (right and left) begin midaxilla and are parallel to the midsternal line. The posterior axillary lines start at the posterior axiallary folds bilaterally and run parallel to the midsternal line. The right and left scapular lines run parallel to the vertebral line. With the patient in the standing position, the scapular lines run through the inferior angle of the scapula (Seidel, Ball, & Dains, 2003). All documentation relating to examination of the chest should reflect these imaginary lines (see Figure 2.1a–c).

Inspection

During the inspection component of the examination, the child should be sitting, if possible. Keep in mind that a younger child may be more comfortable sitting on the parent's lap. Inspection of the chest should occur with little or no clothing depending on the age and gender of the child. A gown should be available to school-age and adolescent children. Additionally, the space should be private, lighting should be of good quality, and the environmental temperature should be comfortable.

The shape and symmetry of the chest should be noted anteriorly, laterally, and posteriorly. The anteroposterior (AP) diameter of the chest should be approximately half the transverse diameter (Seidel et al., 2003). A barrel chest is characterized by horizontal ribs, a somewhat kyphotic spine, and a prominent sternal angle. Pectus carinatum (pigeon chest) is depicted by a prominent protrusion of the sternum. Pectus excavatum (funnel chest) is

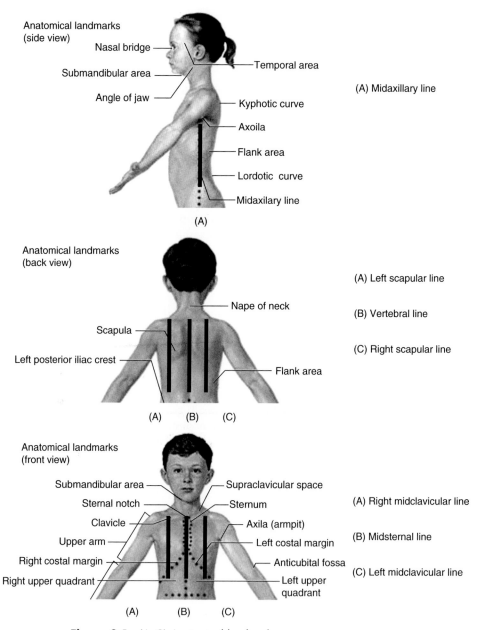

Figure 2.1 (A–C) Anatomical landmarks.

Anatomical landmarks
(side view)

Nasal bridge

Submandibular area

Angle of jaw

Temporal area

Kyphotic curve

Axoila

Flank area

Lordotic curve

Midaxilary line

(A)

(A) Midaxillary line

Anatomical landmarks
(back view)

Nape of neck

Scapula

Left posterior iliac crest

Flank area

(A) (B) (C)

(A) Left scapular line

(B) Vertebral line

(C) Right scapular line

Anatomical landmarks
(front view)

Submandibular area

Sternal notch

Clavicle

Upper arm

Right costal margin

Right upper quadrant

Supraclavicular space

Sternum

Axila (armpit)

Left costal margin

Anticubital fossa

Left upper
quadrant

(A) (B) (C)

(A) Right midclavicular line

(B) Midsternal line

(C) Left midclavicular line

illustrated by an indentation of the sternum (Lippincott, 2007; Seidel et al., 2003).

It is helpful to record a respiratory rate during the inspection portion of the examination. For infants and toddlers, it is useful to measure the respiratory rate before beginning the hands-on portion of the examination because the child is more likely to be fussing or crying during that portion of the examination. For school-age and adolescent children, it is useful to measure the respiratory rate when they do not know you are counting because the child may have a self-conscious response to your measurement; this response may alter the results (Seidel et al., 2003). The respiratory rate should be counted for a full minute. Normal respiratory rates based on age are as follows:

Age	Rate (breaths/min)
Infants	30–40
Toddlers	24–26
Preschoolers	24
School-age children	20
Adolescents	20 (Custer & Rau, 2009)

Next, inspect respiratory effort, respiratory pattern, and chest expansion. Breathing should be relaxed and regular, and chest expansion should be symmetrical. The inspiratory-to-expiratory ratio (I:E ratio) should be 1:2. A list of respiratory patterns along with implications of the patterns are presented in Table 2.1 (Hilman, 1993; Lippincott, 2007; Seidel et al., 2003).

The chest should be inspected for the presence of retractions. The nurse should remember that newborns and infants have a chest wall that is more compliant than older children and adults. Therefore, some mild retractions may be present at baseline at this age. The location of retractions, if present, should be noted and documented. Retractions can be subcostal, substernal, intercostal, suprasternal, or supraclavicular; the higher up on the chest the retraction, the more severe the respiratory distress and the degree of airway obstruction.

Inspection of the respiratory system includes more than an evaluation of the chest. The child's head should be assessed for signs of respiratory distress, such as head bobbing, nasal flaring, an anxious facial expression, or pursed lip breathing (O'Hanlon-Nichols, 1998). Grunting or mouth breathing should be noted. Additionally, skin, nail bed, and lip color should be assessed for cyanosis and pallor. Extremities should be assessed for digital clubbing. Clubbing is an abnormal enlargement and an increase in the angle of the finger (see Figure 2.2) and toe bases. To check for clubbing, ask the child to place both thumbs together (nail beds facing each other). Normally, the nurse will see a diamond shape space between the fingers when the thumbs are in this position. Clubbing eliminates this space

Table 2.1 Breathing patterns.

Pattern	Description	Potential implications
Tachypnea	Abnormally high respiratory rate	Respiratory disease with decreased compliance, fever, anxiety, metabolic acidosis
Bradypnea	Abnormally low respiratory rate	Depression of central nervous system, metabolic alkalosis
Hyperpnea	Unusually deep respirations	Anxiety, exercise, fever, metabolic acidosis
Hypopnea	Shallow breathing	Central nervous system depression, metabolic alkalosis, pain
Apnea	Cessation of respirations for more than 15 seconds or for less if accompanied by bradycardia or cyanosis	
Periodic breathing	At least three respiratory pauses of 3- to 10-second duration with less than 20 seconds of respiration between pauses	Common in preterm infants and sometimes seen in normal full-term infants under 3 months of age
Paradoxical breathing	Seesaw breathing/ thoracoabdominal asynchrony	Can be common in newborns (especially preterm infants) due to the compliant nature of their chest wall; it can also be due to respiratory distress
Kussmaul's breathing	Deep, slow, regular respirations with a prolonged expiratory phase	Ketoacidosis
Cheyne–Stokes breathing	Cycles of increasing and decreasing depths of tidal volumes separated by periods of apnea	Increased intracranial pressure, congestive heart failure
Biot's breathing	Cycles of irregular respiration at variable tidal volumes associated with periods of apnea of varying lengths	Severe brain damage

because the angle of the nail base is greater than 180° (Cox, 2001). Clubbing may be due to chronic hypoxia. However, it can be hereditary, so the nurse should always evaluate the parents' fingers if he/she suspects clubbing.

Palpation

The chest should be palpated for pulsations, tenderness, depressions, and abnormal movements (Seidel et al., 2003). Palpation should be performed with the palm of your hand or the pads of your fingers.

Crepitus is a crinkly sensation that indicates air in the subcutaneous space. It can be present with a chest injury or pneumothorax. In newborns,

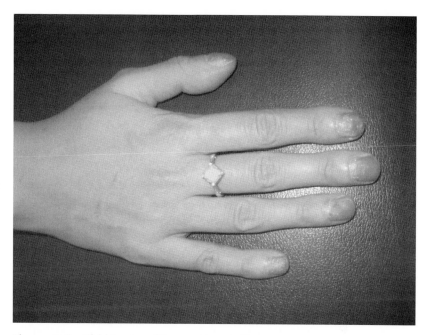

Figure 2.2 Clubbing in a 20-year-old cystic fibrosis patient.

crepitus may be present with a clavicular fracture sustained after a difficult delivery (Seidel et al., 2003). In addition to visualizing chest expansion, it should also be palpated. To do so, posteriorly place thumbs along the spinal process at the level of the 10th rib with palms lightly in contact with the posteriolateral surfaces. During inspiration and exhalation, the thumbs should move symmetrically. This assessment should be repeated anteriorly by placing the thumbs along the costal margin and the xiphoid process. Asymmetrical movement can be due to atelectasis, pneumonia, or pneumothorax (Lippincott, 2007; Seidel et al., 2003).

Tactile fremitus is the palpable vibration of the chest wall that results from verbalization. To check for tactile fremitus, lightly place open palms (fingers should not be touching the back) on the child's back. Ask the child to repeat the word "99" several times. Vibrations produced should be equal on both sides. An increase in vibrations is related to consolidation, such as pneumonia. A decrease in vibrations is related to limited air movement such as pneumothorax (Lippincott, 2007). Tracheal position should be evaluated. To assess for tracheal deviation, place your index finger in the sternal notch and move it gently, side to side, along the upper edges of each clavicle and in the spaces above to the inner borders of the sternocleidomastoid muscles. The trachea should be midline directly above the suprasternal notch (Seidel et al., 2003).

Auscultation

Auscultation is used to assess normal lung sounds and to detect adventitious sounds. Auscultation should be performed using the diaphragm of the stethoscope. The stethoscope should be placed directly on the child's skin. In addition, if old enough, the child should be instructed to breathe with his/her mouth open. It is essential to auscultate the full respiratory cycle (inhalation and exhalation) at each site, systematically moving side to side while comparing the sounds bilaterally.

Lung sounds are characterized by intensity, pitch, quality, and duration. The normal lung sound is not musical and does not have distinct peaks (Pasterkamp, Kraman, & Wodicka, 1997). Normal lung sounds can be further differentiated into vesicular, bronchovesicular, and bronchial/tracheal sounds. Vesicular sounds are low pitched and heard over healthy peripheral lung fields. Bronchovesicular sounds are moderately pitched and heard over the main bronchus. Bronchial/tracheal sounds are high pitched and heard over the trachea and larynx (O'Hanlon-Nichols, 1998).

Adventitious sounds are superimposed on normal lung sounds. Wheezes are high-pitched, whistle-like, musical sounds that are continuous in nature (O'Hanlon-Nichols, 1998; Pasterkamp et al., 1997). Crackles (previously known as rales) are discontinuous sounds that can be classified as fine or coarse. Fine crackles are soft and high pitched. Coarse crackles are louder and lower in pitch (Lippincott, 2007). Crackles resemble the sound of rubbing hair between one's fingers. Crackles are most often heard on inspiration and are not cleared by coughing (O'Hanlon-Nichols, 1998; Pasterkamp et al., 1997). Rhonchi are snorelike, deep sounds usually heard on expiration (O'Hanlon-Nichols, 1998; Pasterkamp et al., 1997). Rhonchi usually clear with coughing. (O'Hanlon-Nichols, 1998).

Percussion

Percussion is a tapping technique used to produce sounds from underlying tissues and organs (O'Hanlon-Nichols, 1998). When percussing the posterior portion of the chest, ask the child to sit with head bent forward and arms folded in front if he is old enough. To percuss the lateral and anterior portions of the chest, ask the child to lift his arms over his head.

Percussion should be performed over the intercostal spaces. To percuss, place the distal joint of your middle finger (use your nondominant hand) firmly on the chest. With the index and the middle finger of your dominant hand, use a quick, sharp, relaxed wrist motion to hit the distal joint of the finger that is resting on the chest. This action will produce a sound. Each site should be percussed about three times. Like auscultation, percussion should be performed systematically and sounds should be compared bilaterally.

Sounds (resonance, hyperresonance, dull, flat, and tympanic) are again characterized by intensity, pitch, quality, and duration. Resonance is heard

Table 2.2 Percussion sounds.

Sound	Intensity	Pitch	Quality	Duration	Example
Resonance	+++	**	Hollow	Long	Normal, healthy lung
Hyperresonance	++++	*/**	Boomlike	Long/longer	Hyperinflated lung
Dull	+/++	***/***	Thudlike	Moderate	Heart or liver
Flat	+	****	Dull	Short	Bone or muscle
Tympanic	+++	****	Drumlike	Moderate	Stomach

+, soft; ++, medium; +++, loud; ++++, very loud;
*, very low; **, low; ***, medium; ****, high.

when percussing over normal lung areas. If an area sounds hyperresonant, it may be due to asthma or a pneumothorax. If an area sounds dull or flat, it may be due to atelectasis or pneumonia. A full description of percussion sounds can be located in Table 2.2 (Cox, 2001; O'Hanlon-Nichols, 1998; Seidel et al., 2003).

If percussion reveals an area of dullness, it should be followed by an assessment of vocal resonance or vocal fremitus. Vocal resonance is the transmission of the patient's voice through lung fields. To assess for vocal resonance, ask the child to say "99" while you auscultate all lung fields with a stethoscope. The sound heard should be muffled. If 99 is heard clearly, it is known as bronchophony and is indicative of a consolidation such as pneumonia. If bronchophony is present, assess for egophony by asking the child to say "E" as you auscultate the abnormal area. If the E sounds like "A," egophony is present and consolidation is likely (O'Hanlon-Nichols, 1998). Another test to determine if consolidation is present is called whispered pectoriloquy. To assess whispered pectoriloquy, ask the child to whisper "1, 2, 3." Normally, it would be difficult to hear what the child is saying. However, if consolidation is present, the numbers will be heard clearly (Lippincott, 2007).

The diaphragm is the primary muscle of breathing. The diaphragm is usually higher on the right because of the liver. To measure diaphragmatic excursion in the older child, ask him/her to inhale deeply and to hold his/her breath. Then, percuss along the scapular line until you reach the lower border (sound changes from resonant to dull when you reach the border of the diaphragm). Mark that point and allow the child to breathe. After a few breaths, ask the child to exhale as much as possible and to hold the exhalation. Percuss up from the marked area and make a mark when the sound changes from dull to resonance. Repeat on the opposite side. Then, measure the distance between the two marks on each side. Diaphragmatic excursion is usually 3–5 cm (Seidel et al., 2003). A decrease in excursion can be related to pain, a mass in the thoracic or abdominal cavity, or paralysis of one of the diaphragms.

REFERENCES

Bhandari, A., & Panitch, H. B. (2006). Pulmonary outcomes in bronchopulmonary dysplasia. *Seminars in Perinatology, 30*, 219–226.

Cox, C. L. (2001). Respiratory assessment. In G. Esmond (Ed.), *Respiratory nursing* (pp. 21–37). London, UK: Harcourt.

Custer, J. W., & Rau, R. E. (2009). *The harriet lane handbook: A manual for pediatric house officers (front cover)*. Philadelphia: Elsevier Mosby.

Driessnack, M. (2010). Overview of growth and development framework. In C. L. Edelman & C. L. Mandle (Eds.), *Health promotion throughout the life span* (pp. 361–377). St. Louis, MO: Mosby Elsevier.

Hilman, B. C. (1993). Clinical assessment of pulmonary disease in infants and children. In B. C. Hilman (Ed.), *Pediatric respiratory disease and treatment* (pp. 57–67). Philadelphia: W.B. Saunders.

Lippincott. (2007). Respiratory system. In A. L. Mosher & M. Foley (Ed.), *Lippincott manual of nursing practice series: Assessment* (1st ed., pp. 77–105). Philadelphia: Lippincott Williams & Wilkins.

O'Hanlon-Nichols, T. (1998). Basic assessment series the adult pulmonary system. *The American Journal of Nursing, 98*(2), 39–45.

Pasterkamp, H., Kraman, S. S., & Wodicka, G. R. (1997). Respiratory sounds advances beyond the stethoscope. *American Journal of Respiratory and Critical Care Medicine, 156*, 974–987.

Seidel, H. M., Ball, J. W., & Dains, J. E. (2003). *Mosby's guide to physical examination* (5th ed.). St. Louis, MO: Mosby.

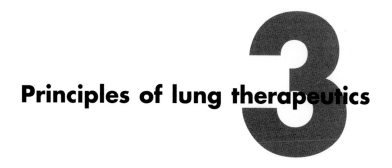

Principles of lung therapeutics

Kathryn Blake, PharmD, BCPS, FCCP

PRINCIPLES OF LUNG THERAPEUTICS

There are a number of classifications of medications utilized in pediatric respiratory medicine disorders. This chapter provides a comprehensive overview (mechanism of action, indication, adverse events, generic and brand name examples, and formulation type) of these common medication categories. Because a number of respiratory medications are administered via inhalation, delivery devices will also be discussed.

BRONCHODILATORS

Short-acting β_2-agonists

Mechanism of action

β_2-agonists bind to and activate the β_2-adrenergic receptor for their pharmacological effects. The β_2-adrenergic receptor belongs to the superfamily of G protein-coupled receptors, which are expressed on membranes in cells in the airways (Barnes, 1995). The β_2-adrenergic receptor spans the cell membrane seven times with the N-terminus located extracellularly and the C-terminus located intracellularly. Activation of the β_2-adrenergic receptor

Nursing Care in Pediatric Respiratory Disease, First Edition. Edited by Concettina (Tina) Tolomeo.
© 2012 John Wiley & Sons, Inc. Published 2012 by John Wiley & Sons, Inc.

initiates the dissociation of the α subunit from the G_s binding protein and stimulation of adenylyl cyclase by the G protein $α_s$ subunit to catalyze the conversion of adenosine triphosphate to cyclic adenosine monophosphate. Activation of protein kinase A by cyclic adenosine monophosphate inhibits myosin light chain kinase phosphorylation and formation of inositol trisphosphate, which promotes Ca^{2+}/Na^+ exchange, causing a decrease in intracellular calcium, leading to smooth muscle relaxation and bronchodilation (Nijkamp et al., 1992). Phosphorylation by protein kinase A (heterologous desensitization) causes rapid receptor desensitization; receptor uncoupling (homologous desensitization) is mediated via G protein receptor kinases and β-arrestin (Barnes, 1995; Billington & Penn, 2003; Lohse, 1993; Shore & Moore, 2003). Short- or long-term agonist exposure of $β_2$-adrenergic receptor causes reduction in receptor density (downregulation) and long-term desensitization (Hardin & Lima, 1999; Lohse, 1993).

The synthetic production of $β_2$-agonists results in a 1:1 racemic mixture of (R)- and (S)-enantiomers (Waldeck, 2002). The pharmacological activity is due to the (R)-enantiomer, and it was originally thought that the (S)-enantiomer was essentially inactive due to the 100- to 1,000-fold potency difference between the (R)- and (S)-enantiomers (Lotvall et al., 2001; Waldeck, 1999). However, animal and *in vitro* studies suggest that the (S)-enantiomer of albuterol could be proinflammatory and could increase bronchial hyperreactivity (Waldeck, 1999), but there is no evidence this is clinically relevant in patients (Kercsmar & McDowell, 2009). Racemic albuterol and levalbuterol provide equivalent bronchodilation and effects on serum glucose and serum potassium at equivalent doses of the (R)-enantiomer (Lotvall et al., 2001). Clinical studies have shown no advantages of levalbuterol over albuterol (Kercsmar & McDowell, 2009).

$β_2$-agonists have anti-inflammatory effects demonstrated *in vitro* that are not apparent by biopsy or clinically even with longer-term administration (EPR 3, 2007; Laitinen, Laitinen, & Haahtela, 1992; Nelson, 1995; Roberts et al., 1999). However, $β_2$-agonists and inhaled corticosteroids may act synergistically at the molecular level (Barnes, 2002).

Common indications

Short-acting $β_2$-agonists are indicated for the treatment of acute bronchospasm with reversible obstructive airway disease or prevention of exercise-induced bronchospasm. Albuterol metered-dose inhaler (MDI) and nebulizer solution are approved for patients aged 4 years and older; pirbuterol MDI is approved for patients aged 12 years and older; levalbuterol MDI is approved for patients 4 years and older; and the nebulizer solution is approved for patients 6 years and older. Albuterol syrup and immediate-release tablets are approved for patients 2 years and older and the extended-release tablets for patients 6 years and older. Metaproterenol syrup and tablets are approved for patients 6 years and older. Terbutaline tablets are approved for patients 12 years and older.

Common adverse effects

Adverse effects associated with acute use

Acute adverse effects are significantly reduced when β_2-agonists are administered by the inhaled route compared to oral administration. The most common adverse effects include tachycardia, tremor, nausea, vomiting, and nervousness.

Other adverse effects can include rhinitis, increased blood pressure, throat irritation, insomnia, headache, hypokalemia, and nightmares. Tolerance to adverse effects generally occurs within several weeks of regular use.

Adverse effects associated with chronic use

There has been concern that β_2-agonists cause worsening asthma, near death, or death with regular or excessive use. After pressurized aerosols were introduced in the late 1950s, the first asthma mortality epidemic occurred in England and Wales between 1961 and 1966 and was associated with the increased use of pressurized β_2-agonist aerosols, primarily isoproterenol (Giuntini & Paggiaro, 1995; Inman & Adelstein, 1969; Sears, 1993). A second epidemic in mortality occurred in New Zealand shortly after the introduction of fenoterol, a full β_2-agonist, in 1976 (Pearce et al., 1995; Sears, 1993), and mortality declined after its withdrawal in 1990 (Beasley et al., 1995; Pearce et al., 1995). Further concerns with short-acting β_2-agonists were raised by an analysis of drug prescription records in Saskatchewan, Canada, from 1978 to 1987, which found that albuterol MDI use was associated with an increased risk of death or near death from asthma (Spitzer et al., 1992).

However, a controlled study of albuterol administered four times daily in asthmatics with milder disease demonstrated no deterioration in asthma control with albuterol use (Drazen et al., 1996). These epidemiological and clinical trial data prompted the recommendation that regular scheduled use of short-acting inhaled β_2-agonists be discouraged and as-needed use be promoted as a way to minimize exposure and to monitor changes in asthma control. It has been further suggested that short-acting β_2-agonist use should be limited in patients with certain genetic polymorphisms in the adrenergic β_2-receptor gene (Israel et al., 2004) and instead, patients should be prescribed alternative bronchodilators such as ipratropium bromide. However, the basis for this recommendation should be confirmed in other studies before being widely adopted in clinical practice.

Generic and brand names

Short-acting β_2-agonists delivered by MDI include albuterol (ProAir HFA, Ventolin HFA, and Proventil HFA), pirbuterol (Maxair Autohaler), and levalbuterol (Xopenex HFA); and by nebulization include albuterol (AccuNeb and various generics) and levalbuterol (Xopenex, and generic).

Oral tablets include albuterol (VoSpire ER and various generics), metaproterenol (various generics), and terbutaline (various generics); and oral syrups include albuterol (various generics) and metaproterenol (various generics).

Formulations

Short-acting β_2-agonists may be administered by inhalation (MDI and nebulization), orally (tablets and syrup), or intravenously.

Long-acting bronchochodilators

Mechanism of action

Long-acting β_2-agonists have the same mechanism for causing bronchodilation as short-acting β_2-agonists but are more lipophilic, which allows greater partitioning into the cell membrane outer phospholipid layer. The long duration of the effect of salmeterol is believed to be due to binding to an exocite, which may permit a nearly continuous stimulation of the β-receptor, while the long action of formoterol is believed to be due to its extreme lipophilicity and high affinity at the β_2-agonist receptor (Anderson, 1993; Rong et al., 1999).

Common indications

Salmeterol is indicated for long-term, twice-daily administration in the maintenance and treatment of asthma and in the prevention of bronchospasm in patients aged 4 years and older with reversible obstructive airway disease, including patients with symptoms of nocturnal asthma. It is to be used only as concomitant therapy with a long-term asthma control medication, such as an inhaled corticosteroid (Salmeterol Prescribing Information, 2010).

Formoterol is indicated for long-term, twice-daily administration in the maintenance and treatment of asthma and in the prevention of bronchospasm in adults and in children 5 years of age and older with reversible obstructive airway disease, including patients with nocturnal asthma, who require regular treatment with inhaled, short-acting β_2-agonists. It is indicated for the prevention of exercise-induced bronchospasm in adults and in children 12 years of age and older when administered on an occasional, as-needed basis (Formoterol Prescribing Information, 2010).

The Food and Drug Administration (as of February 2010) has required that products containing salmeterol or formoterol include the following in the label:

- The use of long-acting β_2-agonists is contraindicated without the use of an asthma controller medication such as inhaled corticosteroid.

Single-agent long-acting β_2-agonists should only be used in combination with an asthma controller medication; they should not be used alone.

- Long-acting β_2-agonists should only be used long-term in patients whose asthma cannot be adequately controlled on asthma controller medications.
- Long-acting β_2-agonists should be used for the shortest duration of time required to achieve control of asthma symptoms and should be discontinued, if possible, once asthma control is achieved. Patients should then be maintained on an asthma controller medication.
- Pediatric and adolescent patients who require a long-acting β_2-agonist in addition to an inhaled corticosteroid should use a combination product containing both an inhaled corticosteroid and a long-acting β_2-agonist to ensure compliance with both medications.

The reason for the Food and Drug Administration issuing these labeling requirements relates to adverse effects that have been noted with chronic daily use of these drugs (see the section "Adverse Effects Associated with Chronic Use").

Common adverse effects

Adverse effects associated with acute use

The adverse effects associated with the acute use of long-acting β_2-agonists are the same as encountered with short-acting β_2-agonists.

Adverse effects associated with chronic use

Salmeterol was introduced into the U.S. market in 1997. A large surveillance study completed prior to marketing compared regularly scheduled use of salmeterol versus albuterol in the United Kingdom and demonstrated fewer worsenings of asthma control, but a greater number of asthma deaths in the salmeterol versus albuterol treated group (Castle et al., 1993). These results prompted the Food and Drug Administration to require the conduct of the Salmeterol Multicenter Asthma Research Trial in 1996 (Nelson et al., 2006). The results from this trial demonstrated a twofold increase in respiratory-related deaths and an over fourfold increase in asthma-related deaths in patients treated with salmeterol versus placebo over 6 months (Nelson et al., 2006). These effects were largely observed in the African American subpopulation. Formoterol has also been associated with increases in exacerbation rates (Mann et al., 2003). After these data were published, the importance of using long-acting β_2-agonists only in conjunction with an anti-inflammatory drug (preferably inhaled corticosteroids) was emphasized in the literature. The *Guidelines for the Diagnosis and Management of Asthma* was revised in 2007 and reflects the fact that long-acting β_2-agonists are to be used only in patients who are not controlled on low to medium doses of inhaled corticosteroids or whose disease is considered severe enough to warrant initial treatment with two mainte-nance therapies (EPR 3, 2007).

Generic and brand names

Salmeterol is available as Serevent Diskus and formoterol is available as Foradil Aerolizer. Both drugs are also contained in several combination inhaler products with inhaled corticosteroids (see the section "Inhaled Corticosteroids").

Formulations

Both salmeterol (as Serevent Diskus) and formoterol (as Foradil Aerolizer) are available only as dry powder inhalers (DPIs). Both MDI and DPI forma-tions are available when these drugs are combined into a single inhaler with an inhaled corticosteroid.

Anticholinergics

Mechanism of action

The parasympathetic (vs. the sympathetic) nervous system is largely responsible for the control of baseline airway caliber. Therefore, anticho-linergic drugs, which are competitive antagonists rather than functional antagonists, will be most useful in those patients whose symptoms are due to excessive cholinergic stimulation. However, it is not possible to predict who these patients are. Because most mediators, such as histamine, aller-gens, and exercise, cause bronchoconstriction only partially through cho-linergic stimulation, anticholinergics will be less effective than β_2-adrenergic agonists and theophylline, which are functional antagonists.

There are five muscarinic acetylcholine receptor subtypes (M1–M5) of which M1, M2, and M3 are expressed in the lung. Each belongs to the superfamily of G protein-coupled receptors. On the airway smooth muscle, acetylcholine activates M3 receptors, which results in the receptors cou-pling with the heterotrimeric G protein G_{q11}. This causes stimulation of phospholipase C and an increase in intracellular calcium and subsequent smooth muscle contraction (Belmonte, 2005). There are about four times more M2 than M3 receptors in airway smooth muscle, and M2 receptors preferentially couple to the G protein $G_{\alpha o/i}$. This action inhibits production and accumulation of cyclic adenosine monophosphate, thus countering the mechanism for β_2-receptor-mediated bronchodilation (Belmonte, 2005). M2 receptors, located on the postganglionic terminal in the airways, inhibit acetylcholine release and stimulate uptake, and thus function as inhibitory feedback receptors (Belmonte, 2005). On airway submucosal glands, stimulation of M3 receptors, located on mucus glands, causes mucus secretion (Belmonte, 2005). Nonselective blockade of M2 and M3 receptors could result in an increased release of acetylcholine (via M2 receptor inhibition on postganglionic terminals), which could overcome the smooth muscle relaxation mediated by the M3 receptor.

Ipratropium bromide is a nonselective antagonist at the M1, M2, and M3 receptors and is a quaternary ammonium compound, which is poorly absorbed across the blood–brain barrier and thus has few systemic effects compared to atropine. Tiotropium bromide, also a quaternary ammonium compound, is an antagonist at the M1, M2, and M3 receptors, but it dissociates from the M2 receptors more quickly, which allows for a more prolonged duration of bronchodilation than seen with ipratropium (Chen, Bollmeier, & Finnegan, 2008). Anticholinergics are effective bronchodilators but do not achieve the same maximal bronchodilation as β_2-adrenergic agonists in asthmatics. Maximum bronchodilation with ipratropium bromide occurs in 1.5–2.0 hours; however, 50% of the eventual maximum occurs within 3–5 minutes and 80% within 30 minutes (Pakes et al., 1980), which is comparable clinically to the time of peak effect (30 minutes) with inhaled β_2-adrenergic agonists. The duration of bronchodilation is 4–8 hours. Tiotropium effects last at least 24 hours. Intensity and duration of effect are dose dependent.

Common indications

Ipratropium and tiotropium are indicated only for relieving bronchospasm associated with, and reducing exacerbations of, chronic obstructive pulmonary disease, including chronic bronchitis and emphysema. However, anticholinergic drugs have been used in the treatment of asthma-like symptoms for over 400 years.

Common adverse effects

Ipratropium and tiotropium are remarkably free of unwanted adverse effects because of minimal systemic absorption. Common adverse effects may include dry mouth, irritated throat, and bitter taste. Anticholinergic drugs may precipitate or worsen narrow-angle glaucoma, mydriasis, acute eye pain, urinary retention, and tachycardia, and may cause paradoxical bronchospasm; allergic reactions may occur. The effects on the eye may be greater for nebulized ipratropium due to ocular exposure with the mist during administration by this route. Patients with peanut or soy allergy should not use combivent MDI (combination of ipratropium and albuterol) as anaphylaxis may occur due to the presence of soya lecithin in the formulation. There is a potential allergic cross-reactivity between soy and other legumes, such as peanuts.

Generic and brand names

The available products include ipratropium bromide (Atrovent HFA, and Combivent [combination of ipratropium and albuterol] as an MDI, and the combination of ipratropium and albuterol (DuoNeb, various generics available) as a solution for nebulization and tiotropium bromide (Spiriva HandiHaler) as a DPI.

Formulations

Ipratropium bromide is available as an MDI and nebulizer solution. Tiotropium bromide is available as a DPI.

INHALED CORTICOSTEROIDS

Mechanism of action

Corticosteroids diffuse across the cell membrane and bind to glucocorticoid receptors in the cytoplasm causing dissociation of molecular chaperone proteins (heat shock protein-90, FL-binding protein) from glucocorticoid receptors allowing the glucocorticoid receptor–corticosteroid complex to be transported into the nucleus. A homodimer of two glucocorticoid receptor–corticosteroid molecules bind to promoter regions (glucocorticoid response elements) of corticosteroid-responsive genes. Gene transcription ensues or, uncommonly, gene suppression, in approximately 10–100 genes, which are directly regulated by corticosteroids (Barnes, 2006). Gene activation is initiated by glucocorticoid–receptor dimer associated histone H4 acetylation or by interaction with cyclic adenosine monophosphate response element binding protein and p300-cyclic adenosine monophosphate response element binding protein associated factor (Barnes, 2006). This action induces histone acetylation, leading to chromatic unwinding allowing DNA to be available for gene transcription (Barnes, 2006). However, there are relatively few anti-inflammatory genes, and most inflammatory genes activated in asthma do not have apparent promoter region glucocorticoid response element sites (Barnes, 2006). Corticosteroids may have their effects largely on chromatin structure and histone acetylation by inhibiting histone acetylase activity and by preventing chromatin unwinding, thus repressing inflammatory genes (Barnes, 2006). Nontranscriptional effects may include reducing messenger RNA (mRNA) stability, leading to a reduction in inflammatory protein expression (Barnes, 2006).

The anti-inflammatory effects of corticosteroids include suppression of inflammatory cytokines and chemokines (IL-3, IL4, IL-6, IL-8, IL-11, IL-13, and IL-16), granulocyte-macrophage colony-stimulating factor, tumor necrosis factor-α, high-affinity IgE receptor, and other molecules.

Corticosteroids also suppress levels and activities of inflammatory cells including eosinophils, basophils, monocytes, mast cells, and dendridic cells. They decrease capillary permeability and plasma exudation, upregulate β_2-receptors on airway smooth muscle but have little effect on the activity of leukotrienes (Negri et al., 2008).

Common indications

All inhaled corticosteroids are indicated for the maintenance treatment of asthma as prophylactic therapy and for patients who require oral corticosteroid therapy for asthma. The minimum approved age for the use of inhalers (pressured MDI and dry powder) and nebulized products are the following: flunisolide (Aerobid), 6 years; mometasone (Asmanex Twisthaler), 4 years; fluticasone (Flovent HFA Inhalation Aerosol and Flovent Diskus), 4 years; budesonide (Pulmicort Flexhaler), 6 years; budesonide for nebulization (Pulmicort Respules), 12 months (to 8 years old); beclomethasone (Q-Var), 5 years; and ciclesonide (Alvesco), 12 years. The combination products of an inhaled corticosteroid plus either salmeterol or formoterol are indicated for maintenance treatment of asthma, and they are not indicated for patients whose asthma can be managed by inhaled corticosteroids with occasional use of inhaled short-acting β_2-agonists. They are also not indicated for the relief of acute bronchospasm. The minimum indicated age for Advair (fluticasone with salmeterol) is 4 years; Dulera (mometasone with formoterol), 12 years; and Symbicort (budesonide with formoterol), 12 years.

Common adverse effects

In large doses, inhaled corticosteroids can cause the same adverse effects as seen with oral use. Systemic adverse effects from inhaled corticosteroids occur due to the portion of the drug that is absorbed orally and that which is absorbed through the lung after inhalation.

Local adverse effects include oral candidiasis, dysphonia, and cough/bronchospasm (EPR 3, 2007). These effects can be minimized by the use of a valved holding chamber with a non-breath-activated MDI (EPR 3, 2007). Prevention of oral candidiasis should include rinsing and spitting after inhalation.

Potential systemic adverse effects include reduction in linear growth, reduction in bone mineral density, disseminated varicella, dermal thinning and increased bruising, increased risk of cataracts or glaucoma, hypothalamic–pituitary–adrenal axis suppression, and impaired glucose metabolism.

Studies of the effects of inhaled corticosteroids on linear growth in children suggest any effects noted with low or medium doses are small and are likely to be reversible (EPR 3, 2007). Children should be maintained on the lowest dose that achieves adequate control of the symptoms. Reduction in growth velocity can occur if asthma is not controlled or if oral corticosteroids are frequently used. There appears to be no differences between inhaled corticosteroids on the effect on linear growth. Children should have height measurements obtained routinely during treatment.

Changes in bone mineral density are unlikely to occur in children treated with low to medium doses (EPR 3, 2007). Although an effect on bone mineral density can be observed in adults, there do not appear to be significant clinical consequences (EPR 3, 2007). Patients with, or risk factors for, osteoporosis should have their bone mineral density measured every 1–2 years (EPR 3, 2007).

The risk for disseminated varicella with inhaled corticosteroids is low, as there is no evidence that the recommended doses are immunosuppressive (EPR 3, 2007).

Dermal thinning and increased skin bruising can occur; the effect is dose dependent. It is not known at what minimum dose these effects would be most likely to occur (EPR 3, 2007).

Ocular effects are not likely with low to medium doses of inhaled corticosteroids, but the risk increases when the lifetime cumulative exposure is above 2,000 mg of beclomethasone dipropionate or equivalent inhaled corticosteroid dosage (EPR 3, 2007). Patients with a family history of glaucoma should have ophthalmic evaluations regularly.

Hypothalamic–pituitary–adrenal axis suppression is unlikely to occur in patients on low to medium doses of inhaled corticosteroids (EPR 3, 2007).

Glucose homeostasis is unlikely to be affected by inhaled corticosteroid doses up to 1,000 µg/day (EPR 3, 2007).

Generic and brand names

Products available as pressurized MDIs include beclomethasone (Q-Var), budesonide (Symbicort—a combination inhaler of budesonide and formoterol), ciclesonide (Alvesco), fluticasone (Flovent HFA and Advair HFA—a combination inhaler with fluticasone and salmeterol), flunisolide (Aerospan HFA and Aerobid), and mometasone (Dulera—a combination inhaler of mometasone and formoterol).

Products available as DPIs include budesonide (Pulmicort Flexhaler), fluticasone (Advair Diskus, a combination inhaler with fluticasone and salmeterol, and Flovent Diskus), and mometasone (Asmanex Twisthaler).

The only product available as a nebulizer solution is budesonide (Pulmicort Respules and generics).

Formulations

Inhaled corticosteroids are available as a pressurized MDI, DPI, and nebulizer solution.

LEUKOTRIENE MODIFIERS

Mechanism of action

Leukotriene production, formed from the 5-lipoxygenase pathway of arachidonic acid metabolism, is initiated when arachidonic acid is released from cell membrane phospholipids by the action of phospholipase A_2. Membrane-bound 5-lipoxygenase, in concert with 5-lipoxygenase-activating protein, converts arachidonic acid to leukotriene A_4, which is converted to leukotriene B_4 by leukotriene A_4 hydrolase or is conjugated with reduced glutathione by leukotriene C_4 synthase to form leukotriene C_4 (Peters-Golden & Henderson, 2007). Leukotriene B_4 and leukotriene C_4 are transported to the extracellular space where leukotriene C_4 is converted to leukotriene D_4 by γ-glutamyltransferase (Anderson, Allison, & Meister, 1982), which is then converted to leukotriene E_4 by dipeptidase (Lee et al., 1983). Leukotriene C_4, leukotriene D_4, and leukotriene E_4 are called cysteinyl leukotrienes. Leukotriene C_4, leukotriene D_4, and leukotriene E_4 are formed primarily in eosinophils, basophils, and mast cells; leukotriene B_4 is found largely in neutrophils, macrophages, and dendridic cells (Peters-Golden & Henderson, 2007). The cysteinyl leukotrienes cause bronchoconstriction, airway hyperresponsiveness, smooth muscle hypertrophy, mucus hypersecretion and mucosal edema, and the influx of eosinophils into airway tissue by binding to and activating two G protein-coupled receptors, cys-leukotriene 1 (CysLT) and cys-leukotriene 2 (Drazen & Austen, 1987; Salvi et al., 2001). The relative affinities of the cysteinyl-leukotrienes for the cys-leukotriene 1 receptor are leukotriene $D_4 \gg$ leukotriene $C_4 >$ leukotriene E_4. Cys-leukotriene 1 receptors are expressed in airway smooth muscle, tissue macrophages, monocytes, and eosinophils, and cys-leukotriene 2 receptors are found in airway macrophages and smooth muscle cells (Lynch et al., 1999; Spahr & Krawiec, 2008).

Leukotriene receptor antagonists (montelukast and zafirlukast) are LTD4 inhibitors at the CysLT1 receptor and exert their beneficial effects in asthma by antagonizing the detrimental effects of the cysteinyl leukotrienes in airways. Leukotriene sysnthesis inhibitors, also called 5-lipoxygenase inhibitors (zileuton), block the formation of leukotrienes at the earliest step by inhibiting the action of the 5-lipoxygenase enzyme. Beneficial effects of leukotriene modifiers (CysLT1 receptor inhibitors and synthsis inhibitors) include improved lung function, reduced β_2-agonist use, attenuated exercise-induced bronchospasm, improved asthma symptoms, reduced use of inhaled corticosteroids, improved quality of life, reduced circulating levels of blood eosinophils, and reduced levels of exhaled nitric oxide (Blake, 1999; Currie & McLaughlin, 2006; Kelly, 2007).

Common indications

Montelukast (an LTD4 inhibitor at the CysLT1 receptor) is indicated for the prophylaxis and chronic treatment of asthma in patients 12 months of age

and older and for the acute prevention of exercise-induced bronchoconstriction in patients 15 years of age and older. It is also indicated for the
relief of symptoms of allergic rhinitis (seasonal allergic rhinitis in patients
2 years of age and older, and perennial allergic rhinitis in patients 6 months
of age and older). Patients with asthma and allergic rhinitis may receive
benefit for both conditions when using montelukast. Zafirlukast (an LTD4
inhibitor at the CysLT1 receptor) is indicated for the prophylaxis and
chronic treatment of asthma in adults and children 5 years of age and older.
Zileuton (a 5-lipoxygenase inhibitor) is indicated for the prophylaxis and
chronic treatment of asthma in adults and in children 12 years of age
and older.

The Guidelines for the Diagnosis and Management of Asthma state that
leukotriene receptor antagonists are indicated as an alternative to low-dose
inhaled corticosteroids for patients with mild persistent asthma and are
recommended as add-on treatment to inhaled corticosteroids after consideration of either increasing the inhaled corticosteroid dose or adding a
long-acting β_2-agonist to inhaled corticosteroid in patients with moderate
to severe persistent asthma (EPR 3, 2007). Despite differences in the mechanism of action, there is no evidence for clinical differences between
5-lipoxygenase inhibitors and leukotriene receptor antagonists (Kelly,
2007).

Common adverse effects

Common but not serious adverse effects include headache, abdominal
pain, pharyngitis, influenza, fever, sinusitis, nausea, diarrhea, dyspepsia,
otitis media, viral infection, and laryngitis.

All the leukotriene modifiers have been associated with the occurrence
of Churg–Strauss syndrome. Occurrence of Churg–Strauss syndrome is
characterized by eosinophilic vasculitis and possible cardiopulmonary
complications (Harrold et al., 2007; Lilly et al., 2002). This syndrome
appears to manifest in individuals with asthma who were previously controlled with oral corticosteroids and who were weaned from their use after
the introduction of a leukotriene modifier or inhaled corticosteroid therapy
(Lilly et al., 2002). No causal association between leukotriene modifiers or
inhaled corticosteroid therapy and the development of Churg–Strauss syndrome has been established. This event is rare but would be considered
serious.

Recently, reports of behavior changes related to leukotriene modifier use
has created concern and prompted warnings to be included in the prescribing information. The labeling for leukotriene modifiers now contains language stating "agitation, aggressive behavior or hostility, anxiousness,
depression, dream abnormalities, hallucinations, insomnia, irritability,
restlessness, somnambulism, suicidal thinking and behavior (including
suicide), and tremor may occur." Analyses from two recent publications
involving over 20,000 patients treated with montelukast found no evidence

of "possibly suicidality related adverse events" nor "behavior-related adverse events" (Philip et al., 2009a, 2009b). In addition, analysis of three recent large asthma trials conducted by the American Lung Association Asthma Clinical Research Centers network in 569 patients treated with montelukast has uncovered no behavioral problems (Holbrook & Harik-Khan, 2008). These events are rare but would be considered serious.

Zileuton can cause liver dysfunction, and liver function monitoring is currently recommended before treatment begins: once a month for the first 3 months, every two to three months for the remainder of the first year, and periodically thereafter for patients receiving long-term therapy (Zileuton Prescribing Information, 2009).

Zafirlukast can also cause liver dysfunction. Periodic serum transaminase testing has not been proven to prevent serious injury, but it is generally believed that early detection of drug-induced hepatic injury along with immediate withdrawal of the suspect drug enhances the likelihood for recovery (Zafirlukast Prescribing Information, 2009).

Generic and brand names

Leukotriene modifiers are available as montelukast (Singulair), zafirlukast (Accolate), and zileuton (Zyflo and Zyflo CR).

Formulations

All leukotriene modifiers are available as tablets for oral ingestion. Montelukast (Singulair) is also available as a chewable tablet and as granules (to be sprinkled on food for young children).

OTHER ANTI-INFLAMMATORY DRUGS AND IMMUNE MODULATORS

Cromolyn

Mechanism of action

The exact mechanisms of action for cromolyn is largely unknown, but it inhibits IgE mediated release of mediators from mast cells and also inhibits the release of mediators from eosinophils, alveolar macrophages, neutrophils, and monocytes (Brogden & Sorkin, 1993). This effect varies depending on the species and the cell type tested (Kelly, 1999a). Cromolyn prevents mast cell degranulation induced by nonimmunologic stimuli, such as phospholipase A, dextran, and polymyxin B. This effect likely involves regulation of intracellular calcium probably by phosphorylation of a specific membrane protein, which inhibits calcium influx into the cell. Other nonspecific effects include inhibition of phosphodiesterase, modification of the vagal reflex, inhibition of irritant receptors, chemotaxis inhibition of inflammatory mediators, and possibly inhibition of inflammatory neuro-peptide release, which induce bronchoconstriction through efferent cholin-ergic pathways (Kelly, 1999a).

Common indications

Cromolyn is indicated for the prophylaxis of asthma symptoms. The solu-tion for nebulization is indicated for patients 2 years and older. It is not indicated for the relief of symptoms from acute bronchoconstriction.

Common adverse effects

Adverse effects include transient bronchospasm, cough, bad taste, and nausea. Bronchospasm is quickly relieved with the administration of an inhaled β_2-agonist.

Generic and brand names

The only available cromolyn products are solution for nebulization (various generics).

Formulations

Cromolyn is available as a solution for nebulization.

Omalizumab

Mechanism of action

Omalizumab is an anti-IgE monoclonal antibody. IgE plays a critical role in the inflammatory process of allergic asthma, and high-affinity receptors for circulating IgE (Fcε-R1) are found on mast cells and basophils. Allergens inhaled into the lung cross-link IgE bound to mast cells and basophils, which causes the mast cells and basophils to degranulate and release pre-formed mediators (histamine and tryptase) and rapidly synthesized medi-ators (bradykinin, prostaglandin E2, prostaglandin F2, and leukotrienes). Omalizumab binds to the Cε3 domain of free IgE in the serum and not to IgE already bound to mast cells. The omalizumab–IgE complex prevents IgE from binding to the Fcε-R1 on mast cells and basophils. Omalizumab also downregulates Fcε-R1 receptor expression on basophils, which further dampens the allergic response (Holgate et al., 2005). Serum IgE levels are not to be measured for monitoring purposes, as most clinical assays do not distinguish between free and bound IgE in the serum (Ruffin & Busch, 2004).

Common indications

Omalizumab is indicated for patients with moderate to severe persistent asthma who have had a positive skin test or *in vitro* reactivity to a perennial aeroallergen and symptoms that are inadequately controlled with inhaled corticosteroids (Omalizumab Prescribing Information, 2010). It is not indicated for other allergic conditions, acute bronchospasm, or for patients less than 12 years of age.

Common adverse effects

The most common adverse reactions are arthralgia and pain. Injection site reactions including bruising, redness, warmth, burning, stinging, itching, hive formation, pain, indurations, mass, and inflammation can occur within 1 hour of injection and may last up to 8 days. Injection site reactions tend to decrease with continued treatment (Omalizumab Prescribing Information, 2010).

Anaphylaxis is a potential adverse effect; thus, patients should be observed for a period of time after dosing. The frequency of anaphylaxis attributed to omalizumab is estimated to be at least 0.2% of patients (Omalizumab Prescribing Information, 2010). Signs and symptoms in these reported cases have included bronchospasm, hypotension, syncope, urticaria, and/or angioedema of the throat or tongue (Omalizumab Prescribing Information, 2010). Anaphylaxis has occurred as early as after the first dose of omalizumab but also has occurred beyond 1 year after beginning regularly scheduled treatment (Omalizumab Prescribing Information, 2010). Symptoms may begin within 2 hours after the dose.

Malignant neoplasms have been reported with omalizumab use and were observed in 20 of 4,127 (0.5%) Xolair-treated patients compared with 5 of 2,236 (0.2%) control patients in clinical studies of adults and adolescents with asthma and other allergic disorders (Omalizumab Prescribing Information, 2010). The observed malignancies in omalizumab-treated patients included breast, nonmelanoma skin, prostate, melanoma, and parotid, which occurred more than once, and five other types, which occurred only once each (Omalizumab Prescribing Information, 2010). An independent panel concluded that these findings did not suggest a neoplastic risk with omalizumab, though most patients were observed for only about 1 year (Corren et al., 2009). However, a 5-year study is in progress to monitor for these effects.

There is a possible increased risk for parasitic (*helminth*) infections with omalizumab treatment. Patients at high risk of geohelminth infection should be monitored during and after stopping omalizumab treatment (Omalizumab Prescribing Information, 2010).

Generic and brand names

The only IgE monoclonal antibody available is omalizumab (Xolair).

Formulations

Omalizumab is available as a lyophilized, sterile powder for subcutaneous injection.

COUGH SUPPRESSANTS

Dextromethorphan

Mechanism of action

Dextromethorphan is the methyl ether *d*-isomer of the codeine analogue levorphanol but lacks typical opiate agonist characteristics aside from its antitussive activity. The exact mechanism of action is in dispute but may have several mechanisms for cough suppressant effect, including glutamate receptor antagonism (specifically, *N*-methyl-D-aspartate receptor), sigma-1 receptor agonism, serotonin pathway agonism, and effects on the cough gating mechanism (Bolser, 2006; Canning, 2009; Bolser, 2009; Eccles, 2009).

Common indications

Dextromethorphan is indicated for the temporary relief of nonproductive cough.

Common adverse effects

Common adverse effects are mild and infrequent and can include dizziness, fatigue, gastrointestinal disturbances, and drowsiness. Dextromethorphan has been associated with serotonergic effects and at higher doses may cause confusion, nervousness, restlessness, dysarthria, irritability, nausea and vomiting.

Some dextromethorphan-containing products contain tartrazine, which may cause allergic-type reactions (including asthma symptoms) in patients with a specific sensitivity (Ardern & Ram, 2001). Although the overall prevalence of tartrazine sensitivity in the general population is low, it may occur in patients who also have aspirin hypersensitivity, though this was disputed in a recent study evaluating tartrazine sensitivity in patients with nonsteroid anti-inflammatory drug sensitivity (Pestana, Moreira, & Olej, 2010).

Beginning in 2007, the Centers for Disease Control issued warnings for the risk of serious injury and fatal overdose from cough and cold products administered to children less than 2 years old. Subsequently, the Food and Drug Administration Nonprescription Drug Advisory Committee and Pediatric Advisory Committee recommended that products containing dextromethorphan, pseudoephedrine, chlorpheniramine, diphenydramine, brompheniramine, phenylephrine, clemastine, and guaifenesin not be used in children less than 6 years old. The Food and Drug Administration issued a Public Health Advisory recommending that nonprescription products (though prescription products also containing these ingredients would be included) not be used in children under 2 years old. Further official rulings from the Food and Drug Administration are expected.

Generic and brand names

There are numerous brand and generic products available without prescription.

Formulations

Dextromethorphan is available in liquid, tablet, softgel, and dissolving film formulations.

Codeine

Mechanism of action

Codeine is a narcotic opioid that acts centrally in the cough center in the medulla by binding primarily to μ-opioid receptors and possibly κ-opioid receptors (Takahama & Shirasaki, 2007). Codeine also has a drying effect on the mucosa of the respiratory tract and increases the viscosity of bronchial secretions.

Common indications

Codeine is indicated for the temporary relief of nonproductive cough.

Common adverse effects

The most serious adverse effects include respiratory depression and arrest, circulatory depression, shock, and cardiac arrest. Codeine can also cause drowsiness, dizziness, confusion, insomnia, nervousness, dysphoria, euphoria, mood alterations, and anxiety. Gastrointestinal effects may include anorexia, nausea, vomiting, and constipation.

Due to histamine release, codeine can cause flushing and pruritus. Anticholinergic effects are infrequent but can include sinus bradycardia, sinus tachycardia, changes in blood pressure, and syncope, as well as dry mouth, blurred vision, or urinary retention. Miosis can occur at therapeutic doses.

Also see the information regarding use in children from the Centers for Disease Control and Food and Drug Administration previously discussed under the section "Dextromethorphan."

Generic and brand names

Codeine-containing cough suppressant products are Schedule V. Numerous brand and generic products are available and distributed at retail without prescription, but only by a registered pharmacist; in some states, a prescription may be required.

Formulations

Products are available as tablets and oral liquids alone or in combination with expectorants and decongestants.

Diphenydramine, promethazine, and other first-generation antihistamines

Mechanism of action

First-generation antihistamines such as diphenhydramine and promethazine have direct suppressive actions on the cough center in the medulla.

Common indications

First-generation antihistamines can be used for the temporary relief of nonproductive cough.

Common adverse effects

The most frequent adverse effects include drowsiness, dizziness, and xerostomia. Central nervous stimulation is more likely to occur in children, and effects can include agitation, insomnia, increased appetite, restlessness, palpitations, muscle spasms, and seizures. Anticholinergic effects can include xerostomia, insomnia, urinary retention, nervousness, mydriasis, xerophthalmia, and blurred vision. Gastrointestinal effects include diarrhea, constipation, and abdominal pain. Quinidine-like anesthetic effects can include sinus tachycardia and cardiac arrhythmias. Blockade of alpha-adrenergic receptors can cause hypotension.

Also see the information regarding use in children from the Centers for Disease Control and Food and Drug Administration previously discussed under the section "Dextromethorphan."

Generic and brand names

Numerous brand and generic products are available without prescription.

Formulations

Products are available as tablets, capsules, gelcaps, orally disintegrating tablets, oral dissolving film, and oral liquids.

EXPECTORANTS

Guaifenesin

Mechanism of action

Guaifenesin induces expectorant effects by increasing sputum volume and decreasing viscosity presumably by decreasing the surface tension of sputum (Woo, 2008). Ciliary action is improved with the flow of less viscous secretions converting a dry, nonproductive cough to a productive cough (Woo, 2008).

Common indications

Guaifenesin is indicated for loosening and thinning phlegm associated with coughs from colds and minor upper respiratory tract infections in order to facilitate clearing of bronchial passages and increasing productive cough.

Common adverse effects

No adverse effects commonly occur with usual doses.

Also see the information regarding use in children from the Centers for Disease Control and Food and Drug Administration previously discussed under the section "Dextromethorphan."

Generic and brand names

Products containing guaifenesin include Mucinex, Robitussin, as well as numerous other store brands and generics. Guaifenesin is also found in numerous combination products with antihistamines, decongestants, dextromethorphan, and other cough and cold products.

Formulations

Guaifenesin is available as tablets, oral liquids, and granules.

DECONGESTANTS

Oral decongestants

Mechanism of action

Oral decongestants reduce nasal blockage by acting directly on α_1-receptors, indirectly by displacing norepinephrine from storage vesicles in the nerve terminal, and/or by inhibiting the reuptake of norepinephrine.

Pseudoephedrine has direct and/or indirect effects, whereas phenylephrine acts directly on α_1-receptors.

Stimulation of postcapillary α_1-adrenergic receptors causes vasoconstriction of postcapillary venules in the nasal mucosa (Johnson & Hricik, 1993). These postcapillary venules are capacitance vessels and can accommodate a relatively large amount of blood. Congestion is caused by increased blood volume, which increases the volume of the nasal mucosa. Stimulation of the α_1-receptors, which are coupled to G proteins ($G_{q/11}$ family), leads to activation of phospholipase Cβ, which results in cleavage of phosphatidylinositol-4,5-bisphosphate into inositol-1,4,5-triphosphate and diacylglycerol (Biaggioni & Roberston, 2009; Hein & Michel, 2007). IP_3 promotes the release of intracellular calcium stores, which increases cytoplasmic concentrations of free calcium and activation of calcium-dependent protein kinases to cause vessel contraction. Diacylglycerol activates protein kinase C and modulates the activity of multiple signaling pathways. α_1-adrenergic receptors may activate other signaling molecules such as pertussis-sensitive G proteins, G_s family, G12-13 family G proteins, phospholipases A_2 via protein kinase C, phospholipase D, and may increase cyclic adenosine monophosphate (Hein & Michel, 2007). These effects shrink swollen nasal mucous membranes to increase nasal airway patency. Sinus drainage is improved and relief from obstructed eustachian ostia may occur.

The only clinically useful oral decongestant available is pseudoephedrine. Phenylephrine is extensively metabolized in the intestinal wall, resulting in low bioavailability; it is unclear if sufficient amounts are absorbed to have a therapeutic effect.

Common indications

Oral decongestants are indicated for the temporary relief of nasal and sinus congestion due to common cold, allergic rhinitis, or sinusitis, or for relief of eustachian tube congestion. They are also indicted for otalgia prophylaxis (due to air pressure changes) during air travel.

Common adverse effects

Common adverse effects from oral decongestant use include headache, increased blood pressure, increased intraocular pressure, insomnia, mydriasis, nervousness, tachycardia, and urinary retention.

Also see the information regarding use in children from the Centers for Disease Control and Food and Drug Administration previously discussed under the section "Dextromethorphan."

Generic and brand names

Oral decongestants are found in many store brand and generic products as well as in numerous combination products with guaifenesin, antihistamines, dextromethorphan, and other cough and cold products.

Formulations

Oral decongestants are available as tablets, oral liquids, and chewable tablets.

Topical decongestants

Mechanism of action

Topical decongestants reduce nasal blockage by directly stimulating the α_1-receptors in the nose by the same mechanism as described for oral decongestants.

Common indications

Topical decongestants are indicated for the temporary relief of nasal and sinus congestion due to common cold, allergic rhinitis, or sinusitis, or for the relief of eustachian tube congestion.

Common adverse effects

The usual adverse effects related to topical use include sneezing, stinging, transient burning, and ulceration of the nasal mucosa.

Topical decongestants should not be used for longer than 3 days due to the risk of developing rhinitis medicamentosa associated with long-term use.

Generic and brand names

Topical decongestants are found in many store brand and generic products.

Formulations

Topical decongestants are available as sprays or drops.

INHALED ANTIBIOTICS

Mechanism of action

Three antiobiotics for administration by inhalation are commonly available: tobramycin, colistimethate sodium, and aztreonam lysine. Tobramycin is actively transported into the bacterial cell and exerts bacteriocidal activity by irreversibly binding to the 30S bacterial ribosome, which inhibits protein synthesis in susceptible gram-negative bacilli and gram-positive cocci. Binding interrupts messenger RNA action, causing production of abnormal, nonfunctional proteins. Tobramycin must achieve intracellular concentrations in excess of extracellular concentrations in order to be bacteriocidal. Tobramycin has a concentration-dependent killing and a post-antibiotic effect against gram-negative aerobic rods and gram-positive organisms.

Colistimethate sodium is bacteriocidal for gram-negative bacteria and acts by binding to bacterial cell membrane phospholipids by displacing calcium and magnesium. This results in increased cell membrane permeability and leakage of cell contents, leading to cell death.

Aztreonam is a synthetic monocyclic beta lactam active against gram-negative aerobic organisms and is stable against most β-lactamases. It acts by binding to penicillin-binding protein-3 of gram-negative rods. The sulfonic acid group promotes acetylation of penicillin-binding protein-3, which is responsible for the development of the septum in cell wall synthesis. Inhibition of the action of penicillin-binding protein-3 prevents cell division and causes the bacterial cell to elongate. Eventual breakage of the cell wall leads to cell lysis and death.

Common indications

Inhaled tobramycin, inhaled colistimethate sodium, and inhaled aztreonam lysine are indicated for the management of cystic fibrosis patients with *Pseudomonas aeruginosa*.

Common adverse effects

Adverse effects common with intravenous administration of tobramycin are significantly less likely to occur with administration by the inhaled route. Neither renal toxicity nor ototoxicity has been reported during clinical trials (Heijerman et al., 2009), and only dysphonia and mild to moderate tinnitus has occurred more often than with placebo in clinical trials; the latter resolved with drug discontinuation. Bronchospasm may occur; pretreatment with an inhaled β_2-agonist may be useful.

Nebulized colistimethate sodium can commonly cause bronchospasm, cough, and throat irritation; inhaled β_2-agonist may be administered prophylactically or for treatment of these effects (Heijerman et al., 2009). Irritated oral mucus membranes and *Candida* superinfection may occur. Colistimethate sodium must be inhaled within 24 hours after reconstitution because when mixed with sterile water, the drug is hydrolyzed into the bases colistin A (polymyxin E1) and colistin B (polymyxin E2) (Heijerman et al., 2009). Polymyxin E1 may cause severe localized airway inflammation and eosinophilic infiltration (Heijerman et al., 2009).

The most common adverse effects with inhaled aztreonam lysine are increased cough, chest tightness, wheezing, pharyngolaryngeal pain, and nasal congestion. As with the other inhaled antibiotics, administration of an inhaled β_2-agonist may be used prophylactically or for treatment of bronchial adverse effects.

Generic and brand names

Inhaled tobramycin is available as TOBI; colistimethate sodium is available as Coly-Mycin M and generic products; and aztreonam lysine is available as Cayston.

Formulations

Tobramycin is available as a solution for nebulization. Colistimethate sodium and aztreonam lysine are available as a powder for reconstitution for subsequent nebulization.

DELIVERY DEVICES (SEE TABLE 3.1)

MDIs (See Figure 3.1)

MDIs are the standard means to deliver drugs to the lungs due to convenience and efficacy; however, they can be difficult to use correctly. MDIs deliver suspensions or solutions of drug mixed with propellants and other chemicals via a pressurized canister with a metering valve. Technique is extremely important for proper use to ensure delivery to the lower airways; significant hand–lung coordination is required. The majority of patients and health professionals (over 60%) have incorrect technique. Reinstruction is frequently needed because correct use declines over periods as short as 6–10 weeks (De Blaquiere et al., 1989; Dolovich et al., 2000). With appropriate technique, approximately 10–25% of the drug is delivered to the lungs (Dolovich et al., 2000). Breath-actuated devices have further simplified the use of MDIs by significantly lessening the degree of coordination needed. However, these devices provide no advantage to patients with good inhaler technique and cannot be used with spacers and holding chambers, which have advantages of their own.

DPIs (See Figure 3.2)

DPIs are available as a variety of devices in which active drug as micronized dry powder with excipient, such as lactose, is inhaled into the lungs (Dolovich et al., 2000). Patients must inspire deeply and forcefully to empty a small holding chamber or capsule of the powder following activation. Once the device is ready for inhalation, the patient should not exhale into the device as moisture will prevent dispersion of the powder. Furthermore, they should not tip the device upside down as the powder can spill from the device. An inspiratory flow of about 60 L/min is important for dispersal of the micronized powder; this flow is about twice that needed for optimal MDI inhalation technique (Dolovich et al., 2000; Kelly, 1999a). Although 60 L/min is a general guide, each device has its own inspiratory

Table 3.1 Aerosol delivery devices.

Device/drugs	Population	Optimal technique
Metered-dose inhaler (MDI) β_2-agonists Corticosteroids Anticholinergics	≥5 years old (<5 with spacer or valved holding chamber [VHC] mask)	Actuation during a slow (30 L/min or 3–5 seconds), deep inhalation, followed by 10-second breath hold Under laboratory conditions, open-mouth technique (holding the MDI 2 in. away from the open mouth) enhances delivery to the lung. This technique, however, has not been shown to enhance clinical benefit consistently compared to closed-mouth technique (inserting the MDI mouthpiece between lips and teeth).
Breath-actuated MDI β_2-agonist	≥5 years old	Tight seal around mouthpiece and slightly more rapid inhalation than standard MDI (see above) followed by a 10-second breath hold
Dry powder inhaler (DPI) β_2-agonists Corticosteroids Anticholinergics	≥4 years old	Rapid (60 L/min or 1–2 seconds), deep inhalation. Minimally effective inspiratory flow is device dependent. Most children <4 years of age may not generate sufficient inspiratory flow to activate the inhaler.
Spacer or VHC	≥4 years old <4-year-old VHC with face mask	Slow (30 L/min or 3–5 seconds) deep inhalation, followed by 10-second breath hold immediately following actuation. Actuate only once into spacer/VHC per inhalation. If face mask is used, it should have a tight fit and should allow at least five inhalations per actuation. Rinse plastic VHCs once a month with a low concentration of liquid household dishwashing detergent (1:5,000 or one to two drops per cup of water) and let it drip dry.
Nebulizer β_2-agonists Corticosteroids Cromolyn sodium Anticholinergics	Patients of any age who cannot use MDI with VHC and face mask	Slow tidal breathing with occasional deep breaths. Tightly fitting face mask for those unable to use mouthpiece. Using the "blow-by" technique (i.e., holding the mask or open tube near the infant's nose and mouth) is not appropriate.

Adapted from the National Asthma Education and Prevention Program (2007). *Expert Panel Report 3: Guidelines for the diagnosis and management of asthma*. Bethesda, MD: U.S. Department of Health and Human Services, Public Health Service, National Institutes of Health, National Heart, Lung, and Blood Institute, publication no. 08-4051. ED, emergency department; SABAs, inhaled short-acting β_2-agonists.

Therapeutic issues

Slow inhalation and coordination of actuation during inhalation may be difficult, particularly in young children and in the elderly. Patients may incorrectly stop inhalation at actuation. There is deposition of 50–80% of the actuated dose in the oropharynx. Mouthwashing and spitting are effective in reducing the amount of drug swallowed and absorbed systemically.

Lung delivery under ideal conditions varies significantly between MDIs due to differences in formulation (suspension vs. solution), propellant (chlorofluorocarbon [CFC] vs. hydrofluoroalkane [HFA]), and valve design. For example, inhaled corticosteroid (ICS) delivery varies from 5 to 50%.

May be particularly useful for patients unable to coordinate inhalation and actuation. May also be useful for elderly patients. Patients may incorrectly stop inhalation at actuation. Cannot be used with currently available spacer/VHC devices.

Dose is lost if patient exhales through device after actuating. Delivery may be greater or lesser than MDI, depending on device and technique. Delivery is more flow dependent in devices with highest internal resistance. Rapid inhalation promotes greater deposition in larger central airways. Mouthwashing and spitting is effective in reducing the amount of drug swallowed and absorbed.

Indicated for patients who have difficulty performing adequate MDI technique.

May be bulky. Simple tubes do not obviate coordinating actuation and inhalation. The VHCs are preferred.

Face mask allows MDIs to be used with small children. However, the use of a face mask reduces delivery to the lungs by 50%. The VHC improves lung delivery and response in patients who have poor MDI technique.

The effect of a spacer or VHC on output from an MDI depends on both the MDI and device type; thus, data from one combination should not be extrapolated to all others. Spacers and/or VHCs decrease oropharyngeal deposition and thus decrease the risk of topical side effects (e.g., thrush).

Spacers will also reduce the potential systemic availability of ICSs with higher oral absorption. However, spacer/VHCs may increase systemic availability of ICSs that are poorly absorbed orally by enhancing delivery to the lungs.

No clinical data are available on the use of spacers or VHCs with ultra-fine particle-generated HFA MDIs.

Use antistatic VHCs or rinse plastic non-antistatic VHCs with dilute household detergents to enhance delivery to the lungs and efficacy. This effect is less pronounced for albuterol MDIs with HFA propellants than for albuterol MDIs with CFC propellants.

As effective as nebulizer for delivering SABAs and anticholinergics in mild to moderate exacerbations; data in severe exacerbations are limited.

Less dependent on patient's coordination and cooperation.

Delivery method of choice for cromolyn sodium in young children.

May be expensive, time-consuming, and bulky; output is dependent on device and operating parameters (fill volume, driving gas flow); internebulizer and intranebulizer output variances are significant. Use of a face mask reduces delivery to the lungs by 50%. Nebulizers are as effective as MDIs plus VHCs for delivering bronchodilators in the ED for mild to moderate exacerbations; data in severe exacerbations are limited. Choice of delivery system independent on resources, availability, and clinical judgment of the clinician caring for the patient.

Potential for bacterial infections if not cleaned properly.

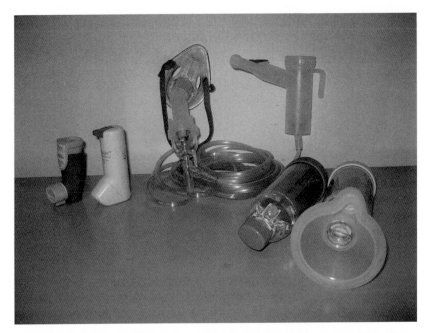

Figure 3.1 Metered-dose inhalers (MDIs), nebulizers, and valved holding chambers. From left to right: MDI, breath-actuated MDI, nebulizer cup with face mask, nebulizer cup with mouthpiece, valved holding chamber with mouthpiece, valved holding chamber with face mask.

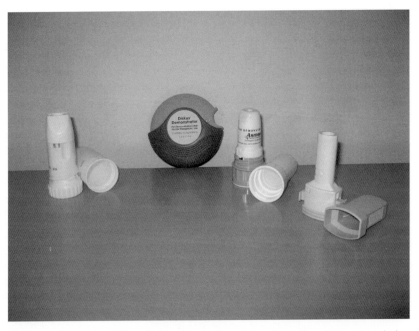

Figure 3.2 Dry powder inhalers (from left to right): Flexhaler, Diskus, Twisthaler, Aerolizer.

flow range for optimal deposition. Compared to pressurized MDIs, DPIs do not require the patient to coordinate activation of the device with inhalation (Kelly, 1999a). A disadvantage of DPIs is that higher inspiratory flows are required for optimal delivery. This makes them unsuitable for some patients, such as young children under 4 years old. Some DPIs (i.e., Diskus) are more robust in terms of the inspiratory flow rate required for drug delivery such that delivery is still effective even at flow rates <60 L/min (Dolovich et al., 2000; Kelly, 1999a).

Nebulizers (See Figure 3.1)

There are two types of nebulizers: jet (those driven by compressed air) and ultrasonic. Jet nebulizers produce an aerosol by having compressed gas delivered up through the bottom of the nebulizer, creating a region of negative pressure, which entrains the solution of drug; air and solution strike a baffle and break into droplets to be inhaled (Dolovich et al., 2000). Larger droplets, which adhere to the sides of the nebulizer, drip back into the nebulizer base to be re-nebulized. A gas flow of approximately 8 L/min is required to generate particles within the respirable range (Dolovich et al., 2000) and either tidal breathing or deep inhalation with a breath hold are acceptable methods for delivery. Ultrasonic nebulizers produce aerosols by a piezoelectric transducer vibrating at a high frequency (1–3 MHz). Ultrasonic nebulizers should not be used for the delivery of suspensions and viscous solutions as mostly water and not drug is nebulized (De Benedictis & Selvaggio, 2003).

A significant amount of drug is wasted during nebulization with only about 10% of the dose placed in the nebulizer reaching the patient's lower airways. Sixty to eighty percent is retained in the nebulizer, 20% exhaled, and 2% is deposited into the mouth (Kelly, 1999b). The use of a face mask is needed for young children, and proper use is required as holding the face mask only 2 cm from the face can reduce delivery by 80% (Everard, Clark, & Milner, 1992). A Cochrane Database Review found similar outcomes for β-agonist treatment of acute mild to moderate asthma exacerbations using an MDI plus holding chamber versus a nebulizer (Cates, Rowe, & Bara, 2002).

Holding chambers (See Figure 3.1)

Spacers and valved holding chambers used with pressurized MDIs offer several advantages including increased pulmonary drug deposition in patients with poor MDI technique, reduced oropharyngeal deposition of the drug, thus decreasing the risks for topical as well as systemic adverse effects, reduced bad taste, and reduced need for coordination (valved holding chambers only) which is required to properly use MDIs (Dolovich et al., 2000; EPR 3, 2007). A spacer is simply an open ended tube or bag that creates a space for the aerosol to expand and allow the propellant to evaporate (Dolovich et al., 2000). A minimum volume of 100 mL and 10–13 cm length is required for a spacer as smaller devices will actually reduce drug delivery (Dolovich et al., 2000). Valved holding chambers (available with masks or mouthpieces) are typically larger, which allows the aerosol to expand and remain in the device until inhaled; exhaled air does not return to the chamber. Thus, multiple inhalations can be used to completely empty the aerosol from the chamber. This is particularly important for children with tidal volumes that do not exceed the volume of the holding chamber (Dolovich et al., 2000). The advantages of spacer devices and valved holding chambers override the extra cost and bulkiness.

INHALER TEACHING DEVICE (SEE FIGURE 3.3)

The In-Check DIAL (http://alliancetechmedical.com) is a training device that can help identify which inhaler is best suited for an individual patient. It is a handheld low-range inspiratory flow measurement device with a dial top that can be set to simulate the resistance of MDIs, breath-actuated inhaler (Autohaler) and DPIs (Flexhaler and Diskus). Resistance adapters

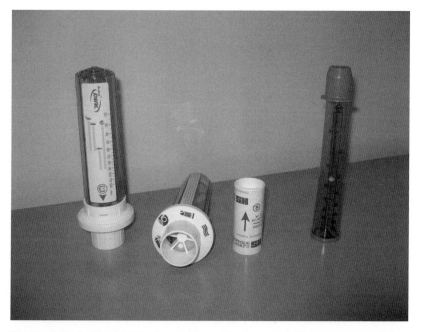

Figure 3.3 In-Check DIAL, disposable mouthpiece, peak flow meter. From left to right: In-Check DIAL (side view), In-Check DIAL (top view/top dial), disposable mouthpiece, peak flow meter.

for the In-Check DIAL are also available for two more DPI devices, the HandiHaler (tiotropium) and the Aerolizer (formoterol).

To use the In-Check DIAL, reset the In-Check DIAL (this is done by holding the device upside down and by tapping the rounded end against one's hand; then, turn the device 180° to return the magnetic weight to the resting position). Next, turn the dial top to the appropriate device (i.e., MDI or Diskus). Attach a disposable mouthpiece (arrow pointing toward the patient) to the top dial. Have the child fully exhale. Then, ask him/her to place his/her lips around the mouthpiece forming a good seal. Instruct the child to inhale using the proper technique for the device selected (i.e., slow deep breath or quick deep breath). Note the inspiratory flow rate opposite the red indicator on the barrel of the DIAL. Compare that inspiratory flow rate with the target flow rate for the selected device (Education/Clinicals, n.d.). Based on how the actual inspiratory flow compares to the target flow rate, coach the child until the proper range is consistently achieved.

The In-Check DIAL measures inspiratory flow rate and allows patients to be trained to use more or less inspiratory force to achieve the necessary flow rate for a particular inhaler. A card that contains a list of flow rates for different inhalers is included. This is the first device that provides an objective measure of a patient's technique and can be used for initial training and for follow-up assessment over time.

PEAK FLOW METERS/FORCED EXPIRATORY VOLUME IN THE FIRST SECOND METERS (SEE FIGURE 3.3)

Peak flow meters are simple, portable, and relatively inexpensive devices (approximately $15–$35) that facilitate accurate and objective self-monitoring of pulmonary function. Variations in brands can give clinically significant different measurements. Therefore, a single device should be used to compare peak expiratory flow (PEF) values over time. Both forced expiratory volume in the first second (FEV_1) and PEF measurements require effort and cooperation on the part of the patient, and patients need to have their technique reevaluated frequently (EPR 3, 2007). Additionally, the accuracy of the device can worsen over time even in patients with technically acceptable maneuvers (EPR 3, 2007). The use of the peak flow meter is described in Chapter 7.

Portable spirometers provide a convenient means for obtaining reliable and reproducible lung function measurements standardized for the patient's age, race, and gender. These devices can measure forced vital capacity, slow vital capacity, and PEF in addition to the forced expiratory volume in 1 second (Tovar & Gums, 2004). The reproducibility between measurements seems to be better than is seen with peak flow meters, allowing for more accurate assessments of lung function over time (Tovar & Gums, 2004).

REFERENCES

Anderson, G. P. (1993). Formoterol: Pharmacology, molecular basis of agonism, and mechanism of long duration of a highly potent and selective beta 2-adrenoceptor agonist bronchodilator. *Life Science, 52*(26), 2145–2160.

Anderson, M. E., Allison, R. D., & Meister, A. (1982). Interconversion of leukotrienes catalyzed by purified gamma-glutamyl transpeptidase: Concomitant formation of leukotriene D4 and gamma-glutamyl amino acids. *Proceedings of the National Academy of Sciences of the United States of America, 79*(4), 1088–1091.

Ardern, K. D., & Ram, F. S. (2001). Tartrazine exclusion for allergic asthma. *Cochrane Database of Systematic Reviews,* (4), CD000460.

Barnes, P. J. (1995). Beta-adrenergic receptors and their regulation. *American Journal of Respiratory and Critical Care Medicine, 152*(3), 838–860.

Barnes, P. J. (2002). Scientific rationale for inhaled combination therapy with long-acting beta2-agonists and corticosteroids. *The European Respiratory Journal, 19*(1), 182–191.

Barnes, P. J. (2006). How corticosteroids control inflammation: Quintiles prize lecture 2005. *British Journal of Pharmacology, 148*(3), 245–254.

Beasley, R., Pearce, N., Crane, J., et al. (1995). Withdrawal of fenoterol and the end of the New Zealand asthma mortality epidemic. *International Archives of Allergy and Immunology, 107*(1–3), 325–327.

Belmonte, K. E. (2005). Cholinergic pathways in the lungs and anticholinergic therapy for chronic obstructive pulmonary disease. *Proceedings of the American Thoracic Society, 2*(4), 297–304.

Biaggioni, I., & Roberston, D. (2009). Chapter 9. Adrenoceptor agonists & sympathomimetic drugs. In G. Katzung Bertram, B. Masters Susan, & J. Trevor Anthony (Eds.), *Basic & clinical pharmacology,* 11e: http://www.accesspharmacy.com.lp.hscl.ufl.edu/content.aspx?aID=4520412.

Billington, C. K., & Penn, R. B. (2003). Signaling and regulation of G protein-coupled receptors in airway smooth muscle. *Respiratory Research, 4*(1), 2.

Blake, K. V. (1999). Montelukast: Data from clinical trials in the management of asthma. *The Annals of Pharmacotherapy, 33*(12), 1299–1314.

Bolser, D. C. (2006). Current and future centrally acting antitussives. *Respiratory Physiology & Neurobiology, 152*(3), 349–355.

Bolser, D. C. (2009). Central mechanisms II: Pharmacology of brainstem pathways. *Handbook of Experimental Pharmacology,* (187), 203–217.

Brogden, R. N., & Sorkin, E. M. (1993). Nedocromil Sodium: An updated review of its pharmacological properties and therapeutic efficacy in asthma. *Drugs, 45*, 693–715.

Canning, B. J. (2009). Central regulation of the cough reflex: Therapeutic implications. *Pulmonary Pharmacology & Therapeutics, 22*(2), 75–81.

Castle, W., Fuller, R., Hall, J., et al. (1993). Serevent nationwide surveillance study: Comparison of salmeterol with salbutamol in asthmatic patients who require regular bronchodilator treatment. *BMJ, 306*(6884), 1034–1037.

Cates, C. J., Rowe, B. H., & Bara, A. (2002). Holding chambers versus nebulisers for beta-agonist treatment of acute asthma (Cochrane Review). *Cochrane Database of Systematic Reviews,* (2): CD000052. Review. Update in: Cochrane

Database Syst Rev. 2003;(3):CD000052. PMID: 12076378 [PubMed—indexed for MEDLINE].

Chen, A. M., Bollmeier, S. G., & Finnegan, P. M. (2008). Long-acting broncho-dilator therapy for the treatment of chronic obstructive pulmonary disease. *The Annals of Pharmacotherapy, 42*(12), 1832–1842.

Corren, J., Casale, T. B., Lanier, B., et al. (2009). Safety and tolerability of omali-zumab. *Clinical and Experimental Allergy, 39*(6), 788–797.

Currie, G. P., & McLaughlin, K. (2006). The expanding role of leukotriene recep-tor antagonists in chronic asthma. *Annals of Allergy, Asthma & Immunology, 97*(6), 731–741. quiz.

De Benedictis, F. M., & Selvaggio, D. (2003). Use of inhaler devices in pediatric asthma. *Paediatric Drugs, 5*(9), 629–638.

De Blaquiere, P., Christensen, D. B., Carter, W. B., et al. (1989). Use and misuse of metered-dose inhalers by patients with chronic lung disease. A controlled, randomized trial of two instruction methods [see comments]. *The American Review of Respiratory Disease, 140*(4), 910–916.

Dolovich, M. A., MacIntyre, N. R., Anderson, P. J., et al. (2000). Consensus statement: Aerosols and delivery devices. American Association for Respiratory Care. *Respiratory Care, 45*(6), 589–596.

Drazen, J. M., & Austen, K. F. (1987). Leukotrienes and airway responses. *The American Review of Respiratory Disease, 136*(4), 985–998.

Drazen, J. M., Israel, E., Boushey, H. A., et al. (1996). Comparison of regu-larly scheduled with as-needed use of albuterol in mild asthma. Asthma Clinical Research Network. *The New England Journal of Medicine, 335*(12), 841–847.

Eccles, R. (2009). Central mechanisms IV: Conscious control of cough and the placebo effect. *Handbook of Experimental Pharmacology, 187*, 241–262.

Education/Clinicals (n.d.). In-Check DIAL, how to reset and use the In-Check DIAL. Retrieved from http://alliancetechmedical.com/index.php?cID=60.

EPR 3. (2007). National Asthma Education and Prevention Program. In *Expert Panel Report 3: Guidelines for the diagnosis and management of asthma*. August 2007. Bethesda, MD: U.S. Department of Health and Human Services, Public Health Service, National Institutes of Health, National Heart, Lung, and Blood Institute. Publication no. 08-4051.

Everard, M. L., Clark, A. R., & Milner, A. D. (1992). Drug delivery from jet nebulisers. *Archives of Disease in Childhood, 67*(5), 586–591.

Formoterol Prescribing Information. (2010). Prescribing information—Formoterol.

Giuntini, C. G., & Paggiaro, P. L. (1995). Present state of the controversy about regular inhaled beta-agonists in asthma. *The European Respiratory Journal, 8*(5), 673–678.

Hardin, A. O., & Lima, J. J. (1999). Beta 2-adrenoceptor agonist-induced down-regulation after short-term exposure. *Journal of Receptor and Signal Trans-duction Research, 19*(5), 835–852.

Harrold, L. R., Patterson, M. K., Andrade, S. E., et al. (2007). Asthma drug use and the development of Churg–Strauss syndrome (CSS). *Pharmacoepidemiology and Drug Safety, 16*(6), 620–626.

Heijerman, H., Westerman, E., Conway, S., et al. (2009). Inhaled medication and inhalation devices for lung disease in patients with cystic fibrosis: A European consensus. *Journal of Cystic Fibrosis, 8*(5), 295–315.

Hein, P., & Michel, M. C. (2007). Signal transduction and regulation: Are all alpha1-adrenergic receptor subtypes created equal? *Biochemical Pharmacology, 73*(8), 1097–1106.

Holbrook, J. T., & Harik-Khan, R. (2008). Montelukast and emotional well-being as a marker for depression: Results from 3 randomized, double-masked clinical trials. *The Journal of Allergy and Clinical Immunology, 122*(4), 828–829.

Holgate, S. T., Djukanovic, R., Casale, T., et al. (2005). Anti-immunoglobulin E treatment with omalizumab in allergic diseases: An update on anti-inflammatory activity and clinical efficacy. *Clinical and Experimental Allergy, 35*(4), 408–416.

Inman, W. H., & Adelstein, A. M. (1969). Rise and fall of asthma mortality in England and Wales in relation to use of pressurised aerosols. *Lancet, 2*(7615), 279–285.

Israel, E., Chinchilli, V. M., Ford, J. G., et al. (2004). Use of regularly scheduled albuterol treatment in asthma: Genotype-stratified, randomised, placebo-controlled cross-over trial. *Lancet, 364*(9444), 1505–1512.

Johnson, D. A., & Hricik, J. G. (1993). The pharmacology of α-adrenergic decongestants. *Pharmacotherapy, 13,* 110S–115S.

Kelly, H. W. (1999a). *Aerosol delivery* (pp. 463–487). New York: Marcel Dekker.

Kelly, H. W. (1999b). Pharmacology of inhaled glucocorticoids: Comparative properties. *Immunology and Allergy Clinics of North America, 19,* 725–738.

Kelly, H. W. (2007). Non-corticosteroid therapy for the long-term control of asthma. *Expert Opinion on Pharmacotherapy, 8*(13), 2077–2087.

Kercsmar, C. M., & McDowell, K. M. (2009). Love it or lev it: Levalbuterol for severe acute asthma—for now, leave it. *The Journal of Pediatrics, 155*(2), 162–164.

Laitinen, L. A., Laitinen, A., & Haahtela, T. (1992). A comparative study of the effects of an inhaled corticosteroid, budesonide, and of a β_2-agonist, terbutaline, on airway inflammation in newly diagnosed asthma. *The Journal of Allergy and Clinical Immunology, 90,* 32–42.

Lee, C. W., Lewis, R. A., Corey, E. J., et al. (1983). Conversion of leukotriene D4 to leukotriene E4 by a dipeptidase released from the specific granule of human polymorphonuclear leucocytes. *Immunology, 48*(1), 27–35.

Lilly, C. M., Churg, A., Lazarovich, M., et al. (2002). Asthma therapies and Churg–Strauss syndrome. *The Journal of Allergy and Clinical Immunology, 109*(1), S1–19.

Lohse, M. J. (1993). Molecular mechanisms of membrane receptor desensitization. *Biochimica et Biophysica Acta, 1179*(2), 171–188.

Lotvall, J., Palmqvist, M., Arvidsson, P., et al. (2001). The therapeutic ratio of R-albuterol is comparable with that of RS-albuterol in asthmatic patients. *The Journal of Allergy and Clinical Immunology, 108*(5), 726–731.

Lynch, K. R., O'Neill, G. P., Liu, Q., et al. (1999). Characterization of the human cysteinyl leukotriene CysLT1 receptor. *Nature, 399*(6738), 789–793.

Mann, M., Chowdhury, B., Sullivan, E., et al. (2003). Serious asthma exacerbations in asthmatics treated with high-dose formoterol. *Chest, 124*(1), 70–74.

Negri, J., Early, S. B., Steinke, J. W., et al. (2008). Corticosteroids as inhibitors of cysteinyl leukotriene metabolic and signaling pathways. *The Journal of Allergy and Clinical Immunology, 121*(5), 1232–1237.

Nelson, H. S. (1995). Beta-adrenergic bronchodilators. *The New England Journal of Medicine, 333*(8), 499–506.

Nelson, H. S., Weiss, S. T., Bleecker, E. R., et al. (2006). The Salmeterol Multicenter Asthma Research Trial: A comparison of usual pharmacotherapy for asthma or usual pharmacotherapy plus salmeterol. *Chest, 129*(1), 15–26.

Nijkamp, F. P., Engels, F., Henricks, P. A., et al. (1992). Mechanisms of beta-adrenergic receptor regulation in lungs and its implications for physiological responses. *Physiological Reviews, 72*(2), 323–367.

Omalizumab Prescribing Information. (2010). Prescribing information—Xolair.

Pakes, G. E., Brogden, R. N., Heel, R. C., et al. (1980). Ipratropium bromide: A review of its pharmacological properties and therapeutic efficacy in asthma and chronic bronchitis. *Drugs, 20*, 237–266.

Pearce, N., Beasley, R., Crane, J., et al. (1995). End of the New Zealand asthma mortality epidemic. *Lancet, 345*(8941), 41–44.

Pestana, S., Moreira, M., & Olej, B. (2010). Safety of ingestion of yellow tartrazine by double-blind placebo controlled challenge in 26 atopic adults. *Allergologia et Immunopathologia, 38*(3), 142–146.

Peters-Golden, M., & Henderson, W. R., Jr. (2007). Leukotrienes. *The New England Journal of Medicine, 357*(18), 1841–1854.

Philip, G., Hustad, C., Noonan, G., et al. (2009a). Reports of suicidality in clinical trials of montelukast. *The Journal of Allergy and Clinical Immunology, 124*(4), 691–696.

Philip, G., Hustad, C. M., Malice, M. P., et al. (2009b). Analysis of behavior-related adverse experiences in clinical trials of montelukast. *The Journal of Allergy and Clinical Immunology, 124*(4), 699–706.

Roberts, J. A., Bradding, P., Britten, K. M., et al. (1999). The long-acting beta2-agonist salmeterol xinafoate: Effects on airway inflammation in asthma. *The European Respiratory Journal, 14*(2), 275–282.

Rong, Y., Arbabian, M., Thiriot, D. S., et al. (1999). Probing the salmeterol binding site on the beta 2-adrenergic receptor using a novel photoaffinity ligand, [(125)I]iodoazidosalmeterol. *Biochemistry, 38*(35), 11278–11286.

Ruffin, C. G., & Busch, B. E. (2004). Omalizumab: A recombinant humanized anti-IgE antibody for allergic asthma. *American Journal of Health-System Pharmacy, 61*(14), 1449–1459.

Salmeterol Prescribing Information. (2010). Prescribing information—Salmeterol.

Salvi, S. S., Krishna, M. T., Sampson, A. P., et al. (2001). The anti-inflammatory effects of leukotriene-modifying drugs and their use in asthma. *Chest, 119*(5), 1533–1546.

Sears, M. R. (1993). Relationships between asthma mortality and treatment. *Annals of Allergy, 70*(5), 425–426.

Shore, S. A., & Moore, P. E. (2003). Regulation of beta-adrenergic responses in airway smooth muscle. *Respiratory Physiology & Neurobiology, 137*(2–3), 179–195.

Spahr, J. E., & Krawiec, M. (2008). Leukotriene modifiers. In M. Castro & M. Kraft (Eds.), *Clinical asthma* (pp. 263–271). Philadelphia: Elsevier Mosby.

Spitzer, W. O., Suissa, S., Ernst, P., et al. (1992). The use of beta-agonists and the risk of death and near death from asthma. *The New England Journal of Medicine, 326*, 501–506.

Takahama, K., & Shirasaki, T. (2007). Central and peripheral mechanisms of narcotic antitussives: Codeine-sensitive and -resistant coughs. *Cough, 3*, 8. PMID: 17620111 [PubMed].

Tovar, J. M., & Gums, J. G. (2004). Monitoring pulmonary function in asthma and COPD: Point-of-care testing. *The Annals of Pharmacotherapy, 38*(1), 126–133.

Waldeck, B. (1999). Enantiomers of bronchodilating beta2-adrenoceptor agonists: Is there a cause for concern? *The Journal of Allergy and Clinical Immunology, 103*(5, Pt 1), 742–748.

Waldeck, B. (2002). Beta-adrenoceptor agonists and asthma—100 years of development. *European Journal of Pharmacology, 445*(1–2), 1–12.

Woo, T. (2008). Pharmacology of cough and cold medicines. *Journal of Pediatric Health Care, 22*(2), 73–79.

Zafirlukast Prescribing Information. (2009). Prescribing information—Accolate.

Zileuton Prescribing Information. (2009). Prescribing information—Zyflo.

Neonatal lung disease: Apnea of prematurity and bronchopulmonary dysplasia

Pnina Weiss, MD, and Concettina Tolomeo, DNP, APRN, FNP-BC, AE-C

NEONATAL LUNG DISEASE

Lung development occurs throughout pregnancy; development includes airway branching and formation of alveoli (gas exchanging units) and pulmonary blood vessels. Alveoli continue to develop after birth. The lungs, respiratory muscles, and nervous control of breathing are less developed in infants than in older children or adults; this predisposes them to respiratory failure. The chest wall of infants is very compliant (less stiff); consequently, they breathe less efficiently than their older counterparts. Their diaphragm is also at a mechanical disadvantage and may be more prone to fatigue. Furthermore, the neurological pathways that control breathing are immature and as a result, infants are more susceptible to apnea, or cessation of breathing.

Developmental immaturity is more pronounced in preterm infants, placing them at an even higher risk of respiratory problems. In 2006, there were approximately 63,000 births in the United States; 1.5% of them were infants less than 1,500 g (Martin et al., 2008). These infants commonly experience apnea of prematurity. They develop respiratory distress syndrome (RDS) and require supplemental oxygen and mechanical ventilation. The support they require produces injury and chronic lung disease, known as bronchopulmonary dysplasia (BPD). In this chapter, two common neonatal problems, apnea of prematurity and BPD, will be explored.

Nursing Care in Pediatric Respiratory Disease, First Edition. Edited by Concettina (Tina) Tolomeo.
© 2012 John Wiley & Sons, Inc. Published 2012 by John Wiley & Sons, Inc.

Apnea of prematurity

Epidemiology

Apnea of prematurity, or the cessation of breathing, is seen commonly in infants less than 37 weeks' postmenstrual age (PMA). The literature clearly defines clinically significant apnea in infants as breathing pauses that last for >20 seconds or for >10 seconds if associated with bradycardia (heart rate less than 80 beats/min) or oxygen desaturation (<80–85% by pulse oximetry) (Committee on Fetus and Newborn, 2003). Apnea of prematurity occurs in over 50% of premature infants and in the majority of infants who are less than 1,000 g at birth (Alden et al., 1972). It has been associated with sepsis, intracranial hemorrhage, vaccine administration (Klein et al., 2008), and severe hyperbilirubinemia (Amin, Charafeddine, & Guillet, 2005). Additionally, a genetic predisposition is likely as there is a higher incidence of apnea of prematurity in infants born to first-degree consanguineous parents compared with other infants (Tamim, Khogali, Beydoun, Melki, & Yunis, 2003).

Apnea of prematurity generally resolves by 36–40 weeks' PMA; however, the more premature the infant, the longer it lasts. In general, the risk of apnea of prematurity seems to resolve by 43–44 weeks' PMA (Ramanathan et al., 2001). Although preterm infants make a disproportionate percent (18%) of sudden infant death syndrome (SIDS), there is no relationship between apnea of prematurity and SIDS (Committee on Fetus and Newborn, 2003).

Pathophysiology

Apnea of prematurity is due to the immaturity of the preterm infant's brain and respiratory muscles (Darnall, Ariagno, & Kinney, 2006). Premature infants have an imbalance in the neural inputs that stimulate breathing and the inhibitory pathways that depress it. Developmental abnormalities in the regulation and production of neurotransmitters such as gaminobutyric acid (GABA), adenosine, serotonin, endorphins, and prostaglandin have been suggested as possible contributing causes to apnea of prematurity (Abu-Shaweesh & Martin, 2008).

Premature infants have blunted respiratory responses to hypoxia (decreased delivery of oxygen to tissues) and hypercapnia (elevated carbon dioxide levels); they do not appropriately increase their breathing efforts in response to either. The impaired response to carbon dioxide is more pronounced in infants with apnea of prematurity (Gerhardt & Bancalari, 1984). Infants, both term and preterm, develop apnea when their larynx is stimulated, which is known as the laryngeal chemoreflex. Preterm infants have decreased tone in their upper airway, which makes them more susceptible to upper airway obstruction. Sleep mechanisms are immature and they have a decrease in their ability to arouse in response to respiratory problems, particularly in the prone position (Bhat et al., 2006).

Apnea of prematurity can be central, obstructive, or mixed. Central apnea is the complete cessation of breathing effort; the brain fails to send the appropriate signals to the respiratory muscles to breathe. Obstructive apnea occurs when the infant's upper airway collapses and air cannot flow in or out of the infant's mouth; however, the infant continues to try to breathe. Mixed apneas have components of both during an episode.

In response to the apnea, infants often become hypoxic and bradycardic. Lung volumes, specifically functional residual capacity (FRC), are low, which predisposes them to hypoxemia when they develop apnea (Tourneux et al., 2008). Hypoxia itself can produce apnea in preterm infants, which may increase the severity and duration of the apneic episode. Bradycardia is also seen with apnea. The mechanism is not well understood. It may be directly produced by the stimulus that causes the apnea or may be due to enhanced sensitivity to vagal nerve stimulation. In addition, hypoxia itself can also cause bradycardia. Apneas are worse during active rather than quiet sleep.

Events that further depress an infant's brain function, such as sepsis or intracranial bleeds, may increase the incidence and severity of apnea. For many years, it was believed that gastroesophageal reflux worsens apnea. However, recent studies do not bear out the association (Di Fiore, Arko, Whitehouse, Kimball, & Martin, 2005). Prone position is associated with an increase in central apneas and a decrease in arousals (Bhat et al., 2006).

Signs and symptoms

Apnea presents with episodes of hypoxemia and bradycardia. It may also be associated with hypotension. Classically, the infant may turn blue, pale, limp, and mottled and makes little or no respiratory effort. Heart rate by cardiac monitoring decreases to less than 80 beats/min. Oxygen saturations by pulse oximetry decrease to less than 85%. Apnea of prematurity may be temporally associated with feeds. Infants may recover by themselves or may require stimulation in order to terminate the episode.

Diagnosis

The diagnosis is made clinically when a lack of respiratory effort is observed along with bradycardia and hypoxemia. In the neonatal intensive care unit (NICU), cardiorespiratory monitoring will pick up bradycardia and hypoxemia. Blood gases are rarely used for diagnosis since cannulation of the artery or vein often causes enough stimulation to terminate the apnea. Secondary causes of apnea should be ruled out such as sepsis and intracranial hemorrhage.

In cases where the diagnosis is more challenging, polysomnography (sleep study) may be used to better delineate the characteristics of the episodes. It can differentiate between central, obstructive, and mixed apneas. During polysomnography, many physiological parameters are monitored: electroencephalogram (EEG), electrocardiogram (ECG), respirations, oxygen saturation levels, carbon dioxide levels, muscle tone, and eye and extremity movements. It can determine the exact duration of an apneic episode and can assess the resultant physiological consequences such as bradycardia, hypoxemia, arousals, and hypercapnia. Monitoring with a pH probe, during the test, can also determine the presence and relationship of gastroesophageal reflux to apnea.

After discharge from the NICU, respiratory monitoring can detect persistent apnea. The most common type of "apnea monitor" is the transthoracic electrical impedance. The apnea monitor has two parts: a belt or electrodes with sensory wires that a baby wears on the chest and a monitoring unit with an alarm. The sensors measure the baby's chest movement and breathing rate, while the monitor continuously records these rates. These monitors are generally effective in identifying and alarming with central apneas; however, apneas are sometimes identified even though the infant is breathing (false positive), and true apneas are not detected because of background "noise," such as cardiac beats (false negative).

Complications

Apnea of prematurity can prolong hospitalization of infants and may require more invasive treatment with positive pressure ventilation and medications. Repeated episodes of hypoxia and bradycardia might cause brain injury. Apnea of prematurity has been associated with impairment in neurological development; infants demonstrate lower scores on Bayley Scales of Infant Development and a higher incidence of cerebral palsy and blindness (Hunt et al., 2004; Janvier et al., 2004). Despite the fact that preterm birth is associated with a higher incidence of SIDS, apnea of prematurity does not seem to be an independent risk factor for SIDS.

Management

Mild episodes of apnea can improve without intervention. More significant episodes may require tactile stimulation—that is, stimulating the infant's limbs, back, or body. Stimulation is a well-recognized treatment for apnea of prematurity. In the past, oscillatory or "bump beds" were used to stimulate the infants. For severe episodes of apnea, the infant may require manual breaths and supplemental oxygen via bag–mask valve ventilation. If the apnea persists, the infant may require support with intubation and positive pressure ventilation. Alternatively, administration of continuous positive airway pressure (CPAP), intermittent positive pressure ventilation, or high-flow gas via nasal cannula may be effective (Pantalitschka et al., 2009). Transfusions with packed red blood cells to treat anemia has been associated with a transient decrease in apneic episodes (Bell et al., 2005).

The mainstay of medical treatment is the use of methylxanthines, primarily caffeine (Bhatt-Mehta & Schumacher, 2003). Methylxanthines stimulate the respiratory and central nervous systems of the preterm infant. In the past, theophylline was widely used. However, caffeine supplanted it as the drug of choice because it is as effective as theophylline but has a longer half-life and fewer side effects. Doxapram, a respiratory stimulant, has been investigated. It is not available in the United States and there is insufficient information about its effects and adverse reactions.

Caffeine is usually discontinued after a period without apnea and bradycardia or at the time when apnea begins to decrease in frequency at 34–36 weeks' PMA. After discontinuing the medication, most NICUs require the infant to have a period of 3–7 days without apnea and bradycardia before discharging the infant to home. However, in some infants, particularly those born less than 28-weeks gestation, the episodes persist longer which may delay discharge. In those cases, home apnea monitors may be used (Committee on Fetus and Newborn, 2003). Monitoring continues until the infants are 43 weeks' PMA or after the cessation of extreme episodes, whichever comes last. The monitors should be equipped with an event recorder, which keeps a record of the events. The information can be downloaded and sent to the primary care provider for review. Of note, home cardiorespiratory monitoring has never been proven to decrease the incidence of unexpected deaths in premature infants.

Nursing care of the child and family

The nursing care of the infant with apnea of prematurity must be systematic and comprehensive. It also requires knowledge of the three different types of apneic episodes described earlier in this chapter—central, obstructive, and mixed.

The first crucial component of care is that the nurse should be able to accurately identify periods of apnea so that the appropriate intervention can be initiated. A monitor (cardiac/apnea/pulse oximeter) should be instituted for all infants diagnosed with apnea of prematurity. The leads must be well placed (in a manner such that they visibly capture the infant's respiratory pattern on the monitor) and the alarms set appropriately (Calhoun, 1996). The heart rate alarm should be based on the infant's baseline heart rate. The respiratory alarm should notify the caregiver when the infant has been apneic for greater than 20 seconds. Typical settings include a low heart rate of 80–100 beats/min with a 20-second apnea delay (Theobald, Botwinski, Albanna, & McWilliam, 2000). Alarm limits should be designed to provide the nurse time to arrive to the bedside and assess the infant.

Assessment of an apneic episode includes color, respiratory rate and effort, oxygen saturation level, heart rate, and position (Theobald et al., 2000). A thorough assessment will help to determine if the apnea is central, obstructive, or mixed. If the infant is having central apnea, the apnea alarm will probably be the first to sound. Heart rate and oxygen saturation alarms may follow if the apneic episode is prolonged and leads to hypoxia and/

or bradycardia. If the infant is experiencing obstructive apnea, the saturation or possibly the heart rate would alarm first as the infant continues to try to breathe. If unsuccessful, the infant will eventually become apneic. In this case, the apnea alarm is a late indicator that the infant is in trouble.

Common triggers for apnea include feeding, suctioning, temperature changes, and immunizations (Calhoun, 1996; Stokowski, 2005; Theobald et al., 2000). The primary intervention for an apneic episode is tactile stimulation, such as foot rubbing (Stokowski, 2005; Theobald et al., 2000). If the infant is not bradycardic or hypoxic, the nurse should observe the infant for a short period of time (approximately 15 seconds) before stimulating the infant to see if he/she will trigger his/her own respirations. If the infant does not spontaneously begin to breathe or if the heart rate or oxygen saturation level drop, the nurse must intervene. If tactile stimulation is insufficient, a more vigorous stimulation, supplemental oxygen, or bag–mask ventilation should be instituted (Stokowski, 2005; Theobald et al., 2000). With obstructive apnea, the infant may require suctioning or repositioning to open his/her airway. Preventive nursing interventions include maintaining a neutral temperature, proper positioning and avoidance of neck flexion, appropriate placement of the nasogastric tube if applicable, slow feedings, avoidance of deep suctioning, and providing periods of undisturbed sleep (Stokowski, 2005; Theobald et al., 2000).

All apnea episodes must be reported and documented. Documentation of apneic episodes is a vital aspect of care. Documentation should include the date and time of the event, the duration of apnea, associated episodes of bradycardia, oxygen saturation level, any precipitating events, and intervention required (Calhoun, 1996).

Apnea of prematurity is also treated pharmacologically with the use of methylxanthines (Calhoun, 1996; Theobald et al., 2000). Therefore, the nurse must monitor the therapeutic and adverse effects of pharmacological therapy. Side effects of methylxanthines include tachycardia, tachypnea, glucose instability, jitteriness, restlessness, tremors, irritability, vomiting, and feeding intolerance (Theobald et al., 2000). Methylxanthines can lead to mild diuresis. Therefore, intake and output should be monitored closely, especially if the infant is on a diuretic (Calhoun, 1996; Gannon, 2000; Theobald et al., 2000).

Theophylline and caffeine are two methylxanthines that have been used in the management of apnea of prematurity. Methylxanthines are thought to stimulate breathing efforts; however, their mechanism of action is not certain (Henderson-Smart & Steer, 2010). A recent review revealed that caffeine and theophylline have similar short-term effects on apnea and bradycardia; however, caffeine is associated with less toxicity, a higher therapeutic ratio, more reliable enteral abosorption, and a longer half-life (Henderson-Smart & Steer, 2010).

Caffeine can be given once a day. It provides stable, predictable plasma concentrations and a wide therapeutic range. Most institutions monitor caffeine levels every 1–2 weeks, while some do not feel monitoring is necessary (Theobald et al., 2000). A therapeutic trough caffeine serum level is 5–25 µg/mL (Gannon, 2000). As previously mentioned, theophylline is not used often because caffeine has increased efficacy and a better safety profile. However, when it is used, it is dosed every 8–12 hours. Serum levels between 7 and 12 µg/mL are generally acceptable (Gannon, 2000). Because theophylline toxicity can occur if levels are slightly higher than the acceptable range, serum levels are checked frequently (Gannon, 2000). Theophylline can affect sleep/wake patterns and can cause gastric irritation. Therefore, it should not be given in the afternoon and stools should be tested for occult blood (Calhoun, 1996; Gannon, 2000; Theobald et al., 2000).

When caring for the infant with apnea of prematurity, it is important to keep the parents informed and well educated. Parents should be updated on their infant's status as well as on changes in therapy. Information regarding apnea of prematurity and its progression is usually welcomed by parents. Knowing that the apnea is likely related to the infant's immaturity and will improve over time can help decrease the parents' level of anxiety. Other educational messages should include positioning, proper feeding techniques, sleep safety measures, avoidance of secondhand smoke, and avoidance of large crowds or exposure to sick contacts. If the infant is experiencing desaturations and/or bradycardia related to positioning, parents should be instructed on the proper positioning that will maintain the infant's airway. Parents should also be instructed to hold their infant semi-upright while feeding and to observe the infant's sucking and breathing patterns during the feed. Premature infants may need to have the bottle removed from their mouth to allow them time to rest between long sucking bursts. At home, parents should also be instructed to feed their infants in an area that is well lit so that they can readily assess the infant's color if an apneic episode occurs (Stokowski, 2005). Parents must be informed that the infant should be maintained in a supine position during sleep and they should avoid having the infant sleep with them in their bed.

Typically, infants are discharged once they are free from apneic episodes for 3–7 days. However, home monitoring can be arranged. The decision to discharge an infant with an apnea monitor is usually institution specific and provider related (Stokowski, 2005). If the infant is discharged home on a monitor, it is important that the parents be informed that the purpose of the monitor is not to prevent SIDS but to provide early recognition of an apneic episode (Stokowski, 2005).

BPD

Epidemiology

BPD is the most common chronic lung disease of infancy (CLDI). It was first described in 1967 by Northway et al. in premature infants who had been exposed to high levels of supplemental oxygen and prolonged mechanical ventilation (Northway, Rosan, & Porter, 1967). Very premature infants are at risk of neonatal RDS and often require support with supplemental oxygen and positive pressure ventilation. BPD occurs primarily in infants who are delivered at a gestational age of less than 30 weeks with a birth weight of less than 1,500 g. BPD occurs in approximately 20% of infants less than 1,500 g (Fanaroff et al., 2007) and one-third of those less than 1,000 g (Walsh et al., 2006). Despite the introduction of antenatal corticosteroids, postnatal surfactant replacement, and more gentle modes of positive pressure ventilation, the incidence of BPD has remained stable throughout the last two decades. Though these interventions have decreased the risk of BPD in older, preterm infants, the younger, more preterm infants are now surviving with an increased incidence of BPD.

The development of BPD has been associated with maternal preeclampsia (Hansen, Barnes, Folkman, & McElrath, 2010), chorioamnionitis (Watterberg, Demers, Scott, & Murphy, 1996), high fluid administration in the early newborn period (Van Marter, Leviton, Allred, Pagano, & Kuban, 1990), patent ductus ateriosus (Brown, 1979), adrenal insufficiency (Watterberg, Gerdes, Gifford, & Lin, 1999), neonatal infections, such as ureaplasma urealyticum (Colaizy, Morris, Lapidus, Sklar, & Pillers, 2007) and cytomegalovirus (Sawyer, Edwards, & Spector, 1987), vitamin A deficiency (Inder, Graham, Winterbourn, Austin, & Darlow, 1998), and intrauterine growth restriction (Bose et al., 2009).

There may be a genetic predisposition to RDS and a subsequent development of BPD. Analysis of twin pairs demonstrates an increased association of BPD in identical versus fraternal twins (Lavoie, Pham, & Jang, 2008). The development of BPD has been correlated with certain genetic polymorphisms or variants (Kwinta et al., 2008; Levit et al., 2009). A family history of asthma has been associated with BPD; however, recent data are not supportive (Evans, Palta, Sadek, Weinstein, & Peters, 1998).

Pathophysiology

Preterm infants have immature lung development. They have a decreased number of branching airways and alveoli. They are deficient in surfactant, which is important for the stability of the alveoli. With insufficient surfactant, the alveoli collapse and develop areas of atelectasis, further impairing gas exchange. As a result, the infants develop respiratory distress and hypoxemia. Prior to the development of surfactant replacement therapy, chest radiographs typically showed a diffuse reticulogranular infiltrate with air bronchograms, and pathology revealed evidence of "hyaline membrane disease."

BPD results from injury induced by the supplemental oxygen and positive pressure ventilation that the preterm infant requires for survival. In addition, there is evidence that immature lungs of the extremely low birth weight infants do not develop normally after birth, which may further limit pulmonary function.

Both supplemental oxygen and mechanical ventilation can cause injury independently; the combination can cause injury and inflammation within minutes (Pierce & Bancalari, 1995). Oxygen can cause damage by the production of reactive oxygen species and free radicals. Mechanical ventilation causes injury because of the swings in both pressure (barotrauma) and volume (volutrauma). The premature infant is at increased risk because it has a poorly developed antioxidant system to protect against the injury (Frank, 1992). In addition, infections may aggravate the underlying inflammation. The inflammation and injury may hinder the postnatal development of the immature lung.

Classic BPD was associated with typical pathological findings, which included inflammation, necrotizing bronchiolitis, parenchymal fibrosis, smooth muscle hypertrophy, squamous metaplasia, loss of ciliated epithelium, and mucus gland and vascular smooth muscle hypertrophy (Northway et al., 1967). Chest radiographs reflected the heterogeneity of disease with areas of patchy consolidation and fibrosis alternating with hyperinflation.

However, a "new" BPD has recently emerged. Infants are now being delivered at earlier gestational ages, such as 23–26 weeks. At this point in development, the lungs and alveoli are poorly developed; they are little more than conducting tubes with only a small amount of functional alveolar tissue available for gas exchange. The pathology of the new BPD reflects less fibrosis and cellular proliferation; there is more evidence of arrested alveolarization and decreased pulmonary blood vessel development (Kinsella, Greenough, & Abman, 2006).

As a result of the pathological changes, infants have a decrease in their lung compliance and an increase in their airway resistance, both of which increase their work of breathing. The scarring and decreased alveolarization produces hypoxemia. Hypercapnia, or an increase in arterial carbon dioxide levels, may result from both the scarring and respiratory muscle fatigue from the increased demands of breathing. Inflammation also leads to increased airways hyperreactivity—airways smooth muscle constricting in response to a variety of stimuli.

Signs and symptoms

Infants with RDS present with tachypnea, retractions, cyanosis, and apnea after birth. Infants in respiratory distress are often put on a trial of high-flow oxygen, CPAP, or intermittent positive pressure ventilation via nasal cannula. If they fail this support or develop apnea, they are often intubated and placed on positive pressure ventilation. Some of the infants may improve quickly and may be weaned off positive pressure and oxygen. However, others demonstrate a persistent need for both. As an infant develops chronic lung disease, chest radiographs often develop a bubbly appearance and irregularly dense areas.

Infants with BPD have evidence of impaired oxygenation and increased work of breathing. Without supplemental oxygen, the infant may experience cyanosis, particularly around his/her mouth and mucus membranes. The increased work of breathing may be reflected in tachypnea, nasal flaring, grunting and retractions (subcostal, intercostal, and/or suprasternal), and tachycardia. In the older infant with BPD, respiratory distress may be accompanied by agitation, irritability, and diaphoresis. In overt respiratory failure, infants may demonstrate apnea and a decreased level of consciousness. Older infants with BPD often have crackles because of pulmonary edema or wheezes because of narrowed, hyperreactive airways. Some have upper airway obstruction because of narrowing in the trachea or larynx; this obstruction may be evidenced by stridor on inspiration.

In the NICU, most young infants with BPD receive nutrition with feeding tubes. However, when oral feeds are instituted, infants with BPD can have difficulty feeding and may experience apnea or dyspnea with feeds. They can also have discoordinate swallowing and often have difficulty gaining weight.

Infants with BPD often have problems with oxygenation and ventilation. Pulse oximetry is widely utilized in NICUs. Blood gases may demonstrate hypoxemia and inadequate ventilation with carbon dioxide retention. An arterial blood gas is the gold standard for determining the arterial oxygen level (PaO_2) and carbon dioxide ($PaCO_2$). Because an arterial blood gas is technically difficult to obtain, a capillary blood gas is often used. An extremity, such as a finger or toe, is pierced with a lancet; the blood is collected into a thin, small capillary tube. Since it reflects a mixture of venous and arterial blood, the capillary blood sample, it is not good for assessing arterial oxygenation. Venous carbon dioxide levels are higher than those in the arterial blood; thus, it may reflect the "worst-case scenario."

A chest radiograph usually demonstrates heterogenous lung disease. There are areas of irregularly dense consolidation and hyperinflation. There may be formation of cysts. If the infant is fluid overloaded, then pulmonary edema and cardiomegaly may be seen. Areas of consolidation may represent superimposed pneumonia or atelectasis.

Diagnosis

The diagnosis of BPD in a child who was born premature and received mechanical ventilation was originally made on the basis of three criteria: supplemental oxygen requirement at 28 days of age, persistent abnormalities on chest radiograph, and tachypnea with crackles or rhonchi (Bancalari, Abdenour, Feller, & Gannon, 1979). However, not all infants met the criteria and, subsequently, the definition was refined to correlate better with pulmonary outcomes. BPD is presently diagnosed in infants less than 32 weeks' gestational age and <1,500 g if they have been on supplemental oxygen for at least 28 days. The severity of disease is stratified by the amount of oxygen that these infants require at 36 weeks' PMA (Jobe & Bancalari, 2001). It is considered mild if no oxygen is required, moderate if less than 30% is required, and severe if greater than or equal to 30% is required (including the need for positive pressure ventilation).

Complications

There are many complications in infants with BPD both related to their prematurity and their lung disease. The complications are greater in those with severe disease. Approximately half of infants with BPD have mild disease and outgrow their need for oxygen by 36 weeks' PMA (Ehrenkranz et al., 2005). In contrast, some with severe disease may require long-term positive pressure ventilation administered via a tracheostomy tube. Infants with BPD demonstrate long-term pulmonary impairment (Bhandari & Panitch, 2006). They have frequent respiratory symptoms, airflow obstruction, and airways hyperreactivity (Kennedy et al., 2000; Northway et al., 1990). However, most long-term studies were done on survivors from the 1980s and 1990s who were born at a mean gestational age of 28–29 weeks. The prognosis of those who were born more premature is unknown. The concern is that the decrease in alveolarization may be irreversible and that these infants may be at risk of chronic obstructive pulmonary disease and pulmonary hypertension in the future.

Infants with BPD are at increased risk for rehospitalization because of respiratory tract infections during their first year of life (Lamarche-Vadel et al., 2004). They have hyperreactive airways and are prone to flare-ups of their BPD characterized by labored breathing, hypoxemia, and wheezing. The exacerbations are usually caused by viral respiratory infections such as respiratory syncytial virus (RSV), rhinovirus, influenza, parainfluenza, and human metapneumovirus. While they may have decreased levels of immunoglobulin because of their prematurity and impaired maternal delivery, they do not seem to have an increase in bacterial pulmonary infections.

Infants with BPD have a higher incidence of tracheal abnormalities, such as subglottic stenosis or edema (from prolonged intubation with endotracheal [ET] tubes) and tracheobronchomalacia, or collapsible airways. The stenosis may be so severe that it may require surgical intervention and tracheal reconstruction.

Infants with BPD are at increased risk for both systemic and pulmonary hypertension. Infants with chronic lung disease and pulmonary hypertension have a high risk of mortality. Many infants with BPD have gastroesophageal reflux. It may be easily diagnosed by recurrent vomiting, or it may be subtle and indicated by failure to thrive, aversion to oral feeds, and arching. Infants with BPD may have hematuria from kidney stones, which are caused by chronic diuretic use. They also demonstrate "soft" neurological signs and irritability. BPD is associated with impairment in IQ, cognitive tests and motor skills, lower academic achievement, and an increased need for special education services (Short et al., 2003).

Management

The goal of management is to support the infant's impaired respiratory status and associated complications, and to provide nutrition in order to allow the infant's lungs to maximally develop and heal. Supplemental oxygen is given in order to prevent hypoxemia. It is important to keep oxygen saturations greater than 91% in order to allow optimal growth and to prevent pulmonary hypertension. However, there is no improved benefit to "hyperoxia," that is, keeping the saturations 95–98% instead of 91–94% (Askie, Henderson-Smart, Irwig, & Simpson, 2003). Hypoxemia may develop during oral feeding, increased activity, sleep, or acute illnesses (Wang et al., 2010); if this occurs, an increased concentration of supplemental oxygen during those periods may be required.

For infants with severe BPD, CPAP or high flow via nasal cannula may be required for a prolonged period. Some of these infants may require a tracheostomy in order to administer either CPAP or positive pressure ventilation. As the infants slowly improve, they are gradually weaned off the positive pressure and supplemental oxygen.

Systemic corticosteroids are often administered to wean infants off the ventilator in the NICU. Corticosteroids, like dexamethasone, improve lung compliance, airways resistance, and gas exchange. However, they must be used judiciously because they have been associated with significant side effects and adverse neurological outcomes. In older infants with BPD, corticosteroids may be used for acute exacerbations of BPD associated with wheezing. Inhaled corticosteroids are of uncertain benefit in early BPD and are not routinely used unless reversible lower airways obstruction, wheezing, or bronchodilator-responsive symptoms are documented.

Inhaled bronchodilators have inconsistent effects in infants with early BPD (Pantalitschka & Poets, 2006). In older patients with BPD, they can be used to treat the bronchoconstriction associated with flare-ups of their reactive airway disease.

Diuretics are widely used for infants with BPD in the NICU. In short-term studies, they improve lung function and compliance. However, they have not been proven to decrease the length of hospitalization, the need for ventilatory support, or long-term outcome (Brion, Primhak, & Ambrosio-Perez, 2000). In general, diuretics are continued until the infants are weaned off supplemental oxygen.

Pulmonary hypertension is an often underappreciated entity in infants with BPD. It can be detected by cardiac echocardiography. However, cardiac catheterization may be required to more accurately assess intracardiac pressures. It is important in patients with pulmonary hypertension to prevent hypoxemia and acidosis, which would increase pulmonary vascular resistance and worsen pulmonary hypertension. Sometimes, the use of pulmonary vasodilators, such as sildenafil or bosentran, are necessary (Krishnan, Krishnan, & Gewitz, 2008).

Systemic hypertension can be diagnosed when the infant's blood pressure is documented to be over the 95 percentile for age. It is important to use the appropriate size cuff and to take the pressure when the infant is quiet. If systemic hypertension is documented, then the cause should be analyzed. In older infants with BPD, it is important to rule out renal artery stenosis, which may have been caused by the presence of an umbilical artery catheter in the early neonatal period. Occasionally, treatment with systemic antihypertensives is necessary.

Nutrition is of paramount importance. Caloric needs are increased because of the infant's increased work of breathing; energy expenditure may be increased by 30% (Gamarra, 1992). Intake may be limited by inadequate oral intake, vomiting from gastroesophageal reflux, and the need to fluid-restrict the infant. Often nasogastric feeds are necessary to ensure adequate calories. In addition, concentrated formulas are often used to minimize the amount of fluid.

Gastroesophageal reflux is very common in infants with chronic pulmonary disease. Small, frequent, or continuous feeds are often necessary. In some cases, gastroesophageal reflux may be aggravated by milk protein intolerance. Elemental hydrolyzed formulas may be used. In addition, use of acid-blocking medications and promotility agents may be necessary. Some infants require surgical placement of gastric feeding tubes and gastrofundoplication.

Infants with BPD are susceptible to severe bronchiolitis with viral illnesses. RSV and influenza are epidemic in the winter months in the northern hemisphere. Palivizumab (Synagis) is a monoclonal antibody to RSV, which has been shown to decrease hospitalizations and moderate/severe exacerbations. Monthly injections are recommended for all infants with BPD who are <2 years of age at the start of RSV season and have received medical therapy (oxygen, diuretics, bronchodilators, and corticosteroids) in the previous 6 months (American Academy of Pediatrics, 2009). For infants who are at least 6 months of age, influenza vaccine is also recommended.

Nursing care of the child and family

The nursing care of the infant with BPD is multifactorial because of the numerous conditions and complications associated with BPD. Moreover, the nursing care is dependent upon the stage (evolving vs. established) and severity of the disease process. However, whether caring for an infant with BPD during the evolving or established phase, the foundation of care should be grounded in the recognition that the infant has all the developmental issues and needs of a well child in addition to those related to his or her chronic lung disease. Furthermore, he or she is a member of a family, and education and support of that family is crucial to the long-term care of that infant at home. Parents should be considered partners in the care of their infant, and parental involvement should be encouraged (Jackson, 1986; Thomas & Speer, 2008).

Evolving phase

During the evolving phase when the infant is experiencing respiratory distress, nursing care of the infant is mainly supportive (Charsha, 2009) and focused on minimizing the potential side effects of therapies required to provide adequate gas exchange. Supportive care includes the administration and monitoring of surfactant, corticosteroids, diuretics, bronchodilators, supplemental oxygen, and positive pressure ventilation therapies that are prescribed (Charsha, 2009).

Surfactant is generally administered within minutes after birth into the ET tube of the infant. The ET tube should be suctioned prior to administration. Furthermore, the infant will require position changes to allow gravity to distribute the product to the lungs (Kee, Hayes, & McCuistion, 2009). Due to a limited ability to regulate cerebral blood flow and the risk of precipitating an intraventricular hemorrhage, very low birth weight (VLBW) infants should not be placed in a head-down position to administer the surfactant but should be rotated side to side during the administration. The nurse or respiratory practitioner must assure that the medication is warmed to room temperature before administration. It should not be artificially warmed and it should not be shaken. Depending on the product being used, surfactant is administered in premeasured aliquots. Crackles may be noted after administration of a synthetic surfactant; however, the infant should not be suctioned for at least 2 hours after administration unless prolonged hypoxemia and/or airway obstruction is present. During and after administration, the infant's respiratory status including inspiratory pressure readings, chest expansion, color, oxygen saturation levels, and arterial blood gases should be monitored closely. Additionally, heart rate, blood pressure, and ET tube patency should be assessed (Kee et al., 2009).

The prolonged use of corticosteroids, especially systemic corticosteroids, are associated with delayed growth, increased blood pressure, osteoporosis, adrenal suppression, and cataracts (Kee et al., 2009). Therefore, these side effects should be monitored for. When given via inhalation, corticosteroids can result in candidiasis. Therefore, if given by a metered-dose inhaler, they should always be used with a holding chamber. Additionally, the infant's mouth should be rinsed after administration.

Diuretic use requires the monitoring of breath sounds, work of breathing, and urinary output, in addition to the monitoring of potential side effects associated with this class of medications. Side effects of chlorothiazide include hypokalemia, hypercalcemia, and hypomagnesemia (Allen et al., 2003; Kee et al., 2009). Furosemide can result in electrolyte imbalances, such as hypokalemia, hyponatremia, hypocalcemia, hypomagnesemia, and hypochloremia (Kee et al., 2009). Metabolic alkalosis can also occur (Allen et al., 2003; Kee et al., 2009). Because of the effect chlorothiazide and furosemide have on potassium, potassium supplements are often prescribed (Allen et al., 2003; Kee et al., 2009).

Spironolactone is a potassium-sparing diuretic. The main side effect of spironolactone is hyperkalemia (Allen et al., 2003; Kee et al., 2009). Infants who are prescribed spironolactone and a potassium supplement should be monitored closely for hyperkalemia. Furthermore, because of the potential electrolyte imbalances associated with the diuretics commonly used in the management of BPD, all serum electrolytes should be monitored on a regular basis (Allen et al., 2003).

If the infant is receiving bronchodilator therapy, the nurse should evaluate the infant's therapeutic response by monitoring the infant's breath sounds, respiratory rate and effort, and oxygen saturation level. The infant receiving bronchodilator therapy should also be monitored for side effects of the medication, including tremors, tachycardia, hyper- or hypotension, dysrhythmias, vomiting, hypokalemia, coughing, wheezing, and bronchospasm (Allen et al., 2003 Kee et al., 2009). In the nonventilated infant, inhaled bronchodilators should always be administered via a face mask, whether given by a metered-dose inhaler or a nebulizer, to help ensure adequate delivery to the airways (Allen et al., 2003).

Infants receiving supplemental oxygen therapy should be monitored with a pulse oximeter. It is important to note that oxygen saturation levels can vary depending on activity level. Therefore, oxygen saturations should be monitored awake, asleep, and during feedings. Saturations consistently above or below the infant's prescribed range should be documented and discussed with the infant's provider.

The goals of oxygen therapy are to promote growth and repair of the immature lungs, to provide adequate exercise tolerance, and to decrease the incidence of pulmonary artery hypertension and right ventricular work load (Allen et al., 2003). The range of optimal oxygen saturation in preterm infants is controversial and is still under study; ranges of 85–95% measured by pulse oximetry have been used. Lower target ranges for oxygen saturation are often advocated to prevent retinopathy of prematurity (ROP) (Carlo et al., 2010).

The target oxygen saturation recommendation for those who are very preterm, with early, immature eyes, and without ROP is 90–94%. For those with ROP or those whose retinal vascularization is complete, target oxygen saturation is 95–99% (Allen et al., 2003). Recent findings have not demonstrated significant differences in rates of severe retinopathy or death among infants born between 24- and 27-weeks' gestation in two oxygen saturation target groups (85–91% and 91–95%). However, death before discharge occurred more frequently and severe retinopathy occurred less often in the lower oxygen saturation group (Carlo et al., 2010). Furthermore, in extremely preterm infants, oxygen saturation levels higher (95–98%) than the standard range (91–94%) have not resulted in significant differences in regard to weight, length, head circumference, or major developmental abnormalities (Askie et al., 2003). Despite the debate, oxygen saturation targets should be monitored closely and individualized for each infant based on his/her condition.

The most common route of supplemental oxygen administration in the nonventilated infant is a nasal cannula. Because the skin of newborns is sensitive, it is important that the nurse or respiratory practitioner monitor for skin breakdown around the cannula site, particularly at the nasal septum and on the infant's face under the cannula tubing. Protective barriers are often used on the face to prevent breakdown. If the infant has a tracheostomy tube in place and is not ventilated, supplemental oxygen is administered via a tracheostomy collar. It is important for the nurse or respiratory practitioner to assure that the infant is receiving proper humidification via the tracheostomy collar to avoid a decrease in ciliary action, injury to the airway epithelium, and retained mucous secretions (Allen et al., 2003; Sherman et al., 2000).

Infants with BPD who require long-term positive pressure ventilation will frequently undergo a tracheotomy procedure. The severity of lung disease is the most significant factor associated with tracheostomy tube placement in preterm infants (Pereira, MacGregor, McDuffie, & Mitchell, 2003). Although the care of an infant with a tracheostomy tube is beyond the scope of this text, a summary of the nursing care will be provided. Tracheostomy tubes should be changed regularly. Changing the tube on a regular basis facilitates parental education and helps to maintain a patent airway. Tracheostomy tubes are usually changed once a week (Sherman et al., 2000). Tracheostomy tube ties should also be changed on a regular basis. Although there is no consensus regarding the frequency for changing tracheostomy tube ties, they are usually changed at least three times a week and whenever soiled. It is imperative that the ties are secured properly to avoid accidental decannulation and skin breakdown. In general, one should be able to fit one finger between the infant's neck and the tracheostomy ties (Sherman et al., 2000). The infant with a tracheostomy tube should be suctioned based on clinical need (presence of secretions, increased work of breathing, a drop in oxygen saturation levels, etc.). If there is no evidence of secretions, the infant should be suctioned at least twice a day to assess for patency of the tracheostomy tube. When suctioning, a premeasured technique is recommended to avoid damage to the airway epithelium (Sherman et al., 2000).

The nursing care of an infant with BPD should include monitoring for complications associated with preterm birth and BPD as well as implementing practices that limit or prevent the occurrence of such complications. Common complications include subglottic stenosis, tracheobronchomalacia, systemic hypertension, pulmonary hypertension and cor pulmonale, growth failure, gastroesophageal reflux, and developmental delay.

Subglottic stenosis can occur after an ET intubation. Symptoms include stridor, hoarseness, apnea and bradycaria, cyanosis, and failure to tolerate extubation (Allen et al., 2003). Thus, making sure the ET tube is properly positioned and taking measures to decrease the infant's level of agitation while intubated are of paramount importance. Tracheobronchomalacia can be acquired or congenital. Symptoms include wheezing that is often unresponsive to bronchodilators (Allen et al., 2003).

The cardiac complications can occur during the evolving phase or the established phase. Indicators include an increase in blood pressure and a decrease in oxygen saturation levels.

The infant with BPD should have an order for daily weight measurement in addition to a weekly length measurement and head circumference. Length can be a predictor of lung growth, which is very important in this patient population. Weight is an important nutritional parameter to monitor; a decrease in weight or poor weight gain can be indicative of other issues, such as increased work of breathing or gastroesophageal reflux. Gastroesophageal reflux can lead to aspiration and bronchospasm (Allen et al., 2003); therefore, the infant should be monitored closely for signs of gastroesophageal reflux and aspiration so that appropriate management can be initiated if required.

Facilitating oral feedings in premature infants is another important nutritional intervention. The nurse should work closely with the occupational therapist to assure this developmental milestone is being addressed. By 28 weeks' gestation, the infant may demonstrate the simple elements of sucking and swallowing. Bursts of sucking may be evident by 32 weeks and a rhythmic suck, swallow, and breathing pattern by 34 weeks. To maximize oral skills and to facilitate transition to oral feedings, it is recommended that perioral stimulation (gentle touch, i.e., hand grasping and facial stimulation) be provided as tolerated at 23 weeks and that nipple readiness is assessed with nonnutritive sucking at 32–34 weeks followed by a transition to nutritive sucking (Liu et al., 2007). Nonnutritive sucking does not involve the flow of nutrients; it occurs at a rate of two sucks per second and is used to satisfy the basic sucking urge. Nutritive sucking involves the intake of nutrition and occurs at a rate of one suck per second that is constant over the course of the feeding (Harding, 2009). Infants with more mature nonnutritive sucking abilities have demonstrated more advanced oral feeding skills (Bingham, Ashikaga, & Abbasi, 2009). Nonnutritive sucking has also been associated with improved weight gain and improved response to pain (Liu et al., 2007).

From a neurodevelopmental perspective, strategies that promote newborn sleep should be implemented. This includes limiting the amount of narcotics and other medications, such as theophylline, which interrupts normal sleep cycles (Liu et al., 2007).

Established phase

Once the infant is stable, continuing care is based on the severity of the disease. Some infants will not require any medications or supplemental oxygen, while others may require numerous medications, including diuretics, bronchodilators, and inhaled steroids, in addition to supplemental oxygen and ventilatory support. During this phase, the nurse should continue to administer the necessary therapies and monitor for therapeutic and adverse effects of the medications/therapies as well as the complications associated with BPD.

Optimal growth and prevention of respiratory infections are critical components of care for infants with BPD. Infants with BPD require calorically dense formulas. However, such formulas can contribute to gastroesophageal reflux and loose stools (Allen et al., 2003). Therefore, the nurse should monitor for symptoms of gastroesophageal reflux and loose stools and report them if they occur.

Early on, infants with BPD usually require continuous enteral feedings in order to decrease their energy expenditure. As the infant's respiratory status improves, bolus feeds can be attempted. Infants receiving enteral feeds should receive oral–motor stimulation in preparation for oral feedings. Once it has been established that the infant's swallow function has matured, the infant can be fed by mouth. When feeding the infant by mouth, the nurse should monitor for oral–motor dysfunction and report it if it occurs. Oxygen saturation levels should also be monitored during feeds as the infant may require supplemental oxygen.

In addition to teaching parents the importance of keeping the infant away from sick contacts and practicing good hand washing, infants with BPD should receive an annual influenza vaccine if they are 6 months of age or older and palivizumab (Synagis) if they are <24 months of age and have received medical therapy within 6 months of the start of RSV season (American Academy of Pediatrics, 2009). The recommended dose of palivizumab (Synagis) is 15 mg/kg once a month, intramuscularly. The first dose should be administered before the start of RSV season and the treatment should continue for a maximum of 5 months. Palivizumab (Synagis) should not be diluted, shaken, or vigorously agitated. Palivizumab (Synagis) is available as single-dose vials (50 mg/0.5 mL and 100 mg/1 mL) and is preservative free (MedImmune, 2009). Therefore, any unused medication should be discarded.

Preparing for discharge

Prior to discharge, it is important to determine the parents' ability and willingness to care for their infant at home as well as the safety and suitability of the home environment (Jackson, 1986). As part of the multidisciplinary team, the nurse is instrumental in identifying family stressors and in advocating for support services such as counseling, sibling support groups, and financial assistance (Jackson, 1986). The nurse also works closely with the care coordinator and medical team to determine the level of services required in the home setting. If skilled nursing services will be involved in the home care of the infant, the family should be provided with anticipatory guidance regarding what the role of the nurse is in the home. If special equipment will be required in the home setting, the home must first be evaluated to determine whether there is enough space for the equipment as well as the appropriate number of electrical outlets to accommodate the necessary equipment. All equipment, supplies, and medications should be secured and in the home prior to discharge (Allen et al., 2003).

Parents learning their infant's care in preparation for discharge should be encouraged to spend as much time at the hospital as possible. This allows them to observe, learn, and participate in all facets of their infant's care. During this time, the role of the nurse should include that of an educator. Nurses must provide thorough and focused education regarding all aspects of the infant's care. Written instructions and materials are also useful for the parents. Documenting the education as well as the parents' level of understanding and ability are crucial in providing continuity of care. Key educational points for the parents are presented in Table 4.1 (Allen et al., 2003; Bakewell-Sachs, 2002; Jackson, 1986). If the infant has a tracheostomy tube in place, it is recommended that parents participate in an "overnight stay" (this is usually divided into 2- to 12-hour or 3- to 8-hour shifts), after having completed all other components of their

Table 4.1   Key educational points for parents going home with an infant who has BPD.

Respiratory assessment—that is, respiratory rate, color, and breathing patterns

Signs and symptoms of infection—that is, temperature, increased work of breathing, change in appetite or behavior, change in color, odor, or quantity of secretions

Fluid balance—that is, assessing intake, monitoring and reporting emesis, monitoring wet diapers and reporting decreases in urinary output, assessing for and reporting edema

Treatments and procedures—that is, airway clearance technique, suctioning, tracheostomy care (cleaning, tracheostomy ties, and tracheostomy changes), preparation of formula, administration of enteral feedings, feeding tube care, care and cleaning of equipment (ventilator, feeding pump, pulse oximeter, etc.), purpose of supplemental oxygen, administration of supplemental oxygen, monitoring of supplemental oxygen

Medication administration—that is, purpose, dose and schedule, how to draw up medication, how to administer medication (oral, inhaled, via nasogastric or gastrostomy tube), side effects, storage, and identifying need for refill

Safety issues—that is, keeping infant away from large crowds, keeping infant away from people who are sick, care of supplemental oxygen (no smoking in the home, store tanks upright, etc.), notifying rescue squad and utility and telephone companies that infant has chronic lung disease and requires special equipment, list of emergency numbers to keep posted by the telephone, CPR training

Anticipatory guidance—that is, developmental issues, potential for rehospitalization

Follow-up—that is, scheduling appointments (primary care provider, pulmonologist, opthomalogist, gastroenterologist, occupational/physical therapy, etc.), obtaining influenza vaccines and palimizumab

Travel—that is, travel bag with necessary supplies (feeding supplies, tracheostomy supplies, suction machine, etc.)

training, in order to demonstrate their ability to care for their infant around the clock (Sherman et al., 2000).

Because gastroesphageal reflux is common in infants with BPD, parents should be instructed on signs and symptoms of gastroesophageal reflux, such as vomiting, irritability and arching after feeding, and failure to thrive. Furthermore, because preterm infants have immature sleep patterns, parents should be provided with anticipatory guidance regarding the fact that these infants have more frequent awakenings over the first few months of life and have less predictable patterns of wakefulness and alertness (Bakewell-Sachs, 2002). Furthermore, infants with BPD have an increased risk for rehospitalization during the first year of life. In a study conducted to describe the rates for rehospitalization during the first year of life among infants with BPD, it was found that 49% of infants were rehospitalized in the first year of life. Those without BPD were hospitalized at a rate of 23% (Smith et al., 2004). Parents should be informed of this fact so that they do not feel they have failed their infant if a readmission becomes necessary. Finally, infants with BPD are at risk of developmental delay. Parents should be provided with the opportunity to learn about premature infant development and behaviors and should be informed of the risk for developmental delay. In a study conducted to examine the effects of BPD and VLBW on the cognitive and academic achievement of a large sample of 8-year-old children, it was found that BPD and duration of supplemental oxygen have long-term adverse consequences on cognitive and academic achievement above and beyond those of being born VLBW (Short et al., 2003).

In addition to the special needs required by infants with BPD, parents should be educated on well child care needs such as feeding, bathing, diaper changes, sleep patterns, development, and immunization schedules (Allen et al., 2003; Bakewell-Sachs, 2002). Developing a daily schedule with the parents for their infant prior to discharge will be helpful as they learn to juggle caring for their infant with their other responsibilities such as work and home life (Allen et al., 2003). Finally, if they have not done so already, parents should identify a primary care provider and preferably meet with that provider before the infant is discharged from the hospital (Bakewell-Sachs, 2002).

REFERENCES

Abu-Shaweesh, J. M., & Martin, R. J. (2008). Neonatal apnea: What's new? *Pediatric Pulmonology, 43,* 937–944.

Alden, E. R., Mandelkorn, T., Woodrum, D. E., Wennberg, R. P., Parks, C. R., & Hodson, W. A. (1972). Morbidity and mortality of infants weighing less than 1,000 grams in an intensive care nursery. *Pediatrics, 50,* 40–49.

Allen, J., Zwerdling, R., Ehrenkranz, R., Gaultier, C., Geggel, R., Greenough, A., et al. (2003). Statement on the care of the child with chronic lung disease of infancy and childhood. *American Journal of Respiratory & Critical Care Medicine, 168*, 356–396.

American Academy of Pediatrics (2009). Policy statement: Modified recommendations for use of palivizumab for prevention of respiratory syncytial virus infections. *Pediatrics, 124*, 1694–1701.

Amin, S. B., Charafeddine, L., & Guillet, R. (2005). Transient bilirubin encephalopathy and apnea of prematurity in 28 to 32 weeks gestational age infants. *Journal of Perinatology, 25*, 386–390.

Askie, L. M., Henderson-Smart, D. J., Irwig, L., & Simpson, J. M. (2003). Oxygen-saturation targets and outcomes in extremely preterm infants. *New England Journal of Medicine, 349*, 959–967.

Bakewell-Sachs, S. (2002). After the NICU. Comprehensive primary care for preterm infants. *Advance for Nurse Practitioners, 10*(41–43), 45–46.

Bancalari, E., Abdenour, G. E., Feller, R., & Gannon, J. (1979). Bronchopulmonary dysplasia: Clinical presentation. *Journal of Pediatrics, 95*, 819–823.

Bell, E. F., Strauss, R. G., Widness, J. A., Mahoney, L. T., Mock, D. M., Seward, V. J., et al. (2005). Randomized trial of liberal versus restrictive guidelines for red blood cell transfusion in preterm infants. *Pediatrics, 115*, 1685–1691.

Bhandari, A., & Panitch, H. B. (2006). Pulmonary outcomes in bronchopulmonary dysplasia. *Seminars in Perinatology, 30*, 219–226.

Bhat, R. Y., Hannam, S., Pressler, R., Rafferty, G. F., Peacock, J. L., & Greenough, A. (2006). Effect of prone and supine position on sleep, apneas, and arousal in preterm infants. *Pediatrics, 118*, 101–107.

Bhatt-Mehta, V., & Schumacher, R. E. (2003). Treatment of apnea of prematurity. *Paediatric Drugs, 5*, 195–210.

Bingham, P. M., Ashikaga, T., & Abbasi, S. (2009). Prospective study of nonnutritive sucking and feeding skills in premature infants. *Archives of Disease in Childhood—Fetal and Neonatal Edition, 95*, F194–F200.

Bose, C., Van Marter, L. J., Laughon, M., O'Shea, T. M., Allred, E. N., Karna, P., et al. (2009). Fetal growth restriction and chronic lung disease among infants born before the 28th week of gestation. *Pediatrics, 124*, e450–e458.

Brion, L. P., Primhak, R. A., & Ambrosio-Perez, I. (2000). Diuretics acting on the distal renal tubule for preterm infants with (or developing) chronic lung disease. *Cochrane Database of Systematic Reviews*, (3), CD001817.

Brown, E. R. (1979). Increased risk of bronchopulmonary dysplasia in infants with patent ductus arteriosus. *Journal of Pediatrics, 95*, 865–866.

Calhoun, L. K. (1996). Pharmacologic management of apnea of prematurity. *Journal of Perinatology & Neonatal Nursing, 9*, 56–62.

Carlo, W. A., Finer, N. N., Walsh, M. C., Rich, W., Gantz, M. G., Laptook, A. R., et al. (2010). Target ranges of oxygen saturation in extremely preterm infants. *New England Journal of Medicine, 362*(21), 1959–1969.

Charsha, D. S. (2009). Gently caring: Supporting the first few critical hours of life for the extremely low birth weight infant. *Critical Care Nursing Clinics of North America, 21*, 57–65.

Colaizy, T. T., Morris, C. D., Lapidus, J., Sklar, R. S., & Pillers, D. A. (2007). Detection of ureaplasma DNA in endotracheal samples is associated with bronchopulmonary dysplasia after adjustment for multiple risk factors. *Pediatric Research, 61*, 578–583.

Committee on Fetus and Newborn (2003). Apnea, sudden infant death syndrome, and home monitoring. *Pediatrics, 111*, 914–917.

Darnall, R. A., Ariagno, R. L., & Kinney, H. C. (2006). The late preterm infant and the control of breathing, sleep, and brainstem development: A review. *Clinics in Perinatology, 33*, 883–914, abstract x.

de Gamarra, E. (1992). Energy expenditure in premature newborns with bronchopulmonary dysplasia. *Biology of the Neonate, 61*, 337–344.

Di Fiore, J. M., Arko, M., Whitehouse, M., Kimball, A., & Martin, R. J. (2005). Apnea is not prolonged by acid gastroesophageal reflux in preterm infants. *Pediatrics, 116*, 1059–1063.

Ehrenkranz, R. A., Walsh, M. C., Vohr, B. R., Jobe, A. H., Wright, L. L., Fanaroff, A. A., et al. (2005). Validation of the National Institutes of Health consensus definition of bronchopulmonary dysplasia. *Pediatrics, 116*, 1353–1360.

Evans, M., Palta, M., Sadek, M., Weinstein, M. R., & Peters, M. E. (1998). Associations between family history of asthma, bronchopulmonary dysplasia, and childhood asthma in very low birth weight children. *American Journal of Epidemiology, 148*, 460–466.

Fanaroff, A. A., Stoll, B. J., Wright, L. L., Carlo, W. A., Ehrenkranz, R. A., Stark, A. R., et al. (2007). Trends in neonatal morbidity and mortality for very low birthweight infants. *American Journal of Obstetrics & Gynecology, 196*(147), e1–e8.

Frank, L. (1992). Antioxidants, nutrition, and bronchopulmonary dysplasia. *Clinics in Perinatology, 19*, 541–562.

Gannon, B. A. (2000). Theophylline or caffeine: Which is best for apnea of prematurity? *Neonatal Network, 19*, 33–36.

Gerhardt, T., & Bancalari, E. (1984). Apnea of prematurity: I. lung function and regulation of breathing. *Pediatrics, 74*, 58–62.

Hansen, A. R., Barnes, C. M., Folkman, J., & McElrath, T. F. (2010). Maternal preeclampsia predicts the development of bronchopulmonary dysplasia. *Journal of Pediatrics, 156*(4), 532–536.

Harding, C. (2009). An evaluation of the benefits of non-nutritive sucking for premature infants as described in the literature. *Archives of Disease in Childhood, 94*, 636–640.

Henderson-Smart, D. J., & Steer, P. A. (2010). Caffeine versus theophylline for apnea in preterm infants. *Cochrane Database of Systematic Reviews, CD000273*(1). DOI: 10.1002/14651858.CD000273.pub2.

Hunt, C. E., Corwin, M. J., Baird, T., Tinsley, L. R., Palmer, P., Ramanathan, R., et al. (2004). Cardiorespiratory events detected by home memory monitoring and one-year neurodevelopmental outcome. *Journal of Pediatrics, 145*, 465–471.

Inder, T. E., Graham, P. J., Winterbourn, C. C., Austin, N. C., & Darlow, B. A. (1998). Plasma vitamin A levels in the very low birthweight infant—relationship to respiratory outcome. *Early Human Development, 52*, 155–168.

Jackson, D. F. (1986). Nursing care plan: Home management of children with BPD. *Pediatric Nursing, 12*, 342–348.

Janvier, A., Khairy, M., Kokkotis, A., Cormier, C., Messmer, D., & Barrington, K. J. (2004). Apnea is associated with neurodevelopmental impairment in very low birth weight infants. *Journal of Perinatology, 24*, 763–768.

Jobe, A. H., & Bancalari, E. (2001). Bronchopulmonary dysplasia. *American Journal of Respiratory & Critical Care Medicine, 163,* 1723–1729.

Kee, J. L., Hayes, E. R., & McCuistion, L. E. (2009). *Pharmacology: A nursing process approach* (6th ed.). St. Louis, MO: Saunders.

Kennedy, J. D., Edward, L. J., Bates, D. J., Martin, A. J., Dip, S. N., Haslam, R. R., et al. (2000). Effects of birthweight and oxygen supplementation on lung function in late childhood in children of very low birth weight. *Pediatric Pulmonology, 30,* 32–40.

Kinsella, J. P., Greenough, A., & Abman, S. H. (2006). Bronchopulmonary dysplasia. *Lancet, 367,* 1421–1431.

Klein, N. P., Massolo, M. L., Greene, J., Dekker, C. L., Black, S., & Escobar, G. J. (2008). Risk factors for developing apnea after immunization in the neonatal intensive care unit. *Pediatrics, 121,* 463–469.

Krishnan, U., Krishnan, S., & Gewitz, M. (2008). Treatment of pulmonary hypertension in children with chronic lung disease with newer oral therapies. *Pediatric Cardiology, 29,* 1082–1086.

Kwinta, P., Bik-Multanowski, M., Mitkowska, Z., Tomasik, T., Legutko, M., & Pietrzyk, J. J. (2008). Genetic risk factors of bronchopulmonary dysplasia. *Pediatric Respiratory, 64,* 682–688.

Lamarche-Vadel, A., Blondel, B., Truffer, P., Burguet, A., Cambonie, G., Selton, D., et al. (2004). Re-hospitalization in infants younger than 29 weeks' gestation in the EPIPAGE cohort. *Acta Paediatrica, 93,* 1340–1345.

Lavoie, P. M., Pham, C., & Jang, K. L. (2008). Heritability of bronchopulmonary dysplasia, defined according to the consensus statement of the national institutes of health. *Pediatrics, 122,* 479–485.

Levit, O., Jiang, Y., Bizzarro, M. J., Hussain, N., Buhimschi, C. S., Gruen, J. R., et al. (2009). The genetic susceptibility to respiratory distress syndrome. *Pediatric Respiratory, 66,* 693–697.

Liu, W. F., Laudert, S., Perkins, B., Macmillan-York, E., Martin, S., & Graven, S. (2007). The development of potentially better practices to support the neurodevelopment of infants in the NICU. *Journal of Perinatology, 27,* S48–S74.

Martin, J. A., Kung, H. C., Mathews, T. J., Hoyert, D. L., Strobino, D. M., Guyer, B., & Sutton, S. R. (2008). Annual summary of vital statistics: 2006. *Pediatrics, 121,* 788–801.

MedImmune (2009). Synagis® (Palivizumab). Package Insert.

Northway, W. H., Jr., Moss, R. B., Carlisle, K. B., Parker, B. R., Popp, R. L., Pitlick, P. T., et al. (1990). Late pulmonary sequelae of bronchopulmonary dysplasia. *New England Journal of Medicine, 323,* 1793–1799.

Northway, W. H., Jr., Rosan, R. C., & Porter, D. Y. (1967). Pulmonary disease following respiratory therapy of hyaline-membrane disease. Bronchopulmonary dysplasia. *New England Journal of Medicine, 276,* 357–368.

Pantalitschka, T., & Poets, C. F. (2006). Inhaled drugs for the prevention and treatment of bronchopulmonary dysplasia. *Pediatric Pulmonololgy, 41,* 703–708.

Pantalitschka, T., Sievers, J., Urschitz, M. S., Herberts, T., Reher, C., & Poets, C. F. (2009). Randomised crossover trial of four nasal respiratory support systems for apnoea of prematurity in very low birthweight infants. *Archives of Disease in Childhood. Fetal and Neonatal Edition, 94,* F245–F248.

Pereira, K. D., MacGregor, A. R., McDuffie, C. M., & Mitchell, R. B. (2003). Tracheostomy in preterm infants: Current trends. *Archives of Otolaryngology—Head & Neck Surgery, 129,* 1268–1271.

Pierce, M. R., & Bancalari, E. (1995). The role of inflammation in the pathogenesis of bronchopulmonary dysplasia. *Pediatric Pulmonology, 19,* 371–378.

Ramanathan, R., Corwin, M. J., Hunt, C. E., Lister, G., Tinsley, L. R., Baird, T., et al. (2001). Cardiorespiratory events recorded on home monitors: Comparison of healthy infants with those at increased risk for SIDS. *JAMA, 285,* 2199–2207.

Sawyer, M. H., Edwards, D. K., & Spector, S. A. (1987). Cytomegalovirus infection and bronchopulmonary dysplasia in premature infants. *American Journal of Diseases in Childhood, 141,* 303–305.

Sherman, J. M., Davis, S., Albamonte-Petrick, S., Chatburn, R. L., Fitton, C., Green, C., et al. (2000). Care of the child with a chronic tracheostomy. This official statement of the American Thoracic Society was adopted by the ATS Board of Directors, July 1999. *American Journal of Respiratory & Critical Care Medicine, 161,* 297–308.

Short, E. J., Klein, N. K., Lewis, B. A., Fulton, S., Eisengart, S., Kercsmar, C., et al. (2003). Cognitive and academic consequences of bronchopulmonary dysplasia and very low birth weight: 8-year-old outcomes. *Pediatrics, 112,* e359.

Smith, V. C., Zupancic, J. A. F., McCormick, M. C., Croen, L. A., Greene, J., Escobar, G. J., et al. (2004). Rehospitalization in the first year of life among infants with Bronchopulmonary Dysplasia. *Journal of Pediatrics, 144,* 799–803.

Stokowski, L. A. (2005). A primer on apnea of prematurity. *Advances in Neonatal Care, 5,* 155–170, quiz 171–174.

Tamim, H., Khogali, M., Beydoun, H., Melki, I., & Yunis, K. (2003). Consanguinity and apnea of prematurity. *American Journal of Epidemiology, 158,* 942–946.

Theobald, K., Botwinski, C., Albanna, S., & McWilliam, P. (2000). Apnea of prematurity: Diagnosis, implications for care, and pharmacologic management. *Neonatal Network, 19,* 17–24.

Thomas, W., & Speer, C. P. (2008). Nonventilatory strategies for prevention and treatment of bronchopulmonary dysplasia—what is the evidence? *Neonatology, 94,* 150–159.

Tourneux, P., Leke, A., Kongolo, G., Cardot, V., Degrugilliers, L., Chardon, K., et al. (2008). Relationship between functional residual capacity and oxygen desaturation during short central apneic events during sleep in "late preterm" infants. *Pediatric Respiratory, 64,* 171–176.

Van Marter, L. J., Leviton, A., Allred, E. N., Pagano, M., & Kuban, K. C. K. (1990). Hydration during the first days of life and the risk of bronchopulmonary dysplasia in low birth weight infants. *The Journal of Pediatrics, 116,* 942–949.

Walsh, M. C., Szefler, S., Davis, J., Allen, M., Van Marter, L., Abman, S., et al. (2006). Summary proceedings from the bronchopulmonary dysplasia group. *Pediatrics, 117,* S52–S56.

Wang, L. Y., Luo, H. J., Hsieh, W. S., Hsu, C. H., Hsu, H. C., Chen, P. S., et al. (2010). Severity of bronchopulmonary dysplasia and increased risk of feeding desaturation and growth delay in very low birth weight preterm infants. *Pediatric Pulmonology, 45,* 165–173.

Watterberg, K. L., Demers, L. M., Scott, S. M., & Murphy, S. (1996). Chorioamnionitis and early lung inflammation in infants in whom broncho-pulmonary dysplasia develops. *Pediatrics, 97,* 210–215.

Watterberg, K. L., Gerdes, J. S., Gifford, K. L., & Lin, H. M. (1999). Prophylaxis against early adrenal insufficiency to prevent chronic lung disease in pre-mature infants. *Pediatrics, 104,* 1258–1263.

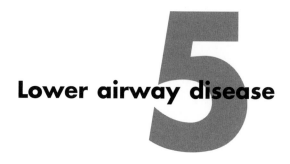

Lower airway disease

Julie Honey, MSN, CPNP, and
Michael Bye, MD, FAAP, FCCP

LOWER AIRWAY DISEASE

Acute respiratory illnesses are common among children. This chapter provides an overview of childhood respiratory illnesses commonly categorized as "lower airway diseases." Despite the title of this chapter, there is no complete agreement among practitioners as to where the lower airway begins. In adults, the lower or small airways usually include those from the 16th generation and beyond. In children, they begin much more proximally. In this chapter, we refer to the "lower airways" as those airways below the thoracic inlet, which is approximately one-third of the way down the trachea. Thus, the "lower airway" diseases covered in this chapter include bronchiolitis, pneumonia, bronchitis, and bacterial tracheitis. We will begin by discussing the common viral and bacterial pathogens commonly associated with lower airway disease in children; then, we will discuss each of the common disease states in detail. Croup and epiglottitis, "upper airway diseases," will be discussed in Chapter 6.

Many different organisms are capable of infecting the lower respiratory tract. The infections they cause will vary in type and severity. Infectious lower airway diseases can be caused by both viral and bacterial pathogens; however, most infections are viral in nature. Respiratory syncytial virus (RSV) is the most common virus causing lower respiratory illness. Influenza, parainfluenza, metapneumovirus, and adenovirus all have the potential to

Nursing Care in Pediatric Respiratory Disease, First Edition. Edited by Concettina (Tina) Tolomeo.
© 2012 John Wiley & Sons, Inc. Published 2012 by John Wiley & Sons, Inc.

cause lower airway disease in children. Together with the myriad rhinoviruses, all of the above-mentioned viruses also have the potential to trigger an asthma exacerbation. Lower respiratory infections can result in numerous complications and they are particularly troublesome for patients with underlying chronic illnesses or compromised immune systems.

Of the bacteria, the most common infecting agents are *Streptococcus pneumoniae, Staphylococcus, Haemophilus influenzae, Chlamydia pneumoniae,* and *Mycoplasma pneumoniae*. Furthermore, *S. pneumoniae* and *Staphylococcus* can cause complications of a preexisting viral infection (Denny, 1999).

One of the most difficult challenges to the clinician is determining whether a given illness is viral or bacterial. Too often the decision is made to treat all children with lower respiratory symptoms with an antibiotic "just in case" a bacterial agent is involved. This practice is not only unnecessary and inappropriate but it can also ultimately be harmful because it can result in the selection of more resistant organisms. For this reason, both the Centers for Disease Control and Prevention (CDCP) and the American Academy of Pediatrics (AAP) are making efforts to reduce antibiotic use in children with lower airway disease.

Clinical features that suggest bacterial infections include an abrupt onset or change in symptoms, toxicity, radiographic findings of lobar consolidation or pleural effusion, and persistence and magnitude of fever. It is critical for practitioners to remember that viral infections remain the most common cause of lower respiratory illnesses. This knowledge must be taken into consideration when making clinical decisions regarding treatment. Treating with an antibiotic just in case will increase the risk of subsequent superinfection with a resistant organism. Bacterial superinfection can occur with some viral infections (especially influenza) 1–2 weeks after the onset of symptoms, when high fevers return with respiratory compromise.

Common viral agents that cause acute lower respiratory infections in children

RSV

RSV is the most common cause of bronchiolitis and viral pneumonia in children under 1 year; it is also the most common cause of acute lower respiratory infections (ALRIs) among children under 3 years of age (Centers for Disease Control [CDC], 2010). Outbreaks occur annually, usually starting in October or November in the Western Hemisphere, and can last up to 6 months. Acute lower airway disease is more common in younger patients, and the morbidity and mortality rates are higher in infants (CDC, 2010). In recent years, it has been estimated that more than 125,000 children under 4 years of age have been hospitalized in the United States for RSV disease during the first year of life (Krilov, 2010). Preexisting lung diseases, such as chronic lung disease of prematurity, increase the likelihood of severe disease. Because there are at least three strains of RSV, reinfection is possible and can result in a more severe illness (Dakhama et al., 2009). RSV infects older children and adults as well, causing a simple URI in otherwise normal subjects and triggering asthma symptoms in those with asthma.

RSV can be confirmed through a nasal wash or swab. Diagnosis can also be assumed through clinical symptoms and presentation. While many children are infected with RSV each year, some will have more serious symptoms requiring hospitalization and sometimes assisted ventilation. The most serious complications facing RSV-infected patients are apnea and respiratory distress. At times, infants under 3 months of age may develop apnea first as the only sign of RSV infection. Additionally, RSV has been linked to death in a number of cases (Poets, 2008).

Infants with recurrent apnea due to RSV infection may require ventilation until the apnea resolves, usually within a few days. Agitation, particularly if not resolved by supplemental oxygen, can be an indication of respiratory insufficiency in infants. In such children, it is mandatory to assess the degree of ventilation, best done with an arterial blood gas. Careful clinical assessment for signs of respiratory distress (nasal flaring, intercostal retractions, grunting, tachypnea, and tachycardia) and monitoring of pulse oximetry is essential when caring for an infant with RSV. A properly performed venous blood gas can give an indication of the degree of ventilation but is generally less accurate than an arterial blood gas.

Parainfluenza

Parainfluenza is another common cause of acute lower respiratory illness in children under 5 years (Dubois & Ray, 1999). The course of illness for parainfluenza is similar to that described above for RSV, and the management of the illness is generally the same. Parainfluenza is also a common cause of acute croup, which is discussed in Chapter 6.

Influenza

Influenza (types A and B) is a major cause of lower respiratory disease in children and can be fatal. Influenza viruses are categorized according to the type of hyaluronidase and neuraminidase they contain. (There are several of each types of enzyme resulting in the viruses being labeled HxNx.) Outbreaks generally occur in the cool winter months and spread quickly. Seasonal influenza rarely survives in the summer months. However, the 2009 H1N1 influenza first appeared in the spring, with the pandemic waning in August of that year. The pandemic then began again that September and persisted into February of the following year.

The clinical presentation of influenza differs from that of RSV or parainfluenza in that the symptoms often appear rapidly and become severe over the first 24 hours. Typically, fever and malaise develop first, followed by the onset of nasal congestion and cough. Although bacterial superinfection can occur at anytime, a more serious viral pneumonia can be seen within the first 2 or 3 days of the illness. Such a viral pneumonia can lead to acute respiratory distress. On the other hand, the bacterial superinfections are more likely to be seen 1–2 weeks after the onset of symptoms. In this scenario, the child is improving or stable when high fevers and varying degrees of respiratory compromise occur. A chest X-ray will often show lobar consolidation. Immune dysregulation by influenza has been suggested as at least part of the reason for this (Heltzer et al., 2009). Diagnosis of influenza can be made with rapid antigen screening and nasal cultures. Treatment is generally supportive as it is with other viral illnesses. Antiviral agents have been proven to be effective in shortening the course and severity of the illness if started within 1–2 days of the symptoms. The seasonal influenza virus has been adept at developing resistance to the commonly used antiviral agents. The 2009 H1N1 virus has not developed such resistance as of this writing. However, it is different from the seasonal influenza in that it causes more morbidity and mortality among young children. It has been recommended that high-risk children be prophylactically treated with antiviral agents if they have been in close contact with a person who has a known case of influenza. Bacterial superinfections should be treated with appropriate antibiotic therapy, keeping in mind the frequency of *Staphylococcus* in this scenario.

Currently, the CDC recommends that all children under the age of 18 receive the influenza vaccine, as this is the most effective way to prevent outbreaks and to protect children from serious consequences of the flu. Vaccination is especially essential for children who are at high risk, such as those with chronic pulmonary, cardiac, hematologic, immunologic, and metabolic conditions. In addition, household members of high-risk children should be immunized, as should all health-care workers and caregivers. High-risk children, or family members of such children, should not receive the live nasal vaccines.

Adenovirus

Adenovirus is a common cause of fever and upper respiratory illnesses in children but can sometimes cause lower respiratory illness as well. Adenoviral pneumonia causes the same type of symptoms as pneumonia from RSV or influenza; however, the symptoms may be more prolonged. Children with adenovirus are more likely to have a persisting fever and conjunctivitis is not uncommon. Adenovirus is also more likely to cause chronic sequelae, including interstitial fibrosis and bronchiectasis. Adenovirus is not susceptible to antiviral agents currently available, and therefore supportive therapy is all that is available for a patient with an ALRI caused by adenovirus.

Human metapneumovirus

Human metapneumovirus (hMPV) is a viral pathogen that causes a wide spectrum of illnesses ranging from asymptomatic infection to severe bronchiolitis. First named in 2001, hMPV tends to affect mainly patients between newborn and 6 years of age. The pathophysiology of the virus is similar to that of RSV and it is found to be the causative virus in 5–15% of infant bronchiolitis. The clinical presentation is similar to that of RSV as well, presenting with symptoms such as rhinorrhea, congestion, cough, tachypnea, and dyspnea (Maranich & Rajnik, 2009). Treatment of a child infected with hMPV is primarily supportive, focusing on adequate hydration and oxygenation. Severe disease can lead to respiratory failure, implying that careful clinical observation is imperative, especially in high-risk infants and children.

Common bacterial agents that cause ALRIs in children

As noted previously, viruses cause the overwhelming majority of lower respiratory illnesses in children; thus, antibiotics should be used sparingly. The most common bacterial agents that cause community-acquired lower respiratory illnesses in children are *S. pneumoniae, Staphylococcus aureus, H. influenzae,* and the "atypical" organisms, *C. pneumoniae,* and *M. pneumoniae.* Given the current overuse of antibiotics, many of these and other organisms have developed resistance to first-line antibiotic treatment. This is especially true with the hospital-acquired organisms, which include *S. aureus* (including the methicillin-resistant strains) and the gram-negative organisms including *Klebsiella, Enterobacter, Acinitobacter,* and *Escherichia coli.* Often, this forces the clinician to use second-generation or multiple antibiotics to treat respiratory illnesses. Table 5.1 provides the common

Table 5.1 Common bacterial pathogens in associated lower respiratory diseases.

Disease	Common bacterial pathogens	Estimated percentage caused by viruses
Pneumonia	*Streptococcus pneumoniae, Staphylococcus aureus, Haemophilus influenzae* type B, *Mycoplasma pneumoniae, Chlamydia trachomatis*	70–80
Bronchiolitis	*C. trachomatis, Chlamydia pneumoniae, M. pneumoniae*	90
Bronchitis	*M. pneumoniae, C. pneumoniae, Bordetella pertussis, H. influenzae*	80

bacterial agents responsible for each of the community-acquired lower respiratory illnesses, as well as the estimated percentage of the illnesses caused by viruses (Dubois & Ray, 1999). These numbers confirm the limited need for antimicrobial treatment in most respiratory illnesses.

Common lower airway diseases in children

As discussed earlier, this chapter will focus on the most common infections that occur below the thoracic inlet. These include bronchiolitis, pneumonia, bacterial tracheitis, and bronchitis. The diagnosis of bronchitis remains controversial in children. Each of these conditions carries with it specific implications and risks, all of which should be considered when caring for an infant or a child with a lower respiratory tract illness.

Bronchiolitis

Epidemiology

Bronchiolitis is an acute illness that usually occurs with an upper respiratory infection where the virus causes inflammation and obstruction of the bronchioles (small airways). It often occurs as a single episode. However, recurrent infections have been reported, often in the first year of life. The initial descriptions of bronchiolitis were of a first episode of wheeze, caused by a virus, in infants under 2 years of age (Everard, 2008). The overlap with asthma is considerable, including signs and symptoms, and the fact that children with RSV bronchiolitis have a higher incidence than the general population of subsequent asthma.

Bronchiolitis commonly affects infants and toddlers; however, it is most severe and troublesome in infants younger than 12 months of age. Infants less than 3 months of age, premature infants (less than 35 weeks' gestation), and infants with chronic lung disease, congenital heart disease, or immune deficiency syndromes who develop bronchiolitis are at higher risk for hospitalization and death (Shay et al., 1999). Factors such as maternal cigarette smoking also increase the severity and perhaps the frequency of the disease. Careful clinical monitoring with early hospitalization to treat the potential morbidity should be the top priority in the management of bronchiolitis.

Preventive medical therapies such as palivizumab (Synagis®) should be considered for high-risk patients. Palivizumab is a monoclonal antibody that has been shown to be effective at decreasing the incidence of serious RSV infection and RSV-related hospitalizations (The ImPACT-RSV Study Group, 1998). However, palivizumab is not advocated for every child. There are specific recommendations for palivizumab administration for infants who were born less than 35 weeks' gestation and for those with congenital airway abnormalities, severe neuromuscular disease, and chronic lung disease (American Academy of Pediatrics [AAP], 2009).

Pathophysiology

Bronchiolitis occurs when viruses invade the mucosal cell lining in the bronchi and bronchioles, resulting in cell death. Cell debris then clogs and obstructs the bronchioles and irritates the airway. The irritated airway swells and develops excess mucus production, which results in airway obstruction. Air becomes trapped distal to the obstructed airways and interferes with gas exchange, leading to decreased oxygenation. Infants and small children are at higher risk of atelectasis.

Signs and symptoms

Bronchiolitis is diagnosed primarily by clinical findings, the age of the child, and the season of the illness. It may be defined as an acute (first) wheezing episode in a child less than 2 years of age, especially during an RSV epidemic. Clinical findings include coryza, wheeze, crackles, and frequent cough. Fever may or may not be present. With progression to respiratory distress, nasal flaring, retractions, tachypnea, and labored breathing may be present. Other findings may include irritability, decreased appetite, and poor sleeping. Post-tussive emesis may consist of thick, clear mucus.

Diagnosis

A diagnosis is primarily made by history and physical exam in the proper season. It is recommended that routine diagnostic studies (chest X-ray, nasal washes/swabs, cultures, and blood gases) not be performed to determine viral infection status or to rule out bacterial infections. Such studies are not generally helpful and result in increased rates of unnecessary admissions, further testing, and unnecessary therapies (Bordley et al., 2004). Chest X-rays may be obtained as clinically indicated when the diagnosis of bronchiolitis is not clear or when a secondary bacterial infection is suspected. Secondary bacterial infections are not common during acute bronchiolitis, and radiographic abnormalities usually represent the underlying disease.

A chest X-ray of a patient with bronchiolitis will generally show nonspecific areas of inflammation. This may be described as peribronchial thickening or increased diffuse markings. These are the same findings seen in the radiograph of a child with acute asthma. As in acute asthma, hyperinflation is not uncommon and areas of atelectasis may be interpreted as infiltrates. Arterial blood gases may be clinically indicated in a patient who is in respiratory distress and in need of further respiratory support. Pulse oximetry is an important measure for children admitted with bronchiolitis.

Complications

The major complications of bronchiolitis are apnea and respiratory failure. Bacterial superinfection is very rare. The long-term morbidity in infants affected by bronchiolitis has been addressed in many studies. As many as

75% of infants who have been hospitalized with RSV have recurrent wheeze and cough episodes in the first few years of life (Young, O'Keeffe, Arnott, & Landau, 1995). While some may be experiencing their first asthma episodes, at these ages, there is no test to distinguish between an asthma episode and a wheeze-associated viral illness. Other than infant pulmonary function testing, which requires sedation in a specialty laboratory, the best way to determine the diagnosis of asthma is through a clinical trial of inhaled beta-agonists. The child with recurrent episodes of wheezing is more likely to have asthma and to respond to therapy. The child with a first episode, in the proper age range, is less likely to respond. If a child does not respond to beta-agonists, the continued use of these treatments is unwarranted.

Management

The basic management of bronchiolitis is to maintain adequate oxygenation and hydration. Hospitalization is necessary for infants with acute bronchiolitis if the above criteria are not able to be maintained at home. Management of the child hospitalized with bronchiolitis includes carefully monitoring their clinical status, maintaining a patent airway, suctioning the nose, maintaining hydration, and providing parent education.

Oxygen therapy is frequently required in the treatment of bronchiolitis. For human beings at sea level, oxygen saturation above 90% is adequate and safe. Infants, however, may have lower reserve, and the ready obstruction of an airway may acutely lower the oxygenation. Thus, it is recommended to consider starting supplemental oxygen when the oxygen saturation is consistently less than 91% and to consider weaning supplemental oxygen when the oxygen saturation is consistently higher than 94% (Bye, 1994).

Albuterol aerosol therapies should not be routinely used as they have not been proven to be helpful in the majority of cases, despite the fact that many of these children will subsequently develop asthma. In the majority of cases, the use of inhalation therapies and other treatments effective for treating asthma will likewise not be efficacious. A meta-analysis of randomized, controlled trials has not shown dramatic effects on clinical scores or hospitalization rates from therapy with nebulized albuterol in children with bronchiolitis (Gadomski & Bhasale, 2006).

Antibiotics, antihistamines, steroids (oral or inhaled), and decongestants should not be routinely used in patients with bronchiolitis as they have not been found to be helpful. Additionally, chest physiotherapy (CPT) and cool mist therapy have not proven to be clinically helpful. There are some data to suggest that inhaled epinephrine may help acutely (Sanchez, Koster, Powell, Wolstein, & Chernick, 1993). It is not clear if this is an action at the nose or in the airways. However, in children with acute respiratory insufficiency who do not respond to albuterol, epinephrine may be tried. Nebulized hypertonic saline may have some benefit in decreasing length of stay (Kuzik et al., 2007).

Careful, frequent clinical assessment of the child is essential to the successful treatment of bronchiolitis. Cardiac and respiratory rate monitoring should be initiated in hospitalized patients. Oxygen saturations should also be monitored to assure oxygenation saturations are at acceptable levels. Premature infants, infants with underlying chronic conditions, and infants less than 3 months of age who contract RSV are at particular risk of severe complications such as apnea or respiratory failure. Furthermore, several studies have reported more severe progression of the disease in children with bronchiolitis who present with low initial oxygen saturations (Wang, Law, & Stephens, 1995).

Nursing care of the child and family
Nursing care focuses on assessing respiratory function, maintaining adequate hydration, and supportive measures. Nursing activities and treatments should be clustered to allow the infant as much rest time as possible and to decrease infant stress. Supportive measures include suctioning of the nose as needed. It is important to remember that coughing is the most effective method of clearing the airway. It is more effective than suction catheters, which have the potential to cause airway edema and laryngospasm.

Contact isolation precautions and frequent hand washing are helpful in preventing the spread of RSV bronchiolitis, as it is highly contagious. Because the virus lives on surfaces, contact with the baby and/or the crib or nightstand will result in the transmission of the virus to the hands of the care provider. This form of transmission can contribute to spreading of the virus to other patients. To prevent spread, it is also important that nurses and other personnel providing care to children with bronchiolitis are not also caring for children with underlying diseases, which put them at high risk for severe RSV disease.

Additionally, the nurse should perform a psychological assessment of the family to observe for signs of fear and anxiety, which can be prominent and worsen with respiratory distress. The nurse can help to reduce anxiety by providing thorough explanations and updates. Emotional security can be promoted by allowing parents to participate in as much of the infants' care as possible.

The nurse should also provide anticipatory guidance for discharge, as symptoms may persist for weeks after discharge. The median duration of illness for children under 24 months with bronchiolitis is 12 days; after 21 days, approximately 18% will remain ill, and after 28 days, 9% will remain ill (Bronchiolitis Guideline Team, Cincinnati Children's Hospital Medical Center, 2005). Discharge instructions should include proper techniques for suctioning the nose and making breathing easier as well as monitoring the clinical status of the child so a health-care provider can be notified if symptoms worsen. Parents should be made aware of the following warning signs: increasing respiratory rate and/or work of breathing as evidenced by accessory muscle use, inability to maintain adequate hydration (specific guidelines should be given based on the age and weight of the patient as to how much liquids should be consumed and how many wet diapers are adequate per day), recurring fever, and a worsening general appearance.

Pneumonia

Epidemiology

Pneumonia is the sixth leading cause of death in the United States, the second most common nosocomial infection, and the leading cause of death from nosocomial infections (CDC, 2010). Approximately 10–20% of all children under 5 years of age in developing countries develop pneumonia each year. Nearly 75% of pneumonia deaths occur among infants under 1 year old (Crawford & Daum, 2008). The risk of death is increased with malnutrition, malaria, and suppressed immunity. According to the World Health Organization, pneumonia is the single largest cause of death in children worldwide. Every year, an estimated 1.8 million children under the age of 5 die from pneumonia, accounting for 20% of all deaths in that age group (Rudan, Boschi-Pinto, Biloglav, Mulhollandd, & Campbelle, 2008).

There are approximately 155 million cases of childhood pneumonia each year in the world. Despite the fact that most pneumonias are easily treated with antibiotics, many children in underdeveloped nations lack access to these medications, contributing to the high mortality rate. Because of the lack of access to medications, malnutrition, crowding, and poor hygiene, pneumonia in developing countries is easily spread and is often fatal.

The overwhelming prevalence of pneumonia warrants its status as a major health concern that needs considerable attention and proper treatment. It can be classified as community-acquired pneumonia (CAP) or nosocomial pneumonia (indicating that the pneumonia developed while the patient was already in a hospital setting). The diagnosis of clinical pneumonia is often given in developing countries to indicate infection of the lower respiratory tract based on signs of fever, cough, and retractions. This is more common when diagnostic measures such as chest X-ray and laboratory studies are not readily available. However, the diagnosis of clinical pneumonia in the United States is becoming increasingly popular and often leads to the unnecessary use of antibiotics and the subsequent antibiotic resistance that is emerging.

Pathophysiology

Pneumonia is an infection of the lung. It indicates either a bacterial or viral infection of the lung parenchyma or interstitium. The etiology of pneumonia depends on many factors including the age of the patient, the setting in which the pneumonia was acquired (hospital vs. community), the vaccination status of the child, relevant exposures such as to contaminated water, host factors such as underlying diseases that predispose to pneumonia, and relevant local epidemiology such as local RSV outbreaks.

However, even with all the relevant information, determining the etiology of the pneumonia is not easy and is often not attempted. Because of the invasiveness and cost of the measures needed to determine the etiology, pneumonia with mild or moderate symptoms is often treated based on current knowledge and generalizations.

The most common causes of bacterial pneumonia in the neonate are Group B B-hemolytic streptococci (GBS), and gram-negative enteric bacilli, such as *E. coli*. Among infants beyond the neonatal period, viruses are the most frequent etiologic agents in CAP, although both viral and bacterial agents can cause pneumonia simultaneously. Among the bacterial agents, Streptococcus pneumonia and *S. aureus* are the most common. *Haemophilus influenzae* type B (Hib) used to be a common causative agent but is much less so due to the development of the Hib vaccine, which is now routinely administered to children in the United States. *M. pneumoniae* is an important consideration among school-age children. Factors that alter an individuals' risk of developing CAP include

- Age (<2 years, >65 years)
- Smoking, including passive smoke exposure in the home
- Underlying pulmonary diseases
- Cardiac diseases
- Malnutrition
- Low birth weight
- Central nervous system dysfunction, with recurrent aspiration
- Immunosuppression
- Lack of immunizations
- Crowding

Signs and symptoms
In children beyond the neonatal period, it may be difficult to distinguish between viral and bacterial pneumonia. Overall, children with bacterial pneumonia may appear to be sicker and have a higher fever; however, this is not always the case. Wheezing is much more common with viral disease and extremely uncommon with bacterial disease. Because a bacterial pneumonia is more likely to be focal, the degree of hypoxemia may be less, but the degree of toxicity may be higher. Cough is generally present but is not always universal, and the production of sputum in a child under the age of 8 is rare. Abdominal pain and emesis are also variable complaints; however, these symptoms are sometimes so severe that diagnosis of the pneumonia is delayed while looking for abdominal conditions as the cause of the fever and pain.

On auscultation, crackles, evidence of pulmonary consolidation, tubular breath sounds, decreased breath sounds, and increased fremitus may be found. However, none of these are specific for pneumonia. With pleural effusion, decreased breath sounds, egophony, and dullness on percussion may be noted in the cooperative child.

General signs of respiratory compromise are present in severe cases and can include shallow breathing, tachypnea, grunting, retractions, and nasal flaring.

Diagnosis

Diagnosis is generally made through history, clinical exam, and chest X-ray. A detailed history should include duration and extent of fever, pain, weight loss, identification of risk factors, and onset of symptoms. Once the diagnosis is made, determining its etiology can be challenging. Often little is done beyond a complete blood count (CBC) and blood culture to determine the cause of the pneumonia. As a result of this, it is estimated that more than 80% of patients who have "nonbacterial pneumonia" receive bacterial antimicrobial treatment (Crawford & Daum, 2008).

If the child is able to produce sputum, a sample can be obtained for culture and sensitivity to identify the causative agent, make the diagnosis, and determine the appropriate treatment. In addition to the culture, the sputum Gram stain can be helpful. A CBC revealing an elevated white cell count and high levels of neutrophils and/or polymorphonucleocytes can be an indication of a bacterial process, but studies have not shown this to be highly specific or sensitive. Serologic studies of the blood and/or urine can be helpful in detecting an acute infection.

Additional diagnostic tests include oxygen saturation level and electrolytes if warranted. Some organisms, particularly *Legionella* species, are associated with the syndrome of inappropriate antidiuretic hormone, resulting in abnormalities in serum electrolytes. In the hospitalized patient, additional tests may include culture of pleural fluid if present and bronchoscopy to assist in the identification of the causative organisms. The latter is reserved for children who are severely ill or who have compromised immune function.

Complications

Complications from pneumonia can be life threatening and require immediate intervention. If the patient is failing to respond to therapy and overall appearance is deteriorating, other causes should be investigated as pneumonia may have been an incorrect diagnosis. Similarly, the patient may not be responding due to improper or insufficient antimicrobial therapy. It is helpful to know the resistance patterns of the common organisms in your area. This information should be readily available from hospital infectious disease specialists.

Sepsis, pleural effusion, and acute respiratory distress syndrome (ARDS) are potential complications of bacterial pneumonia that can cause serious and sometimes fatal outcomes. Although they are not the focus of this chapter, a brief description of these complications and their general management are described in this section. Sepsis, also known as the systemic inflammatory response syndrome (SIRS) is a serious systemic response to bacteremia or another infection. Septic shock is manifested by life-threatening low blood pressure (shock) due to bacteremia. Sepsis can be the result of bacterial infections, most often those that are acquired in a hospital. However, even aspiration pneumonia, which is usually a nonbacterial process, can be associated with the sepsis syndrome. A weakened immune system or a cardiac abnormality puts a patient at higher risk of acquiring sepsis. Because the patient response to sepsis is systemic, careful monitoring for the following signs is imperative: an abnormally high fever, hypothermia, tachypnea, tachycardia, and increased or markedly decreased white blood cell (WBC) count. As sepsis worsens, other organs begin to malfunction and blood pressure may decrease. Septic shock is diagnosed when blood pressure remains low despite intensive treatment. Generally, a suspicion of sepsis is made based on symptoms and should lead to blood cultures and careful evaluation of cardiovascular and respiratory function. However, antibiotics are initiated even when the diagnosis of sepsis is suspected. Oxygen is administered and fluids are given to increase and stabilize blood pressure. Assisted ventilation, whether noninvasive or through an endotracheal tube, is often necessary. In the United States, about 90,000 people die of septic shock each year (Dellinger, 2010).

A pleural effusion is an abnormal collection of fluid in the pleural space resulting from excess fluid production or decreased absorption. Effusions can also develop from direct irritation of the pleural membrane by the underlying pneumonia, resulting in fluid exudation into the pleural space. Pleuritic chest pain, chest pressure, dyspnea, and cough are the most common symptoms of pleural effusion. Cough is usually related to the associated disorder or to compression atelectasis, which accompanies many pleural effusions. Classic physical findings associated with pleural effusions include diminished breath sounds, dullness to percussion, and reduced tactile and vocal fremitus. After the initial stabilization of the patient, the pleural effusion should be confirmed with appropriate radiographic evaluation. The most frequently ordered studies are chest X-ray, ultrasonography, and computed tomography (CT). Chest X-ray is the primary diagnostic tool because of its availability, accuracy, and low cost. It may both confirm the presence of the effusion and suggest the underlying etiology. Bacterial pneumonias are associated with pleural effusions as often as 50% of the time (Duke & Good, 2001). Complicated parapneumonic effusions include empyema (the finding of pus in the pleural space), those with positive pleural fluid cultures or Gram stains, and those in which the microbiology is negative but the patient continues to show signs of infection with fever, severe pain, and leukocytosis. Complicated parapneumonic effusions often require drainage by tube thoracotomy. Some surgeons are now able to evacuate the effusion through video-assisted thoracoscopic surgery (VATS), resulting in a more complete evacuation of the fluid and shorter chest tube time. The patient who has pneumonia with a small amount of pleural fluid present and is clinically responding to

antibiotic therapy (afebrile, no pleuritic pain, minimal oxygen requirements, minimal respiratory difficulty) does not require thoracentesis. By
contrast, rapid accumulation of pleural fluid in a patient with pneumonia
is an indication for immediate thoracentesis.

ARDS is an acute condition characterized by bilateral pulmonary infiltrates and severe hypoxemia resulting from increased alveolar–capillary
permeability. ARDS is considered the pulmonary manifestation of the SIRS
(Gutierrez, Duke, Henning, & South, 2008). Physical findings often are
nonspecific and include tachypnea, tachycardia, and the need for high
inspired oxygen concentrations to maintain oxygen saturation. The patient
may be either febrile or hypothermic. Because ARDS often occurs in the
context of sepsis, associated hypotension and peripheral vasoconstriction
with cold extremities may be present. Examination of the lungs may typically reveal bilateral crackles. No specific therapy for ARDS exists. Systemic
corticosteroids have had varying degrees of success; other anti-inflammatory
agents are being studied. Treatment of the underlying condition is essential, along with supportive care and appropriate ventilator and fluid management. Because infection is often the underlying cause of ARDS, careful
assessment of the patient for infected sites and institution of appropriate
antibiotic therapy are essential. Patients with ARDS often require high-
intensity mechanical ventilation, including high levels of positive end-
expiratory pressure (PEEP) or continuous positive airway pressure (CPAP),
which can lead to further complications. The mortality rate in children with
ARDS can be as high as 40% (Gutierrez et al., 2008).

Pneumothorax is an uncommon complication of pneumonia and is
usually associated with *S. aureus* pneumonia. This complication is first
visible only by chest CT, but it can be seen on a plain chest X-ray as it
develops. However, pneumothorax can be suggested if the child has a
sudden worsening in oxygenation status, with decreased air flow on one
side, and shift of the trachea.

Management

The management of a child with pneumonia varies depending of the age
of the child, the immunologic status of the host, and the severity of the
symptoms. Hospitalization is generally suggested in an infant younger
than 4–6 months of age. Management of pneumonia in older children may
or may not include hospitalization, depending on the severity of the illness
and the ability of the child to maintain adequate oxygenation and hydration. Empiric antibiotic therapy should be initiated promptly if a bacterial
process is suspected. This therapy should, based on the likely organisms,
take into account the patients' age, clinical state, and risk factors. Antibiotic
therapy may need to be adjusted as the identification of causative organisms becomes known and the response of the patient to the therapy is
evaluated.

Additionally, several supportive care measures may be needed. Oxygen
therapy should be used to maintain oxygen saturation above 91%, and

hydration and nutritional support is often necessary in hospitalized patients. If the child develops respiratory distress and the inspired oxygen concentration is high, noninvasive or invasive mechanical ventilation may be warranted. In any patient with pneumonia, whether in the hospital or treated at home, adequate fluid intake should be encouraged, and nonsteroidal anti-inflammatory drugs should be initiated to treat pain and fever.

Additional testing should be performed if a child presents with recurrent pneumonia. Recurrent pneumonia is classified as a child that has had at least two episodes of bacterial pneumonia confirmed on chest X-ray in 1 year, or more than three episodes at any age, with clearing of the X-ray between episodes. The evaluation of a child with recurrent pneumonia often depends on the radiographic picture (Bye, 1994). One should consider performing a bronchoscopy if the infiltrates are always in the same area. To make this determination, it is first important to ensure that the current pneumonia clears radiographically, usually within 6–8 weeks. It is then important to document the location of subsequent episodes. While the decision to conduct further testing should be dependent on the child's presentation, testing should be directed toward conditions that can predispose a child to pneumonia. Thus, further evaluation might include testing for cystic fibrosis, congenital and acquired immunodeficiency, and immotile cilia syndrome.

Nursing care of the child and family
Pneumonia can be a frightening diagnosis both to the child and the child's parents or caretakers. Reassurance and proper teaching is needed to ensure the best possible outcome for the patient and the least amount of stress for the family. The parent or caregiver should be taught the signs to monitor that would indicate poor response to treatment or a worsening condition. Signs that warrant immediate attention include elevated respiratory rate (it is ideal to teach the parents how to take the rate when the child is asleep and give them guidelines for abnormal rates, which will vary with age), persisting fever after 72 hours or a fever that resolves and then returns, cyanosis, tachycardia, confusion, signs of dehydration (dry mucus membranes, absence of tears, and decreased urinary output), difficulty breathing, increased work of breathing, shortness of breath, or respiratory distress. When providing this education, it is important to explain these signs in terms the parents can understand. The family should be told how to contact the health-care provider if needed. Arrangements for proper follow-up should be made before the child leaves the office or is discharged.

Anticipatory guidance should be given to the family to help reduce subsequent infections. Parents should be encouraged to have their children receive a yearly influenza vaccine and the pneumococcal vaccine. They should also be encouraged to practice frequent hand washing and to avoid exposures to smoke and other risk factors.

Bronchitis

Epidemiology

Bronchitis is a commonly diagnosed respiratory problem in children. Most simply, it is an inflammation of the large airways. It usually occurs as part of a viral upper respiratory infection. It can also occur as a component of asthma, cystic fibrosis, immunodeficiencies, immotile ciliary syndrome, and other chronic respiratory conditions. Cough is the primary symptom leading to a diagnosis of bronchitis. Since cough is so common in children, care must be given in making the diagnosis of "bronchitis." In children, a diagnosis of chronic bronchitis is not an acceptable end point and further testing should be performed to evaluate the underlying cause of the cough.

Bronchitis is categorized into acute, recurrent, or wheezy bronchitis; however, the definition of each type remains unclear and controversial. In school-age children, *M. pneumoniae* has occasionally been identified as an organism producing acute bronchitis (Brown, Mutius, & Morgan, 2008). There are no characteristic clinical findings to distinguish this diagnosis from viral bronchitis. Confirmation could only be accomplished with titers or microbiological evaluation of the sputum or bronchoalveolar lavage fluid. Serology is likely more sensitive because of the fastidious nature of *Mycoplasma*. If indicated, treatment with a macrolide antibiotic can be effective. Because titers are not commonly obtained, overtreatment with macrolides has become common in the pediatric outpatient setting.

In the absence of exposure to cigarette smoke, the persistence of bronchitis beyond 2–3 weeks or the recurrence of bronchitis warrants further investigation into the underlying causes. While the definition of recurrent bronchitis is controversial, most clinicians agree that "too many" episodes can be clarified as more than four episodes of productive cough each year with wheezes or crackles. If this criterion is met, alternative diagnosis should be considered.

The presentation of wheezy bronchitis and asthma often overlaps, and the overwhelming majority of these children actually have asthma. An Asthma Predictive Index is helpful in predicting persisting asthma in children with recurrent wheezing. In a child with three or more wheeze episodes a year, the index is positive if a child has one major criteria (parental asthma or eczema) or two or more minor criteria (allergic rhinitis, wheezing apart from colds, and peripheral eosinophilia) (Castro-Rodriguez et al., 2000). Focusing therapy on asthma in these situations is the most helpful approach. Careful considerations should be given to the child who is chronically diagnosed with bronchitis or wheezy bronchitis to evaluate for underlying conditions such as cystic fibrosis.

Persistent bacterial bronchitis has been recently described, as a wet cough in children who may be at risk of developing bronchiectasis without a known underlying disorder (Chang, Redding, & Everard, 2008). Persistent bacterial bronchitis may cause recurrent or protracted wet cough. Its true nature and existence are not well defined as yet.

Pathophysiology

Despite the common trend of pediatric providers to administer antibiotics for bronchitis, most attacks of acute bronchitis are viral. Rhinovirus, RSV, influenza, metapneumovirus, adenovirus, and rubeola virus have all been identified as etiologic agents (Brown et al., 2008). Because bronchitis is usually mild and self-limited, the pathology is ill defined as there is a lack of tissue to study. Mucus gland activity increases and desquamation of the ciliated epithelium occurs. Infiltration of leukocytes into the airway contributes to the purulent appearance of the secretions. Since leukocyte migration is a response to the airway damage, it is not necessarily indicative of a bacterial superinfection and should not be treated as such. Additionally, acute airway inflammation may also be caused by breathing irritants such as chemical fumes, dust, or smoke. Living in an area that has bad air pollution may predispose a child to more frequent episodes of bronchitis. Children may also be more likely to develop bronchitis if they are often around someone who smokes. Of course, all of those factors also increase the likelihood of asthma.

Signs and symptoms

As mentioned, acute bronchitis usually accompanies an upper respiratory infection. Dry cough generally appears 2–4 days after the rhinitis and then evolves into a looser cough with sputum production. Since children do not always expectorate sputum (it is often swallowed), nausea and vomiting following cough spasms can occur. Chest pain is a common complaint in older children as the cough progresses and becomes more frequent and severe. In the early stages of the illness, the chest is generally clear to auscultation; however, as the illness progresses, rhonchi, wheezes, and harsh breath sounds can be heard. Crackles are rare. Chest X-ray is typically normal, although some increased markings can be noted. Symptoms gradually improve and typically disappear within 10–14 days. Symptoms that persist beyond 2 weeks or that worsen over time should be carefully evaluated for an underlying chronic condition or a secondary bacterial infection. Similarly, persisting fever should prompt evaluation. Although much has been made of the color of the secretions, there are no data to support this concern.

Complications

Most children recover completely after acute bronchitis as the illness is generally mild and self-limiting. Some children may develop other complications such as a sinus or ear infection. Rarely, bronchitis may develop into a more serious infection, such as pneumonia. This risk is increased if the child is very young or has other chronic health problems.

Management

If bacterial infection is suspected or confirmed, treatment with appropriate antimicrobial therapy is warranted. Using antibiotics to "prevent" pneumonia is ineffective and will contribute to the development of resistant organisms. Additionally, if the child is very young and the cough is impeding drinking and eating, hospital admission and IV therapy may be indicated to prevent dehydration. Rarely, oxygen support is needed to maintain adequate oxygenation.

Nursing care of the child and family

Nursing care of a child ill enough to be hospitalized with bronchitis should include continuous monitoring of respiratory status, vital signs, and hydration status. Efforts should be made to encourage deep breathing and breathing through pursed lips. Children should be encouraged to expectorate sputum after coughing, and the head of the bed should be elevated to promote easier breathing.

Parents should be educated as to the signs of a worsening respiratory condition and when to take the child back to the health-care provider. Prevention of further symptoms should be discussed. This includes instructing patients regarding the need for immunization for pertussis and influenza to reduce further infection with those potentially harmful organisms. Additionally, parents should be encouraged to avoid other factors that can contribute to bronchitis including exposure to tobacco smoke and air pollutants, such as wood smoke, solvents, and cleaners. In order to limit the spread of the disease, children with acute bronchitis with fever should not attend school or day care. The child should return to school or day care when signs of infection have decreased, appetite returns, and alertness and strength resume.

Bacterial tracheitis

Epidemiology

Bacterial tracheitis is a rare but life-threatening illness characterized by thick membranous tracheal secretions. The secretions are usually infected, as the name would suggest. The secretions are difficult to clear with coughing and can occlude the airway. Bacterial tracheitis is often a complication of croup and affects the same population, with a mean age of 4. Some feel bacterial tracheitis is mimicking croup initially. In one study, it was reported that of the 500 children who were hospitalized for croup at one pediatric hospital over a 32-month period, 2% developed bacterial tracheitis (Tan & Manoukian, 1992). It has also been recognized as a complication of measles.

Pathophysiology

The most common bacterial cause of tracheitis is *S. aureus*. Additionally, Hib (although rare now due to the vaccine), *Moraxella catarrhalis*, *Klebsiella pneumoniae*, and *S. pneumoniae* can cause bacterial tracheitis. Cases usually occur in the fall or winter months, mimicking the epidemiology of viral croup.

Signs and symptoms

Bacterial tracheitis presents with severe upper airway obstruction, often in a child who has had a preceding episode of viral croup. Many, but not all, children present with high fever and systemic toxicity. Bacterial tracheitis is a diffuse inflammatory process of the larynx, trachea, and bronchi.

Diagnosis

Bacterial cultures of the tracheal secretions are needed in order to determine the infecting organism. A CBC will show an elevated WBC count, which is nonspecific and nondiagnostic. Blood cultures are usually negative. A lateral neck X-ray may reveal the subglottic narrowing from the preceding croup and tracheal irregularities. A definitive diagnosis is made through laryngoscopy and tracheoscopy (Asher & Grant, 2008). However, a clinical diagnosis can be made in a child who, after a few days of croup, develops high fever, increasing stridor, and respiratory distress.

Complications

While most children who are properly diagnosed and treated in the early phase of the disease recover completely, serious complications can occur. Toxic shock syndrome, pulmonary edema, and septic shock have all been reported as complications of bacterial tracheitis. A delay in treatment or improper management can result in ARDS and sometimes death from airway obstruction.

Management

Upon initial diagnosis, the child should be admitted to the pediatric intensive care until stabilized. More than half of the children will need to be intubated, and intermittent positive pressure breathing is sometimes needed. In many cases, the endotracheal tube will suffice, as it bypasses the obstruction and allows for adequate ventilation while the antibiotics work and the airway heals. Intubation often lasts from 3 to 11 days.

Antibiotics should be promptly initiated and should cover the above organisms. Gram stain of the secretions may allow narrowing the spectrum of antibiotics. There is no evidence that nebulized epinephrine or corticosteroids relieve the obstruction.

Nursing care of the child and family

Caring for a child with bacterial tracheitis requires the nurse to be attentive to both the child and the family, as it is a stressful and potentially life-threatening illness. Direct nursing care must include maintaining a patent airway, frequent suctioning, monitoring for adequate ventilation, oxygenation, hydration, and nutritional status. CPT may help in clearing the secretions if it is tolerated by the child. The nurse should also be aware of the age-appropriate signs and symptoms of acute respiratory distress and should notify the medical team immediately if the child's condition is worsening. Additionally, the nurse should provide anticipatory guidance to the family as to the expected course of the illness and should try to assist the family by providing answers to the concerns and questions they may have. The family should be reassured that long-term sequelae of tracheitis are very uncommon, as are recurrences of disease.

CONCLUSION

When caring for a child with any of the lower airway diseases described previously, the practitioner must take special care to monitor respiratory status but also must carefully weigh the need for antimicrobial therapy. As has been pointed out many times in this chapter, viral organisms are responsible for a majority of lower airway diseases in children and should be considered first when initiating treatment plans.

Much morbidity and mortality is arising as a result of the developing antibiotic resistance in the pediatric community. An example of the dangers of antibiotic resistance is the spread of methicillin-resistant *Staphylococcus aureus* (MRSA). MRSA was once a concern only for people in the hospital but now is causing infections in healthy people in the community. It is apparent from the above-mentioned discussion and data that in many cases, antibiotic therapy is not warranted and should be avoided to help limit the development of resistant organisms and more severe disease.

REFERENCES

American Academy of Pediatrics (AAP). (2009). Policy statement—Modified recommendations for use of palivizumab for prevention of respiratory syncytial virus infections. *Pediatrics, 124*, 1694–1701.

Asher, I. M., & Grant, C. C. (2008). Infections of the upper respiratory tract. In L. Taussig & L. Landau (Eds.), *Pediatric respiratory medicine* (2nd ed., pp. 453–480). Philadelphia: Mosby.

Bordley, W. C., Viswanathan, M., King, V. J., Sutton, S. F., Jackman, A. M., Sterling, L., et al. (2004). Diagnosis and testing in bronchiolitis: A systematic review. *Archives of Pediatrics & Adolescent Medicine, 158*(2), 119–126.

Bronchiolitis Guideline Team, Cincinnati Children's Hospital Medical Center. (2005). Evidence based clinical practice guideline for medical management of bronchiolitis in infants 1 year of age or less presenting with a first time episode. Guideline 1, pp. 1–12. Retrieved from http://www.cincinnatichildrens.org/assets/0/78/1067/2709/2777/2793/9199/edf8f194-1a56-48f7-8419-7c5e0a168b5d.pdf.

Brown, M. A., von Mutius, E., & Morgan, W. J. (2008). Clinical assessment and diagnostic approach to common problems. In L. Taussig & L. Landau (Eds.), *Pediatric respiratory medicine* (2nd ed., pp. 125–128). Philadelphia: Mosby.

Bye, M. R. (1994). Persistent or recurrent pneumonia. In D. V. Chidlow & D. S. Smith (Eds.), *A practical guide to pediatric respiratory diseases* (pp. 99–103). Philadelphia: Hanley & Belfus.

Castro-Rodriguez, J. A., Holberg, C. J., Wright, A. L., & Martinez, F. D. (2000). A clinical index to define risk of asthma in young children with recurrent wheeze. *American Journal of Respiratory and Critical Care Medicine, 162,* 1403–1406.

Centers for Disease Control (CDC). (2010). Morbidity and Mortality Weekly Report. Respiratory Syncytial Virus Activity—United States, July 2008–December 2009. March 5, 2010, *59*(08), 230–233. Retrieved from http://www.cdc.gov/mmwr/preview/mmwrhtml/mm5908a4.htm.

Chang, A. B., Redding, G. J., & Everard, M. L. (2008). Chronic wet cough: Protracted bronchitis, chronic suppurative lung disease and bronchiectasis. *Pediatric Pulmonology, 43,* 519–531.

Crawford, E., & Daum, R. S. (2008). Bacterial pneumonia, lung abscess, and empyema. In L. Taussig & L. Landau (Eds.), *Pediatric respiratory medicine* (2nd ed., pp. 501–569). Philadelphia: Mosby.

Dakhama, A., Lee, Y. M., Ohnishi, H., Xia, J., Balhorn, A., Takeda, K., et al. (2009). Virus-specific IgE enhances airway responsiveness on reinfection with respiratory syncytial virus in newborn mice. *The Journal of Allergy and Clinical Immunology, 123*(1), 138–145.

Dellinger, P. R. (2010). Septic shock overview. Retrieved from http://emedicine.medscape.com/article/168402.

Denny, R. W. (1999). Acute lower respiratory tract infections: General considerations. In L. Taussig & L. Landau (Eds.), *Pediatric respiratory medicine* (pp. 556–571). St. Louis, MO: Mosby.

Dubois, D. B., & Ray, G. C. (1999). Viral infections of the lower respiratory tract. In L. Taussig & L. Landau (Eds.), *Pediatric respiratory medicine* (pp. 572–578). St. Louis, MO: Mosby.

Duke, J. R., & Good, J. T. (Eds.) (2001). *Frontline assessment of common pulmonary presentations.* Denver: The Snowdrift Pulmonary Foundation. Retrieved from http://www.nlhep.org/books/pul_Pre/pleural-effusion.html.

Everard, M. L. (2008). Respiratory synical virus-associated lower respiratory tract disease. In L. Taussig & L. Landau (Eds.), *Pediatric respiratory medicine* (2nd ed., pp. 491–500). Philadelphia: Mosby.

Gadomski, A. M., & Bhasale, A. L. (2006). Bronchodilators for bronchiolitis. *Cochrane Database of Systematic Reviews,* (3), Art. No.: CD001266. DOI: 10.1002/14651858.CD001266.pub2.

Gutierrez, J. A., Duke, T., Henning, R., & South, M. (2008). Respiratory failure and acute respiratory distress syndrome. In L. Taussig & L. Landau (Eds.), *Pediatric respiratory medicine* (2nd ed., pp. 125–128). Philadelphia: Mosby.

Heltzer, M. L., Coffin, S. E., Maurer, K., Bagashev, A., Zhang, Z., Orange, J. S., et al. (2009). Immune dysregulation in severe influenza. *Journal of Leukocyte Biology, 85*(6), 1036–1043.

The Impact-RSV Study Group. (1998). Palivizumab, a humanized respiratory syncytial virus monoclonal antibody, reduces hospitalization from respiratory syncytial virus infection in high risk infants. *Pediatrics, 102,* 531–537.

Krilov, L. R. (2010). Respiratory syncytial virus (RSV) infection: Differential diagnoses & workup. Retrieved from Winthrop University Hospital http://emedicine.medscape.com/article/971488-overview.

Kuzik, B. A., Al Qadhi, S. A., Kent, S., Flavin, M. P., Hopman, W., & Hotte, S. (2007). Nebulized hypertonic saline in the treatment of viral bronchiolitis in infants. *Journal of Pediatrics, 151*, 266–270.

Maranich, A., & Rajnik, M. (2009). Human metapneumovirus. Retrieved from http://www.emedicine.com/article/972492.

Poets, C. F. (2008). Apnea of prematurity, sudden infant death syndrome, and apparent life threatening events. In L. Taussig & L. Landau (Eds.), *Pediatric respiratory medicine* (2nd ed., pp. 432–433). Philadelphia: Mosby.

Rudan, I. A., Boschi-Pinto, C. B., Biloglav, Z. C., Mulhollandd, K., & Campbelle, H. (2008). Epidemiology and etiology of childhood pneumonia. *Bulletin of the World Health Organization, 86*, 408–416. Retrieved from http://www.who.int/bulletin/volumes/86/5/07-048769.pdf.

Sanchez, I., Koster, J., Powell, R., Wolstein, R., & Chernick, V. (1993). Effect of racemic epinephrine and salbutamol on clinical score and pulmonary mechanics in infants with bronchiolitis. *The Journal of Pediatrics, 122*(1), 145–151.

Shay, D. K., Holman, R. C., Newman, R. D., Liu, L. L., Stout, J. W., & Anderson, L. J. (1999). Bronchiolitis-associated hospitalizations among US children, 1980–1996. *JAMA, 282*(15), 1440–1446.

Tan, A. K., & Manoukian , J. J. (1992). Hospitalized croup (bacterial and viral): The role of rigid endoscopy. *Journal of Otolarynology, 21*(1), 48.

Wang, E. E., Law, B. J., & Stephens, D. (1995). Pediatric Investigators Collaborative Network on Infections in Canada (PICNIC) prospective study of risk factors and outcomes in patients hospitalized with respiratory syncytial viral lower respiratory tract infection. *Journal of Pediatrics, 126*(2), 212–219.

Young, S., O'Keeffe, P. T., Arnott, J., & Landau, L. I. (1995). Infant lung infection airway responsiveness, atopic status and respiratory symptoms before and after bronchiolitis. *Archives of Disease in Childhood, 72*, 16–24.

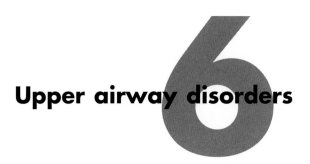

Upper airway disorders

Wendy S. L. Mackey, MSN, APRN-BC, CORLN,
Melissa M. Dziedzic, MSN, CPNP, CORLN, and
Lisa M. Gagnon, MSN, CPNP

ANATOMICAL AND PHYSIOLOGICAL CONSIDERATIONS OF THE PEDIATRIC AIRWAY

A basic understanding of the developmental anatomy of the upper aerodigestive tract is essential to adequately comprehend airway diseases. Fetal weeks 3–8 are vitally important in the embryological development of these structures. This chapter will focus on the laryngeal and tracheal airway, as well as the sinuses.

The larynx is suspended vertically between the epiglottis and the cricoid cartilage. It is situated posterior to the thyroid gland and lies medially between the carotid arteries. The larynx is divided into three compartments (see Figure 6.1):

- *Supraglottis*—begins below the base of the tongue and extends to (but does not include) the level of the true vocal cords; this area houses the epiglottis, aryepiglottic folds, arytenoid cartilages, and false vocal cords
- *Glottis*—true vocal cords, rima glottis, and the glottic slit separating the true vocal cords
- *Subglottis*—extends from just below the true vocal cords to the interior margin of the cricoid cartilage (Becker, Naumann, & Pfaltz, 1989)

Nursing Care in Pediatric Respiratory Disease, First Edition. Edited by Concettina (Tina) Tolomeo.
© 2012 John Wiley & Sons, Inc. Published 2012 by John Wiley & Sons, Inc.

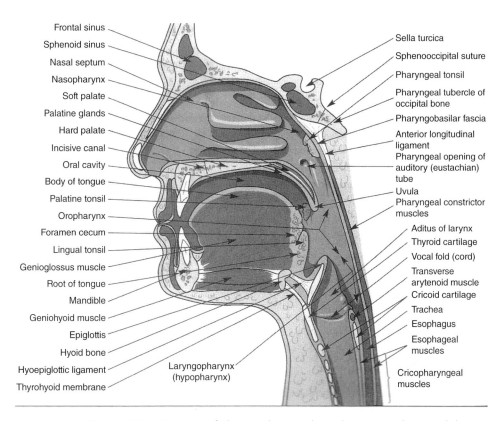

Frontal sinus
Sphenoid sinus
Nasal septum
Nasopharynx
Soft palate
Palatine glands
Hard palate
Incisive canal
Oral cavity
Body of tongue
Palatine tonsil
Oropharynx
Foramen cecum
Lingual tonsil
Genioglossus muscle
Root of tongue
Mandible
Geniohyoid muscle
Epiglottis
Hyoid bone
Hyoepiglottic ligament
Thyrohyoid membrane

Laryngopharynx
(hypopharynx)

Sella turcica
Sphenooccipital suture
Pharyngeal tonsil
Pharyngeal tubercle of
occipital bone
Pharyngobasilar fascia
Anterior longitudinal
ligament
Pharyngeal opening of
auditory (eustachian)
tube
Uvula
Pharyngeal constrictor
muscles
Aditus of larynx
Thyroid cartilage
Vocal fold (cord)
Transverse
arytenoid muscle
Cricoid cartilage
Trachea
Esophagus
Esophageal
muscles
Cricopharyngeal
muscles

Figure 6.1 Anatomy of the oropharynx, hypopharynx, trachea, and larynx. Reprinted from Andresen et al. (2008), with permission from the editors.

The pediatric airway has many unique features that differ depending on the age of the child (Table 6.1). The larynx is significantly higher in infants and in children. The inferior margin of the cricoid cartilage lies at approximately the level of the second or third cervical vertebra in the infant and descends to the sixth cervical vertebra by puberty (Brown, 2000). The larynx is also located more anterior and superior in the neck in the neonate, allowing approximation of the epiglottis and palate. This allows the neonate to be an obligate nose breather for the first several weeks to months of life. This anatomical situation does allow the healthy neonate the ability to both breath and swallow simultaneously, which is not possible as the larynx descends.

The larynx is composed of cartilage and ligaments. There are three large cartilages and three small cartilages (Becker et al., 1989). The larger cartilages include the thyroid, epiglottis, and cricoid cartilage. The thyroid cartilage forms the main skeleton of the larynx; however, it does not assume its adult configuration until adolescence. The epiglottis cartilage protects

Table 6.1 The pediatric airway is different from the adult airway.

Development of supporting airway cartilage and small airway muscles is incomplete until school
age.
The larynx is higher in the child. The cricoid cartilage lies at the level of the third cervical
vertebra in the infant and descends to the sixth cervical vertebra at puberty.
The thyroid cartilage does not assume its adult configuration until adolescence.
The recurrent laryngeal nerve lies just lateral to the trachea. In addition, a pretracheal pad of fat
is generally present in infants.
The articulation between the head and neck is more mobile in infants and the chin may easily
deviate from the midline during surgery.
The airways are smaller (narrower and shorter).

the airway from food, liquids, and saliva during swallowing. The cricoid
cartilage is located inferior to the thyroid cartilage and is the first ring of
the trachea. It is the only rigid circular structure of the airway, which in
turn produces the narrowest fixed point in the pediatric airway. In contrast,
the narrowest portion of the adult airway is at the level of the vocal cords
(Cotton & Willging, 1999). The smaller cartilages include the arytenoid,
corniculate, and the cuneiform. The hyoid bone is the only bone in the
framework of the larynx. It is a landmark in the neck, a movable horseshoe-
shaped bone at the base of the tongue.

The laryngeal muscles are responsible for elevation and depression of
the larynx (extrinsic muscles) as well as movement of the vocal cords
(intrinsic muscles) (Healy, 1989). The development of all supporting airway
cartilage and small airway muscles is incomplete until school age; this may
predispose the infant and young child to malacia.

Physiologically, the role of the larynx is multifactorial. It acts as a valve
during the swallowing process, closing the airway to prevent aspiration
and to allow delivery of food and liquids to the esophagus. During this
process, the vocal cords close and the larynx elevates up against the epiglottis. Second, the larynx allows for vocalization. As air is exhaled from
the lungs, it travels up through the vocal cords, which vibrate, causing
phonation (Brown, 2000). Other aspects of speech are accomplished by
structures higher up as the air is exhaled. Articulation is achieved through
movement of the soft palate, tongue, and lips. Tone and quality of speech
is affected by resonation through the pharynx, sinuses, and nasal passage.
The larynx not only serves as an air passage but also as a filter as it clears
the respiratory tract of secretions through a voluntary cough. The cough
is produced by forcibly closing the glottis.

The recurrent laryngeal nerve and the superior laryngeal nerve are
branches of the vagus nerve (cranial nerve X) that supply innervations of
the larynx (Becker et al., 1989). The recurrent laryngeal nerve is located
just lateral to the trachea and supplies motor innervation to the intrinsic
laryngeal muscles, which are responsible for vocal cord mobility. The left

Table 6.2 Tubular fluid dynamics.

	Tracheal edema (mm)	Resistance	Cross-sectional area (% reduction)
Neonate	1	Increased × 16	75
Teen	1	Triple	44
Adult	1	Double	30

branch of the recurrent laryngeal nerve loops under the aortic arch above the pulmonary artery. The trachea is a flexible cylindrical cartilaginous muscular tube extending vertically from the larynx to its bifurcation (carina) into the right and left mainstem bronchi. Its purpose is to transport warmed, filtered, and humidified air to the lungs for respiration. The trachea is composed of 16–20 C-shaped hyaline cartilage "tracheal rings" (Becker et al., 1989). The posterior wall of the trachea (open part of the C) is composed of smooth muscle and connective tissue that allows the diameter of the trachea to change. The posterior trachea abuts the esophagus and the soft posterior wall allows the esophagus to expand during swallowing. The vagus nerve and the sympathetic system innervate the trachea.

It is no surprise that the larynx and trachea are smaller, both narrower and shorter in infants and in children versus adults. The vocal cords in the newborn infant are 6–8 mm long. The posterior glottis transverse length is approximately 4 mm, and the subglottis has a diameter of about 5–7 mm. The tracheal length is 4 cm long (10–13 cm in an adult), with a diameter of 3.6 mm (25 mm in an adult) (Becker et al., 1989). These measurements leave little margin for obstruction.

Pouseuille's law states that flow within the system is related to the radius of the tube to the fourth power. Resistance is related to the inverse of the radius to the fourth power. One millimeter of tracheal edema will have little effect on the airway of an adult or adolescent; however, it may cause serious airway obstruction and resulting respiratory compromise in an infant or a young child (Table 6.2).

ASSESSMENT OF THE CHILD WITH AIRWAY DIFFICULTIES

Obstruction in the airway can present with a vast spectrum of variability from normal breathing with no symptoms to complete obstruction with apnea, loss of consciousness, cyanosis, and potential death. Evaluation of a child with a suspected compromised airway must first and foremost establish the level of urgency of the situation.

History

In an otherwise nonemergent situation, the initial step in the evaluation of airway disease is a careful history. Presence of respiratory symptoms (stridor, work of breathing, history of cyanosis, or apnea) should be ascertained. A careful history of feeding patterns and growth should also be obtained. Infants and children with more severe airway issues frequently present with feeding difficulties and poor weight gain. Quality of voice/cry, presence of birthmarks, history of traumatic birth, and diagnosis of other health problems or syndromes are key aspects of the history. Furthermore, it is important to establish the child's position of maximum comfort as well as aggravating factors such as excursion, agitation, sleeping, or feeding.

Timing of presentation should be established. It may vary from a prenatal suspicion based on prenatal screening (i.e., tracheal dilation) or prenatal symptoms (i.e., polyhydramnios) to unexpected airway compromise at birth to onset at various postnatal ages. Laryngomalacia, for example, is the most common cause of congenital stridor; however, infants classically present with symptoms at 1 month of age.

Circumstances surrounding the onset of symptoms should be obtained such as recent choking episode, trauma to the head or neck, recent intubation, upper respiratory infection, throat or neck pain, or fever. For example, if signs and symptoms of airway obstruction began following a choking episode, foreign bodies should be considered. Rapidity of progression of symptoms may also be important.

Physical examination

Physical examination should begin with careful inspection of the patient noting the level of consciousness, position, color, respiratory rate, and effort. General inspection will include identification of the presence or absence of structural anomalies, craniofacial malformations, and presence of lesions (masses or hemangiomas). The examination proceeds with auscultation of the nasal cavity, cheeks, neck, and chest.

Stridor/stertor

Stridor is the hallmark physical sign of airway obstruction. Stridor is defined as a harsh, vibratory musical sound of varying pitch produced by turbulent airflow through the airway (Healy, 2000). The quality, pitch, and timing of stridor can elicit valuable information regarding the location of the airway obstruction (see Table 6.3). Other key assessments include quality of respirations, work of breathing, as well as the quality of voice or cry.

Nasopharyngeal obstruction typically produces an inspiratory low-pitched sound known as stertor. Children with nasopharyngeal obstruction

Table 6.3 Location of airway obstruction based on physical assessment.

	Nasal/ nasopharyngeal	Supraglottic/ glottic obstruction	Subglottic obstruction	Tracheal obstruction
Stridor/sterdor	Inspiratory sound Low pitch (stertor)	Inspiratory stridor High pitched	Biphasis stridor Intermediate pitch	Expiratory stridor "Wheeze"
Work of breathing	Mouth breathing with possible distress/apnea	Prolonged inspiration	Prolonged expiration	Prolonged expiration
Voice/cry	Normal to muffled (hot potato)	Weak, hoarse to aphonic	Normal to weak Barky cough	Normal
Examples of airway abnormalities causing obstruction	Nasal congestion Choanal atresia Macroglossia Retrognathia Nasal/oral mass/ tumor	Laryngomalacia Vocal cord palsy/paralysis Laryngeal atresia Laryngeal web/ cyst	Subglottic stenosis Subglottic hemangioma	Tracheomalacia Tracheal stenosis Vascular ring

find it easier to breathe through their mouths. Glottic and subglottic obstruction also presents with inspiratory sounds; however, the sound has a high-pitched quality with a prolonged inspiratory phase.

Subglottic obstruction produces biphasic stridor (stridor on both inspiration and expiration). This stridor has an intermediate pitch.

Tracheal obstruction typically produces expiratory stridor, with more of a "wheezy" sound. Supraglottic, subglottic, and tracheal obstructions all tend to produce a prolonged expiratory phase.

The degree (loudness) of stridor or stertor is not a reliable indicator of severity of obstruction (Papsin, Abel, & Leighton, 1999). Stridor can paradoxically become less obvious as obstruction worsens due to diminishing airflow. The degree of stridor is frequently variable based on activity. Feeding and exertion will typically enhance audible stridor.

Retractions

Retractions can be an excellent indicator of the degree of obstruction (increased retractions denote increased obstruction). However, they do not offer much data in respect to location of the obstruction.

Quality of voice/cry

The quality of voice and cry varies from normal to muffled with oronasopharyngeal obstruction (oropharyngeal obstruction—hot potato voice;

nasopharyngeal obstruction—hyponasal). Laryngeal obstruction naturally affects the voice, ranging from weak to hoarse to aphonia, depending on the location and extent of the obstruction in the larynx. Children with subglottic obstruction will have a normal to weak voice but tend to have a barky (croup-like) cough.

Activity

Many airway lesions will elicit varying symptoms as the child rests, cries, and sleeps. Ideally, it is valuable to assess the child in various positions and states. If possible, attempt further assessment with the child awake or asleep, agitated, during physical exertion, with position changes, and with feedings.

Endoscopy

Endoscopic examination of the patient is the most definitive method of diagnosing a patient with an airway anomaly (Botma, Kishore, Kubba, & Geddes, 2000). Flexible endoscopy allows visualization of the nasal cavity, pharynx, and larynx. Therefore, many etiologies can be ruled in or out based on data from flexible laryngoscopy. It can be performed at the time of initial evaluation, in the office, with the patient awake. This allows for dynamic assessment of the larynx, including vocal cord movement and laryngeal collapse. However, it is not effective in diagnosing lesions below the glottis. It is important to consider that there is a 5% incidence of coexisting lesions in the lower airway when upper lesions are present, and more than 30% have multiple sites of airway abnormalities (Altman, Wetmore, & Mahboubi, 1998). Further endoscopy must also be considered when respiratory symptoms do not match the degree of obstruction identified.

Rigid laryngoscopy and bronchoscopy remain the gold standard for diagnosis of all complex airway lesions. This procedure is accomplished in the operating room with general anesthesia.

Diagnostic imaging

Radiological evaluation of the pediatric airway is an integral component in the diagnostic and therapeutic management of pediatric airway problems. The diagnostic modality is dependent on the suspected site of obstruction (Zawin, 2000):

- Frontal (anteroposterior) and lateral radiographs are the most common imaging studies used to assess the upper airway. They are useful in providing information regarding the size of the adenoids, epiglottic size and shape, radio-opaque foreign body, retropharyngeal profile, as well as subglottic and tracheal anatomy (Contensin, Gumpert, Gaudemar, Chaussain, & Dupont, 1997).

- Computed tomographic (CT) scan and magnetic resonance imaging (MRI) may be obtained to visualize the airway and the surrounding soft tissue structures.
- Airway fluoroscopy is helpful in offering dynamic information about airway caliber and position during different phases of respiration (Altman et al., 1998).
- Video stoboscopy of the vocal cords is helpful in providing information regarding vocal cord anatomy and movement.
- Barium esophagrams are useful in providing information about the esophageal anatomy and peristalsis, diameter, and mucosal integrity. It can identify an extrinsic compression of the airway, foreign body, strictures, and tracheoesophageal fistulas, and may identify gastroesophageal reflux (however, there is a high percentage of false negatives).
- There are various studies that may be employed to rule out laryngopharangeal reflux including pH probe, impedance probe, barrium swallow, and direct visualization (Karkos, Leong, Apostolidou, & Apostolidis, 2006).

ANOMALIES OF THE LARYNX AND TRACHEA

Laryngomalacia

Laryngomalacia is a common condition in infancy in which the soft, immature, cartilage of the supraglottic larynx collapses inward during inhalation, causing airway obstruction.

Epidemiology

Laryngomalacia is the most common anomaly of the larynx and is the most common cause of stridor in infants (Zoumalan, Maddalozzo, & Holinger, 2007). Males are affected twice as frequently as females. The exact etiology of the disorder is unknown. There are three predominant theories that include immaturity or maldevelopment of the cartilaginous structures, extraesophageal reflux, and immaturity of neuromuscular control.

Histologically, the quality of the cartilage in infants with laryngomalacia is the same as those without. As a result, the pathophysiology of the disorder is also poorly understood. There is some evidence that there may be some genetic predisposition in some cases of laryngomalacia. It is also established that infants with gastroesophageal reflux disease may have more severe diseases (Giannoni, Sulek, Friedman, & Duncan, 1998).

Signs and symptoms

The infant with laryngomalacia typically presents with inspiratory stridor and feeding difficulties. Stridor is typically accentuated by feeding, agitation, and supine positioning. Conversely, it may improve when the baby is calm, with neck extended, and in a prone position. The onset of stridor is typically in the first several weeks of life. The severity of the stridor may increase with growth over the next few months as air movement becomes more vigorous. It typically slowly resolves by 12–18 months. Feeding difficulties range from prolonged feeding times with pauses or breaks in feeding, irritability during feeds, and postprandial vomiting, to colic to increased stridor during feeding to failure to thrive in infants with more severe laryngomalacia (Giannoni et al., 1998). The child's cry is typically normal. Respiratory distress, including apnea, cyanosis, retractions, and nasal flaring, is rare. However, some infants will have a more severe form of laryngomalacia, presenting with stridor, severe respiratory distress, and failure to thrive.

Diagnosis

The diagnosis of laryngomalacia is based on the classic history and is confirmed with flexible laryngoscopy (Figure 6.2). The examination will reveal one or more of the characteristic findings of laryngomalacia, including (Richter & Thompson, 2008) the following:

- Omega-shaped epiglottis (elongation and lateral extension) that prolapses posteroinferiorly on inspiration
- Redundant bulky arytenoid mucosa that collapse anteromedially into the airway upon inspiration
- Shortening of the aryepiglottic folds

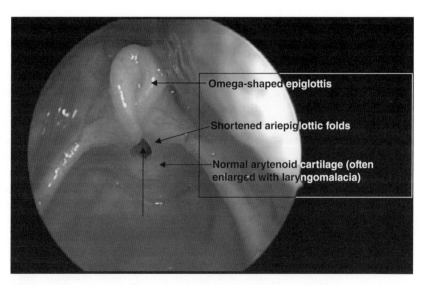

Figure 6.2 Laryngomalacia. Courtesy of Samuel Ostrower, MD.

- Inward collapse of the aryepiglottic folds (cuneiform cartilages) on inspiration
- Anatomy is otherwise normal, including normal structure and function of the vocal cords, and a clear unimpeded airway on expiration.

Management

Most cases of laryngomalacia are managed with careful observation and reassurance. Infants are often evaluated in the office on a monthly basis to monitor respiratory symptoms, weight gain, and feeding tolerance.

The use of antireflux medications, such as a proton pump inhibitor or H2-receptor antagonists, is often helpful in diminishing symptoms, especially in infants with signs and symptoms of gastroesophageal reflux.

Gastroesophageal reflux has been noted in up to 80% of infants with laryngomalacia, many of whom do not exhibit symptoms of reflux (Giannoni et al., 1998). The exposure to acid and pepsin from the reflux of stomach contents can have detrimental effects on the larynx. This may contribute to laryngeal edema, which may exacerbate symptoms of stridor. The use of antireflux medications in infants without clear symptoms of reflux is advocated by some clinicians.

Infants with laryngomalacia who exhibit symptoms of severe respiratory distress and/or failure to thrive will require surgical management. Approximately 10–20% of infants will require surgical intervention to eliminate or bypass the obstruction (Roger, Denoyelle, & Triglia, 1995). Supraglottoplasty is a surgical procedure that involves division of the short aryepiglottic folds. Other revisions to the laryngeal cartilage are sometimes employed, including trimming of the epiglottis, removing the corniculate and cuneiform cartilages, or removing the redundant arytenoid mucosa, all of which may widen the laryngeal inlet (O'Donnell, Murphy, Bew, & Knight, 2007). Tracheotomy may be performed for severe cases not responsive to supraglottoplasty to establish a safe airway.

Complications

Complications are rare as most infants will outgrow the condition within the first 2 years of life. Lower airway lesions may coexist with laryngomalacia and are important to consider and rule out, especially in children with more severe symptoms or atypical history and presentation. Rare complications of severe laryngomalacia include chest deformities, cyanotic attacks, obstructive sleep apnea, pulmonary hypertension, cardiac failure, and failure to thrive (Richter & Thompson, 2008).

Vocal cord disorders

There are a variety of vocal cord issues that children may have. This section will outline the most likely types of problems seen: vocal fold immobility

(VFI), vocal cord paralysis (VCP), vocal cord dysfunction (VCD), and vocal cord lesions.

Immobility, paralysis, and dysfunction

VCP

VCP is the second most common congenital abnormality of the larynx and is responsible for 10% of all congenital airway lesions (Hollinger, Hollinger, & Holinger, 1976). VCP occurs secondary to the dysfunction of the nerve supply to the laryngeal muscles, which differs from VFI (often called vocal cord immobility), which is defined as both paralysis and fixation. Additionally, unilateral VCP differs from bilateral VCP in presentation, etiology, and treatment (Chen & Inglis, 2008).

Epidemiology

Bilateral VCP occurs in 30–62% of all cases of VCP, with spontaneous recovery in 48–62% of these cases (Brigger & Hartnick, 2002). Incidence of bilateral VFI is still low overall with reported estimates at 0.75 cases per million births per year (Murty, Shinkwin, & Gibbin, 1994). When looking specifically at reports of unilateral VFI, research is varied. Two reports found in the literature document rates of 8 and 25% (Cavanaugh, 1955; Schild & Holinger, 1980).

Pathophysiology

Children differ from adults in their causes of bilateral VCP. VCP may occur secondary to the stretching and compression of the vagus nerve or the stretching or compression of the recurrent laryngeal nerves (Chen & Inglis, 2008). The causes of nerve injury may be neurological, traumatic, iatrogenic, or idiopathic.

Twenty-five to thirty percent of VCP is from a neurological cause. One of the most common neurological causes is secondary to Arnold–Chiari malformation with associated myelomeningocele and hydrocephalus. It is thought that the vagus nerve becomes stretched and compressed by the protrusion of the cerebellar tonsils, medulla, and brain stem through the foramen magnum (Chen & Inglis, 2008). With this lesion, the infant or child will usually have bilateral paralysis; however, unilateral paralysis has also been reported. Other less common central nervous system lesions include encephalocele, leukodystrophy, hydrocephalus, and cerebral or nuclear dysgenesis. Amyotrophic lateral sclerosis (ALS) may present in the older child and may cause unilateral or bilateral vocal cord involvement. Perinatal hypoxia or cortical stroke is a rare cause (Jong, Kuppersmith, Sulek, & Friedman, 2000). Muscular dystrophies and peripheral neuromuscular disorders have been reported. Examples include myasthenia gravis, myotonic dystrophy, and Charcot–Marie–Tooth disease.

A traumatic cause may be birth trauma. This is secondary to breech presentation, use of forceps for delivery, or intubation, which can cause stretching or compression of one or both recurrent laryngeal nerves of the neck.

The most common iatrogenic cause is secondary to surgery, including patent ductus arteriosis ligation and repair of tracheoesophageal fistula. Paralysis may occur unilaterally or bilaterally. If unilateral, left VCP is more common, secondary to the longer course of the left recurrent laryngeal nerve. Other cardiac surgeries implicated as causes of VCP include those for tetralogy of Fallot and ventricular septal defect. Vascular rings, aortic arch abnormalities, and patent ductus arteriosis surgeries are more typical for laryngeal paralysis (Jong et al., 2000).

Examples of idiopathic etiologies may include infectious, rheumatologic, or mitochondrial disorders (Rubin & Sataloff, 2007). Most of the infectious etiologies of the past, including poliomyelitis and tetanus, are rare today secondary to immunization. Guillian Barre is still a reported cause.

Signs and symptoms

The most common presenting symptom of bilateral VCP is stridor, which is typically biphasic. Infants will usually have a loud cry. Because the vocal cords are often paralyzed in the paramedian position (abductor paralysis), the voice or cry can be normal. Of note, infants are more likely to present with stridor and dyspnea than with dysphonia or aspiration (Chen & Inglis, 2008). If the cords are paralyzed medially, severe respiratory failure occurs.

Infants with unilateral VCP may present with stridor, or a weak cry (Parikh, 2004). If there is stridor, it will usually be on inspiration, whereas with bilateral paralysis, it is typically biphasic. Symptoms may vary depending on whether the vocal cord is in the paramedian or median position. If the unilateral cord is immobile in the paramedian position, then there is a lack of opposition of the cord and the child may have a weak cry or voice. Over time, the other cord compensates and the child may achieve a more normal voice with time. Feeding difficulties may be present secondary to aspiration or an inability to coordinate the swallow secondary to an incompetent larynx. If there are no feeding or airway problems, the diagnosis may go undetected (Parikh, 2004). Older children and adolescents may present similar to adult patients with a soft or breathy voice disturbances or may have symptoms of dysphagia.

Diagnosis

A full head and neck exam is essential to evaluate for anatomical abnormalities, masses, and/or cranial nerve abnormalities. The child should also be evaluated for any breathing difficulties with particular attention to work of breathing and timing of abnormal respiratory sounds, such as stridor. If suspicion is high for an airway abnormality, then initial consultation of the infant or child with stridor includes airway evaluation with bedside fiberoptic laryngoscopy by an otolaryngologist.

At times, there may be difficulties determining if the VFI is bilateral or unilateral secondary to a crying infant or a limited view of the vocal folds. A confirmatory exam and full evaluation may ultimately be completed by direct laryngoscopy and bronchoscopy in the operating room. The advantage of intraoperative evaluation is the ability to fully evaluate the child for secondary abnormalities such as laryngeal cleft or subglottic stenosis.

Imaging studies such as CT scan or ultrasound are not the standard of care but have been used as diagnostic studies. The utility of the study depends on suspicion of extrinsic lesions or other abnormalities such as central nervous system lesions.

Management

Management differs for bilateral and unilateral VCP. For most cases of bilateral VCP, a tracheostomy will be performed either as a temporary or permanent measure to secure and protect the child's airway. If the cause is thought to be temporary, the child may remain intubated or under close observation, and tracheostomy may be deferred while awaiting spontaneous recovery.

Depending on the etiology, serial airway exams may be performed to evaluate the infant or child for resolution. Neurological and idiopathic causes have the best chance of spontaneous recovery, which, if it occurs, will generally happen in the first 6 months but can occur up to 11 years after diagnosis (Daya, Hosni, Bejar-Solar, Evans, & Bailey, 2000). For this reason, many otolaryngologists will wait before intervening surgically. Moreover, for infants less than 6 months, treating the underlying cause, such as Arnold–Chiari malformation abnormalities or hydrocephalus, by placement of a ventriculoperitoneal shunt may resolve the paralysis in up to 62% of the cases (Parikh, 2004).

For long-term VCP in children, various surgical techniques such as suture lateralization, arytenoidectomy, cordectomy, and posterior cricoid split with cartilage graft have been described in the literature. Outcome measures include rates of decannulation, which may vary. Some of the risks with surgery include voice disturbances, airway issues, and swallowing dysfunction (Bower, Choi, & Cotton, 1994; Gupta, Mann, & Nagarkar, 1997; Hartnick, Brigger, Willging, Cotton, & Myer, 2003; Inglis et al., 2003; Mathur, Kumar, & Bothra, 2004). There is also a theoretical concern of the effect on laryngeal growth (Parikh, 2004).

In most cases of unilateral VCP, the child will not require any airway intervention. Rarely, neonates with significant airway distress from unilateral paralysis may need a tracheotomy. If the infant or child is experiencing significant aspiration or dysphonia, surgical intervention may be recommended. Most commonly, the vocal fold is medialized by the injection of Teflon, gelfoam, or collagen under endoscopy or by external medialization via thyroplasty. Case numbers are small and studies are limited. Teflon has been reported to have an association with granuloma formulation and is not used as frequently (Parikh, 2004).

Complications

For surgical interventions, a variety of complications can occur, including granuloma formulation, scar formation, ongoing voice or swallowing problems, and pneumonia.

VCD

VCD occurs when there is an abnormal movement of the vocal folds in the absence of other diseases. Another term used to describe this is paradoxic vocal fold motion (PVFM).

Epidemiology

PVFM may occur at any age in children; however, the median reported age of presentation is 14. There is a female preponderance in all age groups (Hicks, Brugman, & Katial, 2008). The true incidence may be higher; however, among healthy, physically active adolescents and young adults, there are reports of incidence that range from 8 to 27% (Morris et al., 1999; Abu-Hasan, Tannous, & Weinberger, 2005; Seear, Wensley, & West, 2005).

Pathophysiology

During a symptomatic period, there is paradoxical symmetrical adduction of the vocal folds toward the midline on inspiration. This causes obstruction at the glottic level. There can also be expiratory obstruction with VCD. At asymptomatic times, the vocal fold motion is normal (Christopher & Morris, 2010).

Precipitating factors have been studied to determine etiologic factors in VCD. Upper airway hyperresponsiveness to a variety of triggers has been considered. While there is no absolute certainty in the triggers of the disease, those with VCD have reported such factors as acid reflux, upper airway infections, allergies, sinusitis, and irritants inhaled from accidental or occupational exposure (Hicks et al., 2008). Exercise may be a trigger and has been reported as a precipitating factor in 18% of people with VCD (Morris, Perkins, & Allan, 2006). Another factor thought to be implicated in VCD is significant psychological stress. Those with VCD may have higher levels of anxiety and more anxiety-related diagnoses (Gavin et al., 1998). The stress of competition for athletes may be noted more frequently as a trigger in exercise-induced VCD (McFadden & Zawadski, 1996). Psychiatric disease has been reported as a factor as well. The most common disorder identified was conversion disorder, followed by depression, Munchausen's syndrome, obsessive–compulsive disorder, and adjustment disorder (Lacy & McManis, 2004).

Signs and symptoms

There may be noisy breathing, stridor, wheezing, and/or difficulty breathing, which often occurs on inspiration but can occur on expiration. Cough, chest tightness, throat tightness, and changes in voice have been reported as well, though less commonly (Christopher & Morris, 2010). Symptoms may start and/or end abruptly. Children have presented with asthma-like symptoms and may be diagnosed with exercise-induced asthma. However, they report suboptimal response to bronchodilator therapy.

Diagnosis

Direct laryngoscopy performed at the time of symptoms is the gold standard for the diagnosis of VCD (Morris et al., 2006). Spirometry can be helpful in the diagnosis of a symptomatic child but will not be helpful for children who are asymptomatic at the time of testing. If symptomatic, spirometry will typically reveal a flattened inspiratory loop.

Management

Once the diagnosis is certain, children should be supported and reassured that the condition is benign and self-limiting. Precipitating factors should be identified and avoided. The child may be referred for psychotherapy or psychological counseling and/or speech therapy. Psychotherapy may include biofeedback or hypnotherapy as part of the treatment plan. A speech language pathologist (SLP) can help in the evaluation and treatment of VCD. Therapy usually includes exercises to help abort acute attacks. The SLP can also teach therapeutic exercises to help prevent future episodes.

For exercise-induced VCD, anticholinergic inhalers may be helpful (Doshi & Weinberger, 2006). For acute episodes, there are reports of sedatives and benzodiazepines being used successfully. Bronchodilators, steroids, and other asthma medications show minimal response, though heliox may afford a favorable response. In the event of a very acute onset of symptoms with the appearance of acute respiratory failure, children have been intubated. Often the symptoms quickly resolve and the child is extubated within 24 hours. There are reports of tracheotomy in the literature as well (Christopher & Morris, 2010).

Complications

Complications are secondary to the acute or ongoing treatment of the child before diagnosis, including the overuse of asthma medications, such as corticosteroids. In extreme cases when intubation or tracheotomy is performed, there may be airway or surgical complications to the procedure.

Vocal cord masses and lesions

Most vocal fold lesions are benign in children. This section will briefly discuss two of the more common lesions found in children: vocal cord nodules and recurrent respiratory papillomatosis.

Vocal cord nodules

Epidemiology
Vocal nodules are defined as a bilateral symmetric epithelial swelling of the anterior middle third of the true vocal folds (Seear et al., 2005). They can be found in children of all ages. They occur more frequently in females and in those who have high voice demands, including singers and cheerleaders; young adult patients may be teachers.

Signs and symptoms
Symptoms include chronic hoarseness and episodes of voice loss.

Diagnosis
Diagnosis is typically made by direct laryngoscopy. Ultrasound has recently been reported in the literature as a possible option for diagnosis (Bisetti, 2009).

Management
The main focus of treatment is voice therapy, addressing voice use demands, and minimizing contributing factors. Microsurgical techniques are rarely implemented; however, these may be necessary for suspicious lesions or for those refractory to treatment. If reflux is a contributing factor, a trial of antireflux medication, preferably a proton pump inhibitor, should be considered.

Recurrent respiratory papillomatosis

Epidemiology
Recurrent respiratory papillomatosis (RRP) is a chronic disease that affects children and adults. Incidence of juvenile-onset RRP is reported to affect 1 per 100,000 children younger than 18 years per year (Armstrong et al., 2000).

Pathophysiology
It is caused by human papillomavirus (HPV), with strains 6 and 11 being the most common. It is a somewhat rare disease but is the most common cause of laryngeal neoplasm (Altman, 2007). It is thought that a child becomes infected with the virus at the time of birth; however, the virus may remain latent for any number of years. There has been an association between maternal condylomata acuminata and subsequent RRP in an offspring, though some mothers do not have a report of anogenital or cervical warts (Quick, Watts, Krzyzek, & Faras, 1980; Hallden & Majmudar, 1986). Interestingly, there are many infants who are exposed to HPV during the birthing process but never go on to develop the disease, which speaks to other factors, such as immunity, viral load, and/or genetics that may play a role in the acquisition of the disease.

Signs and symptoms

Children typically present in toddlerhood or as a young adult (Derkay, 2001). Symptoms may include hoarseness/dysphonia, stridor, and/or respiratory distress.

Diagnosis

Diagnosis is typically made by direct laryngoscopy in the office. The warts are typically found in the larynx and are usually on the vocal folds.

Management

The warts may recur frequently, and children often have to undergo repeated laryngoscopy and bronchoscopy with laser excision to maintain their airway and to keep the disease in control. If left unchecked, the warts can grow large enough to obstruct the airway. There is a lot of variability in the course of the disease with some children having procedures monthly and others every few years.

Complications

Distal spread to the trachea is uncommon, but if this occurs, further narrowing of the airway and obstruction of the lung parenchyma can result. It is rare for the papillomas to undergo malignant transformation (Altman, 2007).

Subglottic stenosis

Subglottis stenosis is a narrowing of the subglottic airway, which is housed in the cricoid cartilage and is described as either congenital or acquired.

Epidemiology

Congenital subglottic stenosis is the third most common congenital anomaly of the airway. Males are affected twice as often as females. Occasionally, it can be associated with congenital abnormalities or syndromes such as Down syndrome (Miller, Gray, Cotton, Myer, & Netterville, 1990). Acquired cases of subglottic stenosis can occur at any age but most commonly occur in the early months of life. It is the most common acquired anomaly of the larynx in children. The true incidence of subglottic stenosis is not known, yet the incidence has been reported between 1 and 8% in neonates requiring endotracheal (ET) intubation for any reason (Cotton & Willging, 1999). The incidence has recently increased with the successful management of low birth weight and babies of earlier gestational age. Conversely, the incidence of the congenital form has remained stable. The population primarily affected by this anomaly is premature infants with immature lungs requiring long-term mechanical ventilation via an endotrachial tube. Subglottic stenosis is the most common abnormality requiring tracheostomy in children less than 1 year of age.

Pathophysiology

The cause of congenital subglottic stenosis is unknown. The infant airway is simply narrower than it should be, causing varying levels of respiratory distress. The severity can vary from very mild narrowing to complete atresia of the larynx. The etiology of the congenital anomaly is due to incomplete recanalization of the laryngotracheal structure in the third month of gestation (Healy, 1989). The anomaly can be divided histopathologically into membranous (circumferential submucosal hypertrophy of the subglottic area) and cartilaginous types (small or malformed cricoid cartilage).

A number of pathogenic processes such as trauma, inflammation, or iatrogenic insults may predispose a child to the development of subglottic stenosis. Endotrachial intubation is the most common factor responsible for acquired subglottic stenosis. The relative size of the ET tube in relation to the child's larynx, duration of intubation, motion of the tube, and number of repeated intubations have all been implicated as factors influencing its development (Healy, 1989). Other factors implicated in its development include factors affecting wound healing, laryngotracheal reflux, and infection (historically tuberculosis and diphtheria).

Signs and symptoms

Presentation and severity of symptoms will depend upon the degree of narrowing of the subglottic area. Infants with significant narrowing will have corresponding respiratory distress, including biphasic stridor, croupy cough, retractions, cyanosis, and nasal flaring. Feeding tolerance and appropriate growth can be affected and can be particularly troublesome during respiratory infections. In the most severe cases, it may not be possible for the infant to maintain a safe airway without intubation or tracheostomy.

Infants with mild to moderate subglottic stenosis may be completely asymptomatic with symptoms becoming evident only with an inflammatory process such as an upper respiratory infection. The infant's symptoms will mirror those of infectious laryngotracheobronchitis (croup); inspiratory or biphasic stridor; and croup, like cough with varying levels of respiratory distress. Subglottic stenosis should be suspected if events are recurrent or if they last for periods longer than 3 days, which is typical of laryngotracheobronchitis. Some children are identified due to difficulty with intubation and extubation. Hoarseness may be present in some infants if the scarring extends superiorly to the vocal cords.

Diagnosis

Definitive diagnosis of subglottic stenosis is made with rigid bronchoscopy (Figure 6.3). The stenosis is evaluated in respect to degree of narrowing, length of narrowing, and to rule out any other airway anomalies. The diagnosis is considered when a 4-mm scope (3mm in a neonate) or age-appropriate-sized ET tube cannot pass through the subglottic larynx

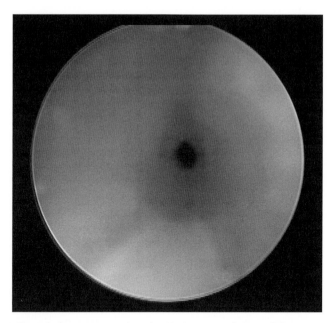

Figure 6.3   Subglottic stenosis (grade III). Courtesy of Samuel Ostrower, MD.

(Healy, 1989). Flexible laryngoscopy is not adequate to evaluate the sub-glottic area but is useful in ruling out VCP or other glottic and supragrottic disorders and is sometimes used during the same procedure as part of a comprehensive airway evaluation.

Radiological studies such as plain films or CT scans of the neck may be helpful in offering details regarding the length of narrowing, structural information about the larynx, and caliber of the airway (Zawin, 2000). Whenever possible, this information is gathered during the bronchoscopy. However, in severe cases where the scopes are not able to pass through the stenotic area, diagnostic imaging can help plan the ultimate intervention.

Subglottic stenosis is typically classified based on the degree of subglot-tic narrowing. Myer and Cotton describe a classification system for grading from I to IV (Myer, O'Connor, & Cotton, 1994). This system describes the stenosis as a percentage of the area that is obstructed (Table 6.4).

Management
Management of the child with subglottic stenosis is multifactorial and must be individualized. Infants and children with milder forms of subglot-tic stenosis (grades I and II) will only require supportive treatment during episodes of upper respiratory infections, and most will completely outgrow the disorder as their airway grows.

There are no medications that will cure subglottic stenosis, yet they may have a supportive role. The use of steroids and/or recemic epinephrine with supplemental oxygen may be indicated during times of increased

Table 6.4   Meyer–Cotton staging of subglottic stenosis.

Staging	Narrowing of subglottic lumen
Grade I	Up to 50%
Grade II	51–70%
Grade III	71–99%
Grade IV	No detectable lumen

symptoms with an inflammatory process or with anticipated/recent extubation (Cotton & Willging, 1999). They may be effective in reducing the edema in the airway and may lessen the need for more invasive treatment. Antireflux medications may also be indicated in any child with signs and symptoms of gastroesophageal reflux to reduce the possible increased insult to the airway.

In more severe cases of subglottic stenosis, surgical intervention is warranted to relieve the obstruction. Many factors are taken into consideration when considering surgical repair of subglottic stenosis. The procedure performed is based on the degree of stenosis, length of narrowing, child's age and weight, presumed etiology, general medical well-being, and coexisting anomalies (Healy, 1989; Hughes & Dunham, 2000).

The cricoid split (anterior laryngotracheal decompression) involves dividing the anterior cricoid ring in an attempt to expand the airway without the need for a tracheostomy. Laryngotracheal reconstruction is a technique that employs cartilaginous grafts (usually from the child's rib or thyroid cartilage) to stent the subglottis anteriorly and/or posteriorly (Koempel & Cotton, 2008). This reconstruction may be performed as a single stage or multiple stage repair based on the severity of stenosis. Cricotracheal resection with primary anastomosis is advocated in children with severe subglottic stenosis. Tracheostomy is performed to ensure a safe airway, bypassing the level of the obstruction, until a definitive repair or appropriate growth of the airway is achieved. Serial dilations of the subglottic area and/or the use of lasers may be useful as primary treatment or in combination with the procedures previously mentioned.

Endoscopic evaluation and treatments and less invasive procedures may be attempted in some less severe cases. This includes CO_2 or KTP laser treatment, dilatation, or balloon laryngoplasty.

Complications

Subglottic stenosis can be life threatening in extreme cases. Furthermore, viral illness and other upper respiratory infections may cause further narrowing of the airway, resulting in significant respiratory distress.

Laryngeal webs

Laryngeal webs are a banding of tissue across the larynx resulting in varying degrees of obstruction.

Epidemiology

The incidence of laryngeal webs is 1/10,000 births. Although laryngeal webs may be an isolated finding, it is commonly associated with other congenital defects, the most prevalent being chromosomal and cardiovascular (McDonald-McGinn, Zachai, & Goldmuntz, 2002). There is a known association of congenital laryngeal webs with velocardiofacial syndrome (chromosome 22q11.2 deletion, also known as DiGeorge syndrome) (Dyce, McDonald-McGinn, & Kirschner, 2002). Approximately a third of children with laryngeal webs will have an additional anomaly in the respiratory tract.

Pathophysiology

Similar to congenital subglottic stenosis, laryngeal webs are the result of failure of laryngeal recanalization in the third gestational month. This can result in either complete occlusion of the larynx by mucosal and submucosal tissue or partial occlusion by a thin, membranous web. Webs may occur in a variety of locations in the larynx, including most commonly the anterior vocal folds, posterior interarytenoid, or in the subglottic or supraglottic areas. Although typically congenital, they may be acquired secondary to a surgical procedure, intubation, or infection (corynebacterium diphtheria or *Bacillus cereus*) (Desuter, Veyckemans, & Clement de Clety, 2004).

Signs and symptoms

Symptoms depend on the location and degree of webbing that is present. Infants typically present with a weak or absent cry (Nicollas & Triglia, 2008). They may have varying levels of stridor and respiratory distress, including retractions, nasal flaring, and cyanosis. These symptoms are not positional.

Diagnosis

Fiber-optic laryngoscopy is useful in identifying a laryngeal web. Rigid laryngoscopy and bronchoscopy is employed for further evaluation of the web and the remaining airway. It assesses the web's location, thickness, and horizontal and vertical extent (Nicollas & Triglia, 2008). The remainder of the airway must also be inspected to rule out other anomalies. Genetic testing may be considered to rule out velocardiofacial syndrome in patients with anterior webs.

Management

Treatment may vary from lysis, excision, dilation, cryotherapy, and CO_2 laser to obliterate the web (Nicollas & Triglia, 2008). Surgical goals are to resolve airway obstruction and to ensure quality vocal function. Thicker webs may require stenting with temporary protection of the airway with tracheostomy. Revision procedures are sometimes indicated in more complicated or posterior webs.

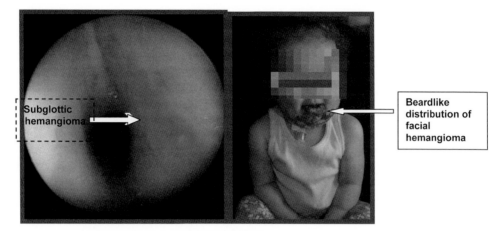

Figure 6.4 Subglottic hemangioma.

Subglottic hemangioma

Subglottic hemangiomas are benign vascular tumors found in the subglottis.

Epidemiology

Hemangioma of infancy is the most common tumor of childhood. There is a 10% incidence in infants. It is seen in all racial groups but is more common in Caucasians. Children with beardlike distribution of hemangioma have a higher incidence of airway involvement (Orlow, Isakoff, & Blei, 1997) (Figure 6.4). Fifty percent of patients with subglottic hemangioma have a concomitant cutaneous lesion, yet only 1–2% of patients with a cuteanous hemangioma also have a subglottic lesion. Laryngeal lesions comprise 1.5% of all congenital anomalies of the larynx (O-Lee & Messner, 2008). Females are affected twice as much as males. Hemangiomas of the tongue, choana, and palate may also cause substantial airway obstruction.

The proliferative phase begins at approximately 1–2 months of age and generally lasts up to 1 year. The involution phase is typically 5–7 years but may last up to 10 years (Bruckner & Frieden, 2006). Multiple skin hemangiomas may be associated with hemangiomas of internal organs, including liver, lungs, intestines, brain, spine, and kidneys. PHACES syndrome may occur in children with facial hemangiomas and involves coexisting abnormalities of the posterior brain (P), segmental facial hemangioma (H), arterial anomalies (A), cardiac defects (C), eye abnormalities (E), and sternal defects (S) (Frieden, Reese, & Cohen, 1996).

Pathophysiology

Subglottic hemangiomas develop as a result of a vascular malformation in the subglottis. They occlude the airway in one of two forms. It may develop in the submucosa of the posterior subglottis, causing anterior posterior obstruction. In other cases, circumferential hemangioma causes substantial narrowing of the entire subglottic airway (Hughes & Dunham, 2000).

Signs and symptoms

Infants are typically asymptomatic in the neonatal period; there is progressive respiratory distress as the lesion grows. Symptoms are similar to those of infectious croup and are manifested as biphasic stridor, barking cough, normal or hoarse cry, and failure to thrive. Approximately half of all children with subglottic hemangioma will have a cutaneous hemangioma of the head or neck (Hughes & Dunham, 2000).

Diagnosis

Rigid bronchoscopy is necessary for the diagnosis of subglottic hemangioma (Figure 6.4). However, flexible endoscopy is important to exclude other laryngeal or upper airway anomalies. Cardiac evaluation and other diagnostic tests should be considered to rule out PHACES syndrome. Plain radiographs demonstrating asymmetric subglottic narrowing may be suggestive of the diagnosis.

Management

Multiple modalities have been used over the years for the treatment of children with subglottic hemangiomas. Treatment is dependent on the child's symptoms, airway involvement, and response to other therapies. Observation is often appropriate for very small lesions that with time resolve with minimal sequelae. However, hemangiomas of the airway often require urgent treatment as persistent growth can lead to life-threatening airway compromise.

Propanolol, an oral nonselective beta-blocker was recently serendipitously discovered to induce early regression of hemangioma in the proliferative phase (Leaute-Labreze, Roque, Hubiche, & Boralevi, 2008). Multiple studies have verified rapid successful treatment, and propanolol is now considered mainstay therapy for children with hemangiomas (Friedlander, 2010; Jephson et al., 2009; Lawley, Siegfried, & Todd, 2009; Truong, Chang, Berk, Heerema-McKenney, & Bruckner, 2010). However, there have been treatment failures reported (Canadas, Baum, Lee, & Ostrower, 2010). Steroids have a long history of effectiveness in the treatment of hemangiomas in the proliferative phase. Unfortunately, they are known to cause significant side effects as well as potential rebound growth upon cessation of therapy (Buckmiller, 2009). Vincristine and interferon have also been used but are also associated with many side effects (Avila et al., 2003; Enjolras et al., 2004). Other options include laser ablation, cryosurgery, or open surgical excision (O-Lee & Messner, 2008). In the most severe cases, tracheostomy is necessary in order to bypass the lesion while awaiting involution.

Tracheomalacia

Tracheomalacia is an abnormal collapse of the tracheal walls due to weakness or floppiness of the trachea. It can be classified as primary (intrinsic) or secondary (extrinsic) (Benjamin, 1984).

Epidemiology

Tracheomalacia is a rare disorder, but the true incidence is unclear. There is no racial or sexual predilection. Primary tracheomalacia is predominantly a congenital disorder but frequently occurs following repair of tracheoesophageal fistula. Therefore, primary tracheomalacia tends to be a disorder of infancy. Most children will have resolution of symptoms by 1–3 years of age, as the tracheal cartilage normalizes and the airway enlarges. Secondary tracheomalacia is most common at birth due to vascular compression but may occur at any age.

Pathophysiology

Primary tracheomalacia is an intrinsic disorder due to an abnormality in the wall of the airway (Healy, 2000). Bernoulli's law of tubular fluid dynamics can explain this. As velocity increases through a constant area, the pressure on the wall of the lumen decreases. In children with tracheomalacia, the posterior mucosal wall of the trachea collapses into the airway as a result of this phenomenon, causing airway obstruction.

Secondary tracheomalacia refers to an extrinsic disorder causing an external compression on the trachea. Vascular rings encircle and compress the esophagus and trachea, resulting in tracheomalacia (Shah et al., 2007). The most common lesions include anomalous subclavian artery, double aortic arch, right aortic arch, and innominate artery compression (Mahboubi, Harty, Hubbard, & Meyer, 1996). Compression may also occur due to an expanding mediastinal tumor, cyst, or lymphadenopathy.

Signs and symptoms

Patients with tracheomalacia present with varying levels of respiratory distress. Patients exhibit expiratory stridor (wheeze-like) secondary to an insufficient tracheal lumen. As with laryngomalacia, the noisy breathing is frequently not present until 4–8 weeks of age, as airflow increases. Other symptoms mimic those of other airway obstruction and are naturally based on the degree of tracheal obstruction. Patients with mild to moderate tracheomalacia are sometimes mistakenly diagnosed with bronchiolitis or asthma; however, these children are differentiated as they are typically "happy wheezers" (airway wheeze; lungs are normally clear throughout), with normal growth and disposition despite persistent noisy breathing. The child's voice and cry are usually normal.

Diagnosis

Definitive diagnosis of tracheomalacia is made with bronchoscopy. The tracheal wall is visualized collapsing during inspiration and/or expiration.

Infants with vascular rings will have tracheal compression with pulsation. Furthermore, other lesions can be diagnosed or excluded under direct visualization.

Airway fluoroscopy can also be helpful in confirming the diagnosis. CT scan or MRI may be helpful in identifying the source and location of compression in children with secondary tracheomalacia, but the scan will not reveal the dynamic nature of the lesion (Zawin, 2000). Echocardiography is indicated in any child with cardiac involvement or a concern for vascular rings. Esophagoscopy and swallow studies may offer additional information regarding esophageal compression, disorders of the esophagus, and reflux.

Management

For the majority of children with primary tracheomalacia, watchful waiting is the best treatment. Bronchodialators are ineffective for children with tracheomalacia. The child will outgrow symptoms with maturation of the tracheal rings and growth of the airway. Systemic steroids may be indicated during episodes of airway inflammation with respiratory illnesses.

Children with severe airway compromise may require continuous positive airway pressure (CPAP). This can be accomplished with a face mask, ET tube, and, for severe tracheomalacia, a tracheostomy. The ET tube or tracheostomy will allow delivery of CPAP and may also act as a stent in some children, depending on the location of the malacia. Surgical correction of the compressing lesion is indicated in children with secondary tracheomalacia.

Nursing care of the child and family

Laryngeal and tracheal conditions

Children with airway disease may be at risk for potentially devastating and life-threatening situations. Paramount to the care of a child with airway disease is the education and the support of the child's family. It is imperative that the caregivers have the appropriate knowledge, education, support, and resources to care for their child. Of course, the depth of education and support to the family is dependent on the severity and chronicity of the child's disease. All families should receive detailed information regarding their child's condition; appropriate treatment including therapies, medications, and surgery; exacerbating situations; and when to seek medical attention.

Many children with laryngeal and tracheal conditions require lengthy hospitalizations. This often poses many stressors to the family including, but not limited to, anxiety/fear regarding their child's diagnosis and future, financial burdens, time off from employment, marital strain, separation from family life/other children, and guilt. Ensuring appropriate support of the family by providing consistent nursing care and providers as well as access to social work, religious supports, support groups, and counseling is essential. Families must also have a sense of control in caring for their child during lengthy hospitalizations. Unfortunately, many families feel overwhelmed in the hospital setting and are not sure of their role with their child in this environment. Nurses should empower parents to continue to provide love and care for their child and encourage them to be involved in the plan of care and decision making.

Successful transition from the hospital to the home is often dependent on the family's ability to provide essential care to their child along with a safe and healthy living environment. Many of these children will require continued complex care and/or assessment in the home setting. Nurses are instrumental in teaching families and caregivers the skills required to care for their child once they transition to the home setting. Professional nursing care often accompanies the child into the home setting as some children will require nursing services in the home setting, either via skilled home visits or private duty. Nurses play an essential role in caring for not only the child but also for the family of children with laryngeal and tracheal anomalies—from diagnosis to discharge and providing education, support, advocacy, encouragement, insight, and excellent nursing assessment and care.

UPPER AIRWAY INFECTIONS

Laryngotracheobronchitis (Croup)

Laryngotracheobronchitis, commonly known as croup, is caused predominantly by viral illnesses and is the most common cause of upper airway obstruction in children (Sobol & Zapata, 2008).

Epidemiology

The incidence of croup is estimated to be 1.5–6.0% and most commonly affects children age 6 months to 5 years, but can affect children up to the age of 12. Boys are affected 1.5 times more than girls (Knutson & Aring, 2004). Croup can occur at any time of the year; however, there is a seasonal variability with most cases occurring in the fall and winter (Roosevelt, 2007). Parainfluenza virus type I is the most common causative organism, responsible for 50–70% of cases. Other viral pathogens include parainfluenza types II and III, respiratory syncytial virus, adenovirus, influenza viruses A and B, and, less commonly, varicella, herpes simplex virus, measles, and enteroviruses. *Mycoplasma pneumoniae* may also be the causative organism in school-age children, though still relatively uncommon. In remote cases, bacteria such as staphylococcus and streptococcus are possible organisms and can cause a significant bacterial tracheitis (see Chapter 5), which is far more serious and can cause considerable airway obstruction, often requiring intravenous antibiotics and possible

intubation. Fungi and atypical bacteria are extremely uncommon pathogens for croup, and, if found to be the source of the infection, then consideration for an underlying immune deficiency should be made (Sobol &
Zapata, 2008).

Pathophysiology

The virus is transmitted via the inhalation route infecting the epithelial
cells of the mucosa in the larynx and trachea, and subsequently results in
swelling and inflammation. The subglottis is the narrowest part of the
pediatric airway and the only region of the airway bounded by a complete
cartilaginous ring; any swelling in this area can result in significant airway
obstruction. Even 1 mm of edema in the normal pediatric subglottis reduces
its area by more than 50% (Sobol & Zapata, 2008).

Signs and symptoms

The child with viral croup will typically present with a low-grade fever,
hoarse voice, cough, and coryza over the first 24–72 hours. There is a classic
"barky" cough notable, which intensifies at night. Most cases of croup are
mild; however, progression to inspiratory or biphasic stridor may occur
with increasing respiratory distress. Children tend to prefer to sit upright
and demonstrate an improvement in their symptoms in this position.
While most children have mild cases of croup, in some cases, respiratory
distress can become moderate to severe with the child developing nasal
flaring, intercostal and suprasternal retractions, and tachypnea. The severity of the symptoms is related to the degree of narrowing of the larynx and
trachea due to inflammation and swelling (Kliegman, 2007).

Diagnosis

Diagnosis is typically made by clinical history and exam; however, in some
cases, radiograph confirmation is necessary. The classic finding visualized
on the anteroposterior neck radiograph is the "steeple sign" (Figure 6.5),
although this is only seen about 50% of the time (Knutson & Aring, 2004).
This is due to the swelling and inflammation of the airway at the subglottic
region.

Management

The treatment of croup is directed toward reducing inflammation of the
airway. In most cases, children will only need supportive measures which
include fluids, antipyretics, rest, and letting the child assume a position of
comfort. Historically, pediatric providers advised parents to either provide
warm mist typically in the form of shower steam in a closed-door environment or alternately to provide cool mist or air by bringing the child out in

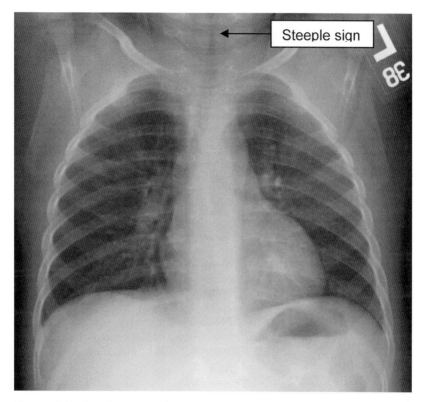

Figure 6.5 Steeple sign on chest X-ray (AP view).

the cold. Theoretically, cool air results in vasoconstriction of the airway with a resultant decrease in inflammation, soothes inflamed mucosa, and thins mucus; warm, humidified air may also soothe the inflamed mucosa, which in turn decreases coughing due to mucosal irritation, eases symptoms, and may allow for an easier air exchange and improvement of symptoms (Knutson & Aring, 2004). More recently, Scolnik et al. (2006) completed a randomized controlled study on the use of humidified mist for children with moderate croup, which showed no significant benefit.

If croup results in stridor at rest and/or a trip to the hospital, other therapies have proven to be beneficial. Use of corticosteroids has been studied and has been shown to have a clinical benefit within 6 hours of administration (Klassen, 1997). Steroids can be given in a variety of forms, including oral, intramuscular, or nebulized form. A single dose of 0.6 mg/kg of dexamethasone has been shown to be equally effective to the same dose delivered by intramuscular injection and has, in general, become the standard of care for children with moderate croup (Rittichier & Ledwith, 2000). Researchers have also looked at the potential for a lower dose of oral dexamethasone to 0.15 mg/kg with one study showing equal efficacy to higher dosing (Geelhoed & Macdonald, 1995). Nebulized budesonide has been compared to oral dexamethasone for the treatment of croup, and comparatively, both therapies were found to have similar decreases in croup scores and can be a consideration for treatment (Klassen et al., 1998). In addition, nebulized vaponephrine, otherwise known as racemic epinephrine, had been used for many years as a standard therapy for moderate to severe croup and continues to be used today. It works by decreasing mucosal edema by vasoconstriction and by reducing bronchial and tracheal secretions. Onset of action is typically within 10–30 minutes and generally lasts about 2 hours. Children given vaponephrine are observed in the emergency department for 3 hours after administration to ensure they do not experience a rebound effect when the beneficial effects of the medication subside (Kliegman, 2007). Heliox, a mixture of oxygen and helium, has also been used for children with severe croup in an effort to avoid intubation. This mixture of gas allows for easier diffusion of oxygen across the narrowed compromised airway (McGarvey & Pollack, 2008). In almost all cases, prompt appropriate treatment of croup results in excellent outcomes, and in very few cases, hospitalization or a more critical airway intervention such as intubation will be necessary.

If a child is not responding to routine therapy for croup, other diagnoses must be considered, including epiglottitis, bacterial tracheitis, airway burns, and structural lesions, which may have become more obstructive with laryngotracheobronchitis. Furthermore, with instances of recurrent croup, gastroesophageal reflux may be a contributing factor.

Complications

Complications from croup are very rare. In some instances, pneumonia develops. Most children do very well with standard therapy, but in the event croup becomes severe and respiratory failure develops, there is potential for complete airway obstruction and respiratory arrest.

Epiglottitis

Epiglottitis, also known as supraglottitis, is an acute and very serious illness due to infection of the epiglottis and adjacent structures (Rafei & Lichenstein, 2006).

Epidemiology

There has been a significant decline in the incidence of epiglottitis since the routine administration of the *Haemophilus influenzae* type B (Hib) vaccine in 1998. In fact, the incidence has reduced by nearly 80–90% for infection with invasive Hib disease. Previously, children aged 2–6 years were most likely affected, though there have been reported cases in children less than 1 year old and in older children (Kliegman, 2007). Epidemiology is changing and there has been a shift to the median age of the child to ages 6 and 7 (Gorelick & Baker, 1994). A recent retrospective study on the review of epiglottitis admissions revealed that epiglottitis is still a significant problem. Interestingly, it was identified that infants less than 1 year are the current population affected. The study noted a shift toward an older adult population, with males affected more than females (Shah, 2010).

Pathophysiology

In the past, the most likely causative organism was Hib. Hib infection is still reported as the etiology in both unimmunized and immunized children; however, in most cases now, childhood epiglottitis is more likely caused by other pathogens such as streptococci, staphylococci, and *Candida albicans* (Rafei & Lichenstein, 2006).

Signs and symptoms

A characteristic of this disease is acute onset. Classically, children present with a rapid onset of high fever, sore throat, drooling, muffled or "hot potato" voice, significant airway obstruction, and may appear toxic. They have stridor and usually do not cough. They often prop themselves forward in a tripod position to optimize air exchange with obvious mouth breathing and neck extension (Kliegman, 2007).

Management

If a child presents with symptoms consistent with epiglottitis, airway protection and preparation for securing the airway is essential. Children should be allowed to presume their position of comfort, and there should be avoidance of any interventions, such as an oral exam with tongue depressor or venipuncture, which may provoke or aggravate the child and may cause laryngospasm and severe obstruction.

The airway exam is often coordinated with the anesthesia and otolaryngology team and typically occurs in the operating room. Upon direct laryngoscopy, a cherry red epiglottis is often visualized. Once a secure airway has been established, intravenous antibiotics against B lactamase-producing pathogens should be initiated. Intravenous steroids may be used for management of airway inflammation. A complete blood count and blood culture should be obtained to determine the causative organism. If a lateral neck radiograph is performed, the enlarged epiglottis may appear as a "thumbprint." Children remain intubated for a few days until the infection is under control, inflammation reduces, and the child can safely maintain his or her airway (Rafei & Lichenstein, 2006).

Complications

Childhood epiglottitis has the potential for progression into deep neck space infections, respiratory failure, and death if left untreated.

Nursing care of the child and family

Upper airway infections

The child with an upper airway infection will require frequent respiratory assessment to evaluate for increased work of breathing or distress. Observing the child from across the room before approaching him or her is helpful for determining the actual degree of distress. For infants and toddlers, it is helpful to wait before approaching them to conduct a physical examination. Examining the younger child in the parent's/caregiver's lap can make the child feel more relaxed.

When conducting the assessment, the nurse should look for evidence of increased work of breathing, such as retractions, nasal flaring, and unusual positioning to support his or her airway. The nurse should also auscultate the lung fields for adventitious breath sounds, such as stridor, wheezing, crackles, or rhonchi, and should pay particular attention to the phase of respiration. Monitoring vital signs is also important. Often, the first sign of increased respiratory distress is tachypnea. Monitoring hydration status is essential because dehydration can lead to thickening of mucus and decreased airway clearance. Thus, intake and output should be monitored throughout the day.

The psychosocial support of the child and family is essential. The child is typically most comforted by his or her parents or primary caregivers and will benefit from their continued presence if possible. Furthermore, allowing familiar items such as pictures or a favorite blanket will help to comfort the child.

Education is also essential. The nurse should provide education and information to the parents/caregivers about their child's status. Additionally, the nurse should keep in mind that the preschool child will benefit from simple explanations, whereas the school-age child or adolescent will likely respond well to education about the illness and reason for hospitalization.

SINUSITIS AND RHINITIS

Every child seems to have a runny, congested nose sometime throughout the year. This commonly occurs from the fall to spring season. Parents become quite concerned over these symptoms and frequently seek medical attention and advice to address them. Pediatric rhinitis and sinusitis are largely responsible for many upper respiratory symptoms in children.

Anatomy of the nasal cavity and sinuses

The nasal skeleton consists of the nasal bones, the paired lateral cartilages, and the septal cartilage. The septum divides the nasal cavity into two halves. The lateral wall of the nose has three projecting divisions of bones known as turbinates, specifically the inferior, middle, and superior turbinate. The space below each turbinate is called a meatus. The middle meatus plays an essential role in the ventilation and mucociliary clearance of the sinuses, as all the sinuses, with the exception of the sphenoid and posterior ethmoid air cells, open into this meatus. The osteomeatal complex is a culmination of all the openings of the sinus ostia. Its patency or lack thereof, is responsible for many sinus symptoms and the development of sinusitis.

There are four pairs of sinuses that are air-filled bony cavities within the skull. They are lined with the same respiratory epithelium that lines the nose as well as the trachea, bronchi, and the eustachian tubes. This is specifically called pseudostratified ciliated columnar epithelium and, as we will further discuss, is the reason sinusitis and rhinitis are associated with lower airway and middle ear disorders and illnesses.

Each pair of sinuses forms at varying time frames during the course of a child's development. This information is essential to keep in mind when caring for a child with a suspected sinusitis as a sinus can only be responsible for symptoms if it is already developed and pneumatized. The maxillary and ethmoid sinuses are the only two that are formed at birth but are not aerated until 3–4 months of age. The ethmoid sinuses do not exist as a single cavity as the others but consists of several air cells. It typically reaches its adult size by the age of 12 years. The maxillary sinus continues to grow into puberty and by adulthood is the largest sinus with a volume of 15 mL. The sphenoid sinuses begin to form between 3 and 5 years of age and are fully developed at 7–8 years of age. The frontal sinuses are rudimentary before the age of 7 years and continue to develop into adolescence. It is not uncommon to see either a unilateral absence or complete absence of the frontal sinus without negative implications.

Sinusitis

Epidemiology

The epidemiology of sinusitis parallels that of the common cold (Mandell, Bennett, & Dolin, 2010). Upper respiratory illnesses occur in children on the average of six to eight times per year with 5–13% of these progressing into a secondary bacterial infection of the paranasal sinus (American Academy of Pediatrics Subcommittee on Management of Sinusitis and Committee on Quality Improvement, 2001). This makes sinusitis a frequent pediatric illness and a cause for many office visits. Due to the anatomical contiguity of the paranasal sinus with the nose, the term rhinosinusitis is often used to describe a sinus infection.

The definition of sinusitis has been subdivided by the American Academy of Pediatrics' "Clinical Practice Guideline: Management of Sinusitis." This guideline specifies the diagnosis, evaluation, and treatment of children between the ages of 1 and 21 years. The definitions are described below:

- *Acute Bacterial Sinusitis.* Bacterial infection of the paranasal sinuses lasts less than 30 days, in which symptoms resolve completely.
- *Subacute Bacterial Sinusitis.* Bacterial infection of the paranasal sinuses lasts between 30 and 90 days, in which symptoms resolve completely.
- *Recurrent Acute Bacterial Sinusitis.* Episodes of bacterial infection of the paranasal sinuses, each lasting less than 30 days and separated by intervals of at least 10 days during which the patient is asymptomatic.
- *Chronic Sinusitis.* Episodes of inflammation of the paranasal sinuses lasting more than 90 days. Patients have persistent residual respiratory symptoms, such as cough, rhinorrhea, or nasal obstruction.
- *Acute Bacterial Sinusitis Superimposed on Chronic Sinusitis.* Presence of residual respiratory symptoms with the development of new respiratory symptoms. When treated with antimicrobials, these new symptoms resolve, but the underlying residual symptoms do not.

Pathophysiology

When presented with a child with a suspected sinusitis, consider the pathophysiological factor that may be contributing or causing the illness. Infections within the sinus develops because of either a blockage of the "main river" that drains the sinus, specifically the osteomeatal complex, impaired function of the cilia that "sweeps" the sinus to prevent bacterial invasion, or changes in the quality of the secretions, which can "plug up" the sinus and hamper the function of the cilia.

Ostial obstruction can be related to mucosal swelling or mechanical obstruction. Mucosal swelling can be related to viral upper respiratory illnesses, allergic inflammation, inflammation from gastroesophageal reflux disease, cystic fibrosis, immune disorders, immotile cilia, facial trauma, exposure to cigarette smoke, or rhinitis. Mechanical obstruction includes choanal atresia, deviated septum, nasal polyps, foreign body, turbinate hypertophy, adenoid hypertrophy, and tumors.

Most cases of acute bacterial sinusitis are frequently considered to be bacterial complications of viral upper respiratory infections (Wald, 2008). Viral infections affect ciliary function and cause obstruction of the sinus ostia. This is due to the resulting inflammation and changes in the secretions, which interrupt drainage from the osteomeatal complex predisposing the child to the development of sinusitis (Lusk, 2010). The principle bacterial pathogens for acute sinusitis include *Streptococcus pneumoniae,* affecting 30% of children, and nontypeable *Haemophilus influenzae* and *Moraxella catarrhalis*, each accounting for 20% of cases in children (American Academy of Pediatrics Subcommittee on Management of Sinusitis and Committee on Quality Improvement, 2001). Other less common bacterial species include group A streptococcus, group C streptococcus, viridans streptococci, *Peptostreptococcus* spp., other *Moraxella* spp., and *Eikenella corrodens* (Wald, 2008). *Staphylococcus aureus* and anaerobic bacteria are seen more often in chronic sinusitis (Wald, 2008).

Gastroesophageal reflux disease is common in children suffering from recurrent or chronic sinusitis. Most children who demonstrate evidence of gastroesophageal reflux disease in addition to their symptoms of sinusitis have shown an improvement in their sinus symptoms once their gastroesophageal reflux disease was adequately treated (Phipps, Wood, Gibson, & Cochran, 2000). The exact cause and effect of gastroesophageal reflux disease and sinusitis is unclear. Research suggests that it is due to nasopharyngeal reflux affecting the sinus mucosa directly causing inflammation and edema and impaired mucociliary clearance. This leads to obstruction of the osteomeatal complex and to subsequent infection.

Allergic rhinitis has also been implicated in the etiology of sinusitis in children. Because of this association, it has been suggested that any child with recurrent acute or chronic sinusitis undergo an allergy evaluation with testing for perennial and seasonal allergies, especially dust mite, mold, animal dander, and pollen, which tend to be responsible for many symptoms of allergic rhinitis.

Otontogenic sinusitis can occur due to a periapical abscess or periodontitis of the upper teeth that can extend into the sinus cavity and cause a maxillary sinusitis (Wald, 2003). This is more typical in the adolescent population and can cause symptoms of acute sinusitis in addition to complaints of halitosis or purulent oral drainage from a potential oroantral fistula. Treatment would include drainage of the abscess and operative closure of the oroantral fistula. The child would also require antibiotic therapy.

Signs and symptoms

Uncomplicated viral upper respiratory infections are collaboratively agreed to last 5–7 days in duration. Symptoms usually resolve by the 10th day or are exhibiting significant improvement by that time. When respiratory symptoms persist beyond that point without evidence of improvement, a secondary bacterial infection is felt to have developed. Symptoms of bacterial sinusitis in children are different from those in adults and are difficult at times to distinguish from those of the common cold or rhinitis. They tend to be more nonspecific.

Fever can be present in association with purulent nasal discharge for at least 3–4 days. Headache may be identified in a child with a significant sinusitis, either above or behind the eye. Complaints of a headache should be explored in great detail as it is not uncommon for children's complaints of headaches to be frequently misdiagnosed as a "sinus headache," which results in inappropriate sinus treatment (Senbil, Yavuz Gurer, Uner, & Barut, 2008). Facial pain and facial tenderness is an unusual complaint of children. In highly symptomatic children, they may actually complain of a feeling that their face feels "funny" or "heavy" or like "there is someone sitting on their face."

A cough is frequently described in a child with acute or chronic sinusitis. Cough receptors are present in the pharynx, paranasal sinuses, stomach, and external auditory canals. Because of this, the source of the cough should be viewed holistically (Boat & Green, 2007). Lower respiratory stimuli include excessive secretions and an inflammatory response to upper respiratory infections or allergic processes. Chronic sinusitis, in particular, is responsible for complaints of a chronic cough, especially at night. The cough may or may not be productive and may not present with obvious signs of acute sinusitis (Pratter, 2006).

Additional signs and symptoms that can be seen and reported includes nasal congestion; malodorous breath; hyposmia/anosmia; ear pressure or fullness; fatigue; irritablitiy; snoring; hyponasal speech; mouth breathing; nasal discharge; purulent anterior or posterior nasal discharge that can also be evident in the orophayrnx; decreased appetite; erythematous, pale, and/or boggy nasal mucosa; and, rarely, maxillary dental pain.

On nasal examination, mucopurulent discharge emanating from the middle meatus may be appreciated.

Diagnosis

The diagnosis of acute sinusitis is often difficult and is based on a careful, thorough history and physical examination. Although a sinus aspiration and culture is considered to be the "gold standard" of diagnosis, this procedure is very painful and unreasonable in the pediatric population. Intranasal cultures are not indicative of the bacterial origin of acute sinusitis and are therefore not recommended (Brook et al., 2000).

The American Academy of Pediatrics Subcommittee on Management of Sinusitis and Committee on Quality Improvement Panel (2001) noted that diagnostic imaging is not necessary to confirm a diagnosis of clinical sinusitis in children less than or equal to 6 years of age. Plain sinus radiographs are not felt to be highly diagnostic as they are felt to be technically difficult to perform, especially in young children, making the accuracy of the images not definitive as they can be abnormal in children with mild upper respiratory illnesses. Their diagnostic value is further limited by their poor sensitivity and specificity (Brook et al., 2000). On the other hand, CT scans of the paranasal sinuses are advised for children with persistent and chronic symptoms, particularly if surgical intervention is being considered. A CT scan of the head may be indicated when signs and symptoms of sinusitis are accompanied by increased intracranial pressure, meningeal irritation, proptosis, toxic appearance, limited extraocular movements, or focal neurological deficits.

Anterior rhinoscopy is critical and can be performed with a nasal speculum or otoscope. The examination should encompass notation of the nasal turbinates, septum, quality of the mucus, and for obvious nasal polyps or bleeding. Transillumination is a diagnostic technique that has limited diagnostic use and requires unique expertise. A nasal endoscopy should be completed to investigate the presence of nasal polyps, hypertrophy of the inferior turbinates, septal deviations or spurs, and adenoid hypertrophy.

Allergy testing using either in vivo skin testing or *in vitro* blood tests should be considered in children with recurrent or chronic sinusitis to explore allergic contributing factors. Quantitative immunoglobulins including IgG subclasses should be completed as well to evaluate immunologic deficiencies. Evaluating for cystic fibrosis with a sweat chloride test is also advisable, particularly if nasal polyps are identified.

Due to the association of gastroesophageal reflux disease, a diagnostic laryngoscopy should be completed to investigate for evidence of reflux disease in the supraglottic region with the presence of cobblestoning, erythema, and inflammation. If debilitating symptoms of gastroesophageal reflux are reported and clinical evidence of gastroesohageal reflux disease is appreciated, referral to a gastroenterologist may be considered for a more in-depth evaluation with endoscopy.

A nasal mucosal biopsy can be completed to investigate ciliary function and structure. As this procedure requires sedation, it is often completed simultaneously with another surgical procedure in the operating room.

Management of acute sinusitis

Treatment of acute sinusitis is almost always medical. The goal of therapy is to restore normal mucociliary function, to eradicate the infection, and to improve the child's symptoms and quality of life. The American Academy of Pediatrics' "Clinical Practice Guideline: Management of Sinusitis" developed an algorithm for the care of children between the ages of 1 and 21 years of age with acute sinusitis, which is summarized subsequently.

Amoxicillin is recommended for children who have mild–moderate sinusitis who do not attend day care or have recently been treated with an antibiotic. This can either be dosed at 45 or 90 mg/kg/day divided in twice-a-day dosing. For children who are allergic to penicillin, other appropriate antibiotic choices include cefuroxime (30/mg/kg/day) in two divided doses or cefpodoxime (10 mg/kg/day) once a day. First-generation cephalosporins, such as cephalexin and cefadroxil do not provide adequate coverage against *H. influenzae* and should not be prescribed. Trimethoprim–sulfamethoxazole and erythromycin sulfisoxazole is not recommended due to pneumococcal resistance. While azithromycin is a frequently prescribed antibiotic, the Food and Drug Administration (FDA) has not included this medication for sinusitis (American Academy of Pediatrics

Subcommittee on Management of Sinusitis and Committee on Quality Improvement, 2001). The American Academy of Pediatrics Guidelines continues to endorse the use of azithromycin (10 mg/kg/day on day 1 and 5 mg/kg/day for the following 4 days once a day) and clarithromycin (10 mg/kg/day divided twice a day) for children with severe drug allergies.

Children being treated for acute sinusitis should demonstrate signs of clinical improvement within 48–72 hours. If a child fails to improve or actually worsens, the treatment plan should be reevaluated as the antibiotic selected may be ineffective or the child's initial diagnosis may have not been accurate. Children who do not improve on the initial treatment regime should have their therapy changed to high-dose augmentin. Dosing includes 80–90 mg/kg/day of amoxicillin and 6.4 mg/kg/day of clavulanate in twice-a-day dosing. For those children allergic to amoxicillin, cefdinir, cefuroxime, or cefpodoxime should be used. Ceftriaxone is frequently used either intravenously or intramuscularly with a single dose of 50 mg/kg/day if the child is very ill and unable to tolerate the oral medication. There is no standardized treatment course regarding the duration of therapy once an appropriate antibiotic is started. Empiric recommendations are for 10, 14, 21, or 28 days depending on the clinician's judgment (Wald, 2003).

Additional management strategies

Supplemental therapies are frequently advised in addition to appropriate antibiotics. While there has been no generalized acceptance of any of these treatments, many are recommended for children to address the debilitating and annoying symptoms accompanying the acute infection.

Nasal decongestants (afrin/neosynephrine)

These nasal decongestants are frequently used to provide temporary relief of nasal discharge and congestion. They can be highly efficacious. They are also addictive because of their immediate benefit. Therefore, their usage is limited to 3–5 days to avoid the complication of rhinitis medicamentosa. This is a rebound congestion that is progressive with continued use and actually worsens the congestion and sinus pressure.

Mucolytic agents

These medications aid in decreasing the viscosity of nasal secretions to expedite clearance from the nasal cavities. This helps to lessen the congestion and pressure the child is experiencing.

Nasal saline spray or saline irrigations

The use of nasal saline spray or saline irrigations can be adjusted to either a normal saline concentration or a hypertonic saline concentration for more aggressive irrigation. These are tremendously advantageous for the child with acute sinusitis. They are successful in mechanically clearing secretions, loosening crusted debris and mucus, and liquefying secretions. They can specifically address occlusions of the osteomeatal complexes, which are critical to reopen and to allow normal ventilation and drainage of the sinus cavities. They also promote vasoconstriction of nasal blood flow to reduce inflammation. At times, various additives into the sinus irrigations may be recommended, such as Pulmicort, Bactroban, baby shampoo, and various antibiotics or antifungal agents.

Antihistamines
Antihistamines are generally not advised for the child with acute sinusitis. They can actually worsen symptoms of sinusitis as they can dry nasal and sinus secretions preventing mucous clearance and aggravating sinus pressure and congestion. At times, a child may already be on an antihistamine for baseline allergic rhinitis. In such cases, the antihistamine can he held temporarily during the sinusitis treatment.

Topical nasal steroids
While nasal steroids clearly benefit a patient with allergic rhinitis by decreasing nasal mucosal inflammation, they are not recommended for use in a child with acute sinusitis as there is limited support for its use in the literature.

Oral decongestants (Pseudoephedrine/Phenylpropanloamine hydrochloride)
These decongestants constrict blood vessels in the nares to reduce nasal congestion. Presently, these medications are not advised in children due to their potentially toxic side effects, including cardiac stimulation, hypertension, and neurological complications (Brook et al., 2000).

Herbal and complementary therapies
Many families practice the use of herbal and complementary remedies; thus, the nurse or the nurse practitioner should always inquire about their use. Herbal and complementary therapies include a wide variety of treatments, including various soups, teas, as well as herbal and nutritional supplements, such as vitamin C preparations, zinc lozenges, echinacea, garlic, and eucalyptus oil. Families may seek additional holistic care from acupuncturists, chiropractors, homeopathics, naturopathics, and therapeutic touch therapists. While nurses and nurse practitioners are not able to specifically endorse these therapies as little research has been done regarding their benefits and there is no specific FDA approvals, it can oftentimes be comforting to families to supplement the prescribed medical therapies.

Management of chronic sinusitis/recurrent sinusitis

Antibiotics are used for children with chronic or recurrent sinusitis that is due to the occurrence of an acute exacerbation. Prophylactic antibiotics were considered in the past in the prevention of these exacerbations, but due to recent concerns of antibiotic resistance, their use is highly controversial. Systemic steroids have a place in the treatment of chronic and recurrent sinusitis, particularly in providing relief of the persistent complaints of sinus pressure and congestion. Intravenous antibiotics are sometimes used as an alternative to sinus surgical treatment. A study by Don, Yellon, Casselbrant, and Bluestone (2001) found that intravenous antibiotic therapy for the management of chronic sinusitis was an effective alternative to an endoscopic sinus surgical procedure. Nebulized intranasal antibiotics have also been used in the treatment of chronic sinusitis, but mostly in the adult population, with inconsistent results.

For children with associated allergic rhinitis that is precipitating their chronic or recurrent sinusitis, various oral or intranasal antihistamines, intranasal steroids, leukotriene receptor antagonists, or anticholinergic sprays may be used to supplement their care. These medication therapies should always be accompanied by environmental strategies for allergen avoidance and at times, if found appropriate, by immunotherapy. When children have gastroesophageal reflux disease as an etiologic factor to their sinusitis, appropriate medication therapy should be combined with an antireflux diet. Potential medications include proton pump inhibitors and H2 blockers. Food avoidance includes caffeine-containing foods and beverages, fatty foods, spicy foods, chocolate, citrus foods and beverages, and tomatoes. Children should not be allowed to eat right before bed and should make their final meal of the day at least 2–3 hours before bed. When these therapies are unable to control the allergic rhinitis or gastroesophageal reflux disease effectively, then a referral to a gastroenterologist or an allergist may be appropriate.

Surgical treatment

Children with chronic sinusitis who fail medical therapy may be candidates for surgical intervention. This includes the possibility of an adenoidectomy and/or a functional endoscopic sinus surgery (FESS). The adenoids can act as a reservoir for bacteria and can result in recurrent or chronic sinus infections due to the proximity of the adenoids to the sinus ostia (Ramadan, 1999). They have also been implicated as a source of biofilms acting as a repository for bacterial seeding (Lusk, 2010). A study by Ramadan (1999) found that endoscopic sinus surgery was better than an adenoidectomy for the treatment of refractory sinusitis in a select group of children.

Endoscopic sinus surgery has become a primary method of surgical therapy for chronic sinusitis following an adenoidectomy for those patients whose symptoms persist, although at times they may be completed simul-taneously. Absolute indications for endoscopic sinus surgery include (1) complete nasal airway obstruction in children with cystic fibrosis due to massive polyps, (2) antrochoanal polyps, (3) intracranial complications, (4) mucoceles, (5) orbital abscesses, (6) traumatic injury to the optic canal, (7) dacrocystorhinitis due to sinusitis and resistance to medical treatment, (8) fungal sinusitis, (9) some meningoencephaloceles, and (10) some neo-plasms (Lusk, 2010). There was a long-standing concern of altered facial growth in children undergoing endoscopic sinus surgery, but a study by Bothwell, Piccirillo, Lusk, and Ridenour (2002) found no evidence that endoscopic sinus surgery affected facial growth.

Complications

Complications of sinusitis occur more frequently in children than in the general adult population (Hengerer & Klotz, 2003). These complications are related to the anatomical relationship of the sinus to the other structures of the head, neck, and chest.

Orbital complications

A medial subperiosteal abscess of the orbit is the most common serious complication of sinusitis in children (Pereira, Mitchell, Younis, & Lazar, 1997). The presence of ethmoid sinusitis is largely responsible for the development of orbital complications, particularly a medial subperiosteal abscess. This is due to a direct and hematogenous spread of the infection from the ethmoid sinus to the orbit through the paper-thin bony plates separating the ethmoid from the orbit. Further classification of periorbital and orbital complications include preseptal inflammation, which is limited to the eyelid, and postseptal inflammation, which involves the structures of the orbit (American Academy of Pediatrics Subcommittee on Management of Sinusitis and Committee on Quality Improvement, 2001).

CT scanning is the preferred method of diagnosis of this complication. Symptoms can be limited to the tissues of the eyelid, causing periorbital edema and erythema. Progression of symptoms indicative of extension into the orbital structures can include fever, tenderness, proptosis, chemo-sis of the conjunctiva, diplopia, impaired visual acuity, and/or impaired ocular mobility.

Treatment of mild periorbital cellulitis requires treatment with antibiot-ics and nasal decongestants. If symptoms fail to improve after 24–48 hours, the child requires an admission for intravenous antibiotics and topical nasal decongestants. An opthamological evaluation should be included in the treatment plan. If a subperiosteal abscess is diagnosed, surgical drain-age is indicated. Many times, children may only present with symptoms over a course of 2–4 days before being diagnosed with a subperiosteal abscess, making prevention of this serious complication a challenge (Sinclair & Berkowitz, 2007).

Intracranial complications

Intracranial spread of infection from the frontal, ethmoid, or sphenoid sinuses can produce further complications, including meningeal irritation and infection, brain abscess, and peridural abscess (Hengerer & Klotz, 2003). Chronic sinusitis is the most common predisposing factor for the development of intracranial complications. The frontal sinus is largely responsible for most of these complications due to a frontal sinusitis. Infection may spread hematogenously or by direct extension. The abscess may be present over an exended period of time before treatment (Altman, Austin, Tom, & Knox, 1997). Since the frontal sinusitis does not begin to develop until the age of 6–7 years or older, complications of bony spread of the sinus infection over the frontal area only occurs in the older pediatric age group.

The symptoms of intracranial extension may be nonspecific with only a frontal headache. But when signs of sinusitis are accompanied by lethargy, progressive headache, decreased appetite, loss of interest, and altered consciousness, intracranial complications should be suspected. At times, a history of sinusitis may be absent in a child with intracranial complications (Altman, Austin, Tom, & Knox, 1997). Therefore, one should always keep it on their list of differentials.

Pott's puffy tumor is a rare clinical complication characterized by a subperiosteal abscess associated with osteomyelitis of the frontal bone that results in soft tissue swelling on the forehead and a doughy pitting edema (Karaman, Hacizade, Isildak, & Kaytaz, 2008). Once intracranial complications are suspected, appropriate imaging with either a CT scan or MRI should be performed to evaluate possible complications. Treatment includes intravenous antibiotics and surgical drainage.

Nasal polyps/antrochoanal polyps

Nasal polyps are an atypical complication associated with chronic sinus disease in children. They are more commonly seen in children with cystic fibrosis. Because of this, all children who present with nasal polyps should undergo testing for cystic fibrosis. Allergies can also be responsible for nasal polyps in the older pediatric population. Medical therapy includes steroids (nasal and /or oral), antibiotics, and saline irrigations (Chan, 2010). Surgical excision is indicated for children who have failed medical management and are becoming increasingly symptomatic.

Antrochoanal polyps originate in the antrum of the maxillary sinus and frequently extend into the middle meatus through the maxillary ostium. They are common in children (Lee, 2003). These polyps require surgical excision.

Nursing care of the child and family

Caring for children with sinusitis, especially chronic sinusitis, and their families requires much time, teaching, and support. For episodic acute sinusitis, once appropriate antibiotic therapy is provided, symptoms generally improve within 48–72 hours. But for children with chronic sinusitis, there is a greater need for continued education and reinforcement of the treatment plan. Children and families are often discouraged with the persistence of symptoms, and frequently, the treatment plan needs to be modified to the child's symptoms and response to the original plan of care. When working with children with chronic sinusitis, one needs to respect the sensitivity of these children to their own symptoms. They know the status of their sinuses better than anyone.

Daily sinus irrigations can make a significant difference in enhancing mucociliary transport, vasoconstriction, and promoting drainage and effective ventilation. Families frequently need reinforcement regarding this critical maintenance therapy as many times, once the acute symptoms clear, they become lax about this routine.

If associated precipitating diagnoses are identified, nursing care strategies in the care of these diagnoses should be emphasized. If specific allergens are identified, the family and child needs to have an individualized environmental avoidance treatment plan devised for them that is easy to follow. If gastroesophageal reflux disease is identified, specific food avoidances should be outlined for the child and his or her family, particularly for the adolescent who requires intensive reinforcement. Medication adherence should also be highlighted, especially in regard to completing the full course of antibiotic therapy.

Children and families need to be cognizant about proper hand washing as this can help lessen acute exacerbations. Finally, nurses are in a key position to gain the child's and the family's trust. This trust allows the child and the family to openly communicate with the nurse and to inform the nurse of any use of alternative therapies.

Rhinitis

Pediatric rhinitis encompasses diseases that result in inflammation of the nasal epithelium and can be associated with symptoms of sneezing, rhinorrhea, and nasal congestion. Rhinitis can be divided into two general categories: allergic and nonallergic rhinitis.

Allergic rhinitis is known to be an inflammation of the nasal passages due to an allergic reaction to airborne substances. There are two types of allergic rhinitis, called seasonal allergic rhinitis and perennial allergic rhinitis.

Seasonal allergic rhinitis occurs due to exposure to airborne allergens that have a seasonal pattern, such as in the spring, summer, and early fall, when airborne plant pollens are at their highest levels. Trees usually pollinate in March and in April, grasses in the late spring and summer, and ragweed during the last 2 weeks in August until the first frost. In the warmer climates and in the southern United States, trees may pollinate in the winter months. Also, consideration should be made for unique flora within individual regions that can contribute to allergy symptoms at different points in time.

Perennial allergic rhinitis occurs all year and is usually due to airborne allergens in the home. Therefore, patients experience symptoms throughout the year due to pet exposure, like dog and cat dander, cockroaches, mold, or dust mites. Dust mites are found in the highest concentrations in indoor areas and accumulate in bedding, mattresses, upholstered furniture, and carpets. Primary pets responsible for perennial allergic rhinitis are cats and dogs. Contrary to popular belief, nonallergic breeds of cats and dogs do not exist (Lasley, 2000). Cat and dog allergens remain in a room or home even when they are not physically present.

Nonallergic rhinitis occurs less frequently in children and encompasses a group of nasal diseases that is responsible for rhinitis symptoms without an allergic or immunologic cause. This can be further subdivided into anatomical and nonanatomical causes.

Nonanatomical causes

Atrophic rhinitis in an uncommon cause of rhinitis, especially in the pediatric population. It is associated with progressive atrophy of the nasal mucosa and underlying bone, which results in enlarged nasal cavities that become filled with foul-smelling crusts. It can also result from granulomatous nasal infections, chronic sinusitis, radical nasal surgery, trauma, and irradiation (Dykewicz, 2003). Drug-induced rhinitis results from various medications that cause nasal symptoms as an adverse effect. Typical medications in this category include some antihypertensives, ACE inhibitors, beta blockers, aspirin and other nonsteroidal anti-inflammatory medications, and oral contraceptives. While these may not be common in the pediatric population, they may be seen in some older adolescents. Some foods can cause rhinitis effects, in particular, beer, wine, and other alcoholic beverages. Gustatory rhinitis, which is a cholinergically mediated syndrome, precipitates a watery rhinorrhea that occurs immediately after the ingestion of certain foods, specifically hot and spicy foods.

Rhinitis medicamentosa results from prolonged use of topical nasal decongestants and causes debilitating rebound nasal congestion. When topical intranasal decongestants are used longer than 3–4 days, the patient experiences a rebound congestion that promotes a repeated cycle of reuse that only makes the congestion worse. Hormonal rhinitis can occur due to the hormonal changes of pregnancy or puberty or thyroid diseases, specifically hypothyroidism. Vasomotor rhinitis, also referred to as idiopathic rhinitis, causes persistent year-round nasal disease in response to environmental conditions. Symptoms include rhinorrhea, nasal congestion, and postnasal drip with minimal sneezing, pruritis, or ocular symptoms.

Infectious rhinitis causes nasal symptoms resulting from either bacterial or viral causes. The most common viral etiology is the common cold. Rhinovirus accounts for 30–40% of infections, coronavirus for at least 10%, and respiratory syncytial virus, influenza virus, parainfluenza virus, and adenovirus together for about 10–15% (Wald, 2003). Bacterial etiologies include streptococcal infection, pertussis due to *Bordatella pertussis*, diphtheria from *Corynebacterium diphtheriae*, *Chlamydia trachomatis*, and congenital syphilis.

Nonallergic rhinitis with eosinophilia syndrome (NARES) is characterized by year-round symptoms of rhinorrhea, nasal congestion, sneezing, pruritis, and occasional loss of smell. Nasal smears demonstrate eosinophils, but patients lack evidence of allergic disease by skin testing or by serum levels of IgE to specific environmental allergens. This is more commonly seen in adults and is not usually seen in young children.

Anatomical causes

Adenoidal hypertophy is a common cause of persistent rhinitis in young children, causing nasal obstruction with mouth breathing, snoring, and hyponasal speech with persistent rhinitis. Cerebrospinal fluid (CSF) rhinorrhea can be assessed after a significant head trauma or following intracranial surgery and causes a clear, watery unilateral rhinorrhea and. Choanal atresia is the result of a bony or membranous obstruction between the nose and the pharynx. It can be unilateral or bilateral and results in nasal obstruction. Nasal foreign bodies are a frequent occurrence in children where various items are lodged within the nasal cavity causing unilateral nasal obstruction and an eventual purulent foul smell, and, at times, bloody nasal drainage.

Granulomatous nasal lesions create nasal obstruction and chronic rhinitis and are seen in children with Wegener's granulomatosis and sarcoidosis. Nasal polyps can be unilateral or bilateral and are identified as grayish, grapelike-appearing sacs. As previously stated, they are not common in young children and, when seen, should carry a high index of suspicion for cystic fibrosis, particularly in children less than 10 years of age (Lee, 2003). The nasal congestion can become quite pronounced with nasal polyps and results in anosmia and a hyponasal speech. Septal deviation and turbinate hypertrophy are common and can cause varying degrees of nasal congestion and chronic rhinitis depending on the significance of the abnormality. Septal deviations can occur during delivery, can be due to positioning *in utero*, can occur congenitally, or can occur with facial trauma. Tumors, albeit rare etiologies of rhinitis, should always be in the differential, especially with the appearance of an unusual nasal mass or lesion. The most common malignant neoplasm in children includes rhabdomyosarcomas (Lusk, 2010). Others include neurofibromas, inverting papillomas, squamous cell carcinoma, sarcoma, lymphoma, and olfactory neuroblastoma. Also, congential lesions can include dermoid cysts, teratomas, gliomas, encephaloceles, hemangiomas, and meningoceles. In adolescent boys in particular, one needs to be alerted to the possibility of juvenile angiofibroma when there is a complaint of nasal congestion and significant nosebleeds.

Epidemiology

Allergic rhinitis affects 20–40% of children (Boat & Green, 2007). Vasomotor rhinitis occurs with the same frequency as allergic rhinitis (Weber, 2008). If one parent has allergies, the risk is 25–40% that their child will also develop allergic disease, and if both parents have allergies, the risk increases to 50–70% (Lasley, 2000).

Infectious rhinitis affects young children at a greater frequency than adults. A child can suffer 6–21 upper respiratory illnesses per year, which can vary with age, the number of siblings, and daycare arrangements (Wald, 2003).

Pathophysiology

Allergic rhinitis represents an inflammatory condition of the nasal mucosa as a result of an exaggerated immunoglobulin E (IgG)-mediated immune response to inhalant allergens (Luong & Roland, 2008). Allergens such as pollens are deposited on the nasal mucosa. A chain of immunologic reactions take place causing the release of histamine and other inflammatory substances. These directly act on nasal mucosal cells and nerve endings, producing localized symptoms of nasal discharge, nasal congestion, sneezing, and nasal pruritis. This reaction is also referred to as an early or immediate phase of the allergic reaction. Following the early phase, there is a quiescent period of a few hours followed by a late-phase reaction, which takes place about 4–8 hours later (Lasley, 2000). Additional inflammatory cells infiltrate the nasal mucosa, and once they are activated, there is a release of chemical mediators and a perpetuation of chronic inflammation and nasal hyperreactivation resulting in symptoms of nasal congestion and rhinorrhea.

The pathophysiology of rhinitis medicamentosa, nasal polyps, and NARES is not known. Hormonal rhinitis involves hormone-induced intranasal vascular engorgement and mucosal hypersecretrion. Vasomotor rhinitis is felt to be due to a reaction of the nasal mucosa to nonimmunologic stimuli such as strong odors, like perfumes, solvents or bleach, irritants, such as cigarette smoke, dust, and exhaust fumes, and changes in temperature or humidity.

Infectious rhinitis starts with a bacterial or viral agent that reaches the nasal mucosa by either direct contact with an infected source or via droplet inhalation.

Signs and symptoms

Symptoms related to a common viral rhinitis typically last 7–10 days. Symptoms include nasal congestion; nasal discharge that can be serous, mucoid, or purulent; sneezing; cough; sore throat; conjunctival inflammation; myalgia; malaise that affects appetite and sleep; and possible fever. The nasal and pharyngeal mucosa is erythematous, and the cervical lymph nodes may be enlarged and tender. The outer nares frequently become excoriated from persistent nasal discharge.

The classic symptoms of allergic rhinitis include rhinorrhea, nasal congestion, sneezing, postnasal drip, and nasal itching. Children will often complain of a sore throat from the postnasal drainage and present with a hyponasal speech from congestion, fatigue, decreased appetite, and, at times, poor growth. A chronic cough related to postnasal drainage and irritation of the larynx is also frequently encountered. There are many unique findings in patients with allergic rhinitis, which can also less commonly be evident in children with nonallergic rhinitis and sinusitis. Allergic shiners are darkened circles underneath the eyes from venous dilation and engorgement. Dennie–Morgan lines from periorbital edema causes folds underneath the eyes. The "allergic salute" is the appearance of a transverse nasal crease across the bridge of the nose as children frequently rub their noses in an upward motion in response to nasal itching and rhinorrhea. Nasal turbinates commonly have a pale, bluish, edematous appearance. Cobblestoning in the posterior oropharynx from lymphoid hyperplasia can be identified from postnasal discharge. Chronic mouth breathing results in a high, arched, narrow palate, a marked overbite, or dental malocclusion. Patients with perennial allergic rhinitis present with more nasal congestion and complaints of obstruction rather than sneezing and pruritis.

Diagnosis

Diagnosis of rhinitis always begins with a thorough history and physical examination to sort through the specific etiology of the child's symptoms. For infectious etiologies, diagnostic testing is not always warranted due to the self-limited nature of the disease process. Nasal cultures can be obtained if a bacterial source is suspected, and rapid diagnostic techniques can be utilized for respiratory synyctial virus, parainfluenza virus, and influenza virus. The diagnosis for CSF rhinorrhea would include checking for glucose as CSF contains glucose, or analysis for beta-2 transferrin, which is a CSF protein.

There are various diagnostic techniques available for allergic rhinitis, predominantly for children over 1 year old. Percutaneous (prick or puncture) skin testing provides immediate results. They can be limited in that children need to temporarily hold allergy medications prior to testing to prevent the risk of false-negative results, specifically montelukast and first and second-generation antihistamines. Intradermal testing is another method of testing but is not preferred over percutaneous testing. Radioallergosorbent tests (RASTs) or enzyme-linked immunosorbent assay (ELISA) are *in vitro* tests that measure specific IgE antibodies directed against an allergen. This method of testing has advantages over percutaneous testing as patients can remain on their allergy medications. It is also preferred for patients who suffer from severe dermatitis or dermatographism.

Measurement of total serum IgE or blood eosinophils are generally not useful as they may or may not be elevated in patients with allergic rhinitis. Nasal smears for eosinophils are suggestive of allergic rhinitis, but, as previously stated, they can also be elevated in patients with NARES. Nasal endoscopy is invaluable in assessing and diagnosing a child with rhinitis and can identify anatomical and nonanatomical etiologies.

Management

Treatment of the common cold is largely symptomatic. Acetaminophen and ibuprofen can address fevers and myalgias. Hydration is important to liquefy secretions, and normal saline sprays and irrigations can help clear secretions and relieve congestion. There are various medications available to treat influenza, including antiviral medications such as amantadine, rimantadine, zanamivir, and oseltamivir.

Treatment for vasomotor rhinitis can be difficult as it is challenging to find the right medication to address the child's specific complaints. Oral decongestants, topical anticholinergics, topical nasal steroids, topical azelastine, ipratropium, and saline irrigations are typically the best modalities to consider.

Treatment of rhinitis medicamentosa must first include discontinuing the use of the nasal decongestant. Topical intranasal steroids and oral steroids are typically used to relieve the subsequent rebound congestion, which can take a prolonged period of time. Reassurance and support must be provided to the patient to continue the treatment plan.

Gustatory rhinitis is effectively managed with topical anticholinergics and decongestants. For patients with NARES, intranasal steroid sprays are the most effective.

The mainstay for the treatment of allergic rhinitis, both for seasonal and perennial, includes environmental avoidance strategies, pharmacological management, and immunotherapy.

Environmental avoidance strategies

Environmental avoidance strategies are an essential adjunct for all allergic rhinitis therapies. This entails actions designed to help the child avoid the allergen or to limit significantly their exposure to it. Strategies for environmental avoidance are discussed in Chapter 7. Additional nonpharmacological treatment includes saline sprays and irrigations that can reduce congestion and improve mucociliary flow.

Pharmacological management

In addition to environmental considerations, medication therapy is frequently used to address debilitating allergy symptoms. The pharmacological treatment plan must be tailored to each individual child based on his or her specific symptoms and the severity of symptoms. The child should be reevaluated frequently to determine the effectiveness of the treatment plan and to allow for revisions based on the assessment. The specific classes of medications that are available include oral and intranasal antihistamines, oral and intranasal decongestants (discussed in Chapter 3), oral and intranasal steroids, intranasal anticholinergics, intranasal cromolyn, and oral leukotriene receptor antagonists (discussed in Chapter 3). Each class of medications has its own unique mode of action. The above listed medications can be used individually or in a variety of combinations.

Oral antihistamines are histamine H1-receptor antagonists that prevent histamine from causing the histamine-mediated inflammatory effects. They address allergy symptoms of rhinorrhea, sneezing, pruritis, and conjunctivitis. They have little to no effect on nasal congestion. They can be used on a daily basis or as needed, pending contact with a known allergen, either taken before or with the exposure. There are two subclasses of oral antihistamines: the first-generation and the second-generation antihistamines. The first-generation antihistamines are discussed in Chapter 3. The second-generation antihistamines are less sedating and have a longer duration of action, allowing once- or twice-a-day dosing. These include desloratadine, loratadine, fexofenadine, cetirizine, and levocetirizine. Intranasal antihistamines, specifically azelastine and olopatadine, can cause drowsiness and at times have issues with their bitter taste. They are unique in that they can relieve some complaints of nasal congestion.

Intranasal steroids provide multiple benefits that include relief of sneezing, pruritis, rhinorrhea, nasal inflammation and edema, and congestion. Medications in this class include beclomethasone dipropionate, budesonide, flunisolide, fluticasone, fluticasone furoate, mometasone furoate, and triamcinolone acetonide. They are typically used once a day and can take 2–4 days before their effects are appreciated. They have the best results when used consistently. Studies have been completed on the effect of growth suppression with the use of intranasal steroids, and overall, there is agreement that there appears to be no growth suppression when they are used at their prescribed doses. Also, local side effects of nasal septal irritation, epistaxis, and rarely, septal perforation are rectified by advising patients to direct the nasal spray away from the septum and toward the lateral nasal cavity in the direction of the ear on the same side.

When children present with severe symptoms of allergic rhinitis, a short course of oral steroids can be extremely beneficial to gain control of their symptoms until the maintenance medications can reach their peak effect. Intranasal anticholinergics, specifically ipratropium bromide, are very effective against rhinorrhea and have no effect on other nasal symptoms. Intranasal cromolyn is a mast cell stabilizer that prevents the release of histamine from mast cells. It is available over the counter and works by decreasing sneezing, pruritis, and rhinorrhea with some effect on nasal congestion. They require dosing four times a day but can also be used preventatively prior to exposure to a known allergen.

Immunotherapy

The final mode of therapy for allergic rhinitis includes immunotherapy, which is directed to alter the immune response to a specific allergen. Children who fail to achieve adequate symptom control with medications and allergen avoidance should be considered for immunotherapy, especially when symptoms are severe and cause many complications for the child. At times, children are unable or unwilling to take daily medications. Immunotherapy involves weekly or twice weekly subcutaneous injections of the allergens to which the child is allergic. This results in a stimulation of the production of IgG antibodies against the offending allergens and blocks the antigen from triggering an allergic response. The child and his or her family must be strongly committed to immunotherapy as it can take 3–5 years of therapy before a maximum benefit is appreciated (Dykewicz, 2003).

Complications

Rhinitis can lead to the development of acute sinusitis as swelling of the nasal mucosa and the accumulation of mucus may block the sinus ostia. Otitis media can occur from subsequent eustachian tube dysfunction, which causes negative middle ear pressure and accumulation of fluid and prevents the drainage of secretions (Ruckenstein, 2001). Asthma can be precipitated by rhinitis. The "unified airway model" hypothesizes that the upper and lower airways are an integrated system with similar physiological and pathophysiological mechanisms (Luong & Roland, 2008). Children with rhinitis, especially chronic rhinitis, develop lymphoid hyperplasia of the upper airways. Obstructive sleep apnea can occur when allergic rhinitis is poorly managed. Anosmia can occur due to nasal obstruction and a hyponasal speech can develop.

Nursing care of the child and their family

Education is the mainstay of nursing care for children with rhinitis and their families. Education can help to achieve better adherence to the treatment plan. Taking a child and family through the plan in a step-by-step fashion is essential. This is particularly true with allergy avoidance as many patients can be overwhelmed by having to change their living situation.

REFERENCES

Abu-Hasan, M., Tannous, B., & Weinberger, M. (2005). Exercise-induced dyspnea in children and adolescents: If not asthma then what? *Annals of Allergy, Asthma & Immunology, 94*, 366–371.

Altman, K., Wetmore, R., & Mahboubi, S. (1998). Comparison of endoscopy and radiographic fluoroscopy in the evaluation of pediatric congenital airway abnormalities. *International Journal of Pediatric Otorhinolaryngology, 44,* 43–46.

Altman, K. W. (2007). Vocal fold masses. *Otolaryngology Clinics of North America, 40*(5), 1091–1108.

Altman, K. W., Austin, M. B., Tom, L. W. C., & Knox, G. W. (1997). Complications of frontal sinusitis in adolescents: Case presentations and treatment options. *International Journal of Pediatric Otorhinolaryngology, 41,* 9–20.

American Academy of Pediatrics Subcommittee on Management of Sinusitis and Committee on Quality Improvement. (2001). Clinical practice guideline: Management of sinusitis. *Pediatrics, 108*(3), 798–807.

Andresen, H., Cyr, M., Guadagnini, J., Hickey, M., Higgins, T., Huntoon, M. et al. (2008). General history, risk factors and normal physical assessment. In L. Harris and M. Huntoon (Eds.), *Core curriculum for otorhinolaryngology and head-neck nursing* (2nd edition, p. 64). New Smyrna Beach, FL: Society of Otorhinolaryngology and Head-Neck Nurses.

Armstrong, LR, Preston, EJ, Reichert, M, Phillips, DL, Nisenbaum, R, Todd, NW, et al. (2000). Incidence and prevalence of recurrent respiratory papillomatosis among children in Atlanta and Seattle. *Clinical Infectious Diseases, 31*(1), 107–109.

Avila, L., Gutierrez, J., Diaz, M., Encinas, J., Luis, A., Rivas, S., et al. (2003). Severe complications in the treatment of vascular anomalies. *Pediatrics, 16,* 169–174.

Becker, W., Naumann, H. H., & Pfaltz, C. (1989). Ear nose and throat diseases. In W. Becker, H. Naumann, & C. Pfaltz (Eds.), *Ear, nose and throat diseases* (pp. 386–454). New York: Thieme Medical.

Benjamin, B. (1984). Tracheomalacia in infants and children. *Annals of Otolarygology Rhinology Laryngology, 93,* 438–442.

Bisetti, M. S. (2009). Non-invasive assessment of benign vocal fold lesions in children by means of ultrasonography. *International Journal of Pediatric Otorhinolaryngology, 73*(8), 1160–1162.

Boat, T. F., & Green, T. P. (2007). Chronic or recurrent respiratory symptoms. In R. Kliegman, R. Behrman, H. Jenson, & B. Stanton (Eds.), *Nelson textbook of pediatrics* (18th ed.). Chapter 381. Philadelphia: Saunders.

Bothwell, M. R., Piccirillo, J. F., Lusk, R. P., & Ridenour, B. D. (2002). Long-term outcome of facial growth after functional endoscopic sinus surgery. *Otolaryngology-Head and Neck Surgery, 126*(6), 628–634.

Botma, M., Kishore, A., Kubba, H., & Geddes, N. (2000). The role of fibreoptic laryngoscopy in infants with stridor. *International Journal of Pediatric Otolaryngology, 55,* 17–20.

Bower, C. M., Choi, S. S., & Cotton, R. T. (1994). Arytenoidectomy in children. *The Annals of Otology, Rhinology, and Laryngology, 103*(4, Pt 1), 271–278. Abstract.

Brigger, M. T., & Hartnick, C. J. (2002). Surgery for pediatric vocal cord paralysis: A meta-analysis. *Otolaryngology Head Neck Surgery, 126*(4), 349–355.

Brook, I., Gooch, W. M., Jenkins, S. G., Pichichero, M. E., Reiner, S. A., Sher, L., et al. (2000). Medical management of acute bacterial sinusitis recommendations of a clinical advisory committee on pediatric and adult sinusitis. *The Annals of Otology, Rhinology, and Laryngology, 109*, 2–20.

Brown, O. (2000). Structure and function of the upper airway. In R. Wetmore, H. Muntz, T. McGill, W. Postic, G. Healy, & R. Lusk (Eds.), *Pediatric otolaryngology: Principles and practice pathways* (pp. 679–688). New York: Thieme.

Bruckner, A., & Frieden, I. (2006). Infantile hemangioma. *Journal of the American Academy of Dermatology, 55*, 671–682.

Buckmiller, L. (2009). Propranolol treatment for infantile hemangiomas. *Current Opinions in Otolaryngology Head and Neck Surgery, 17*(6), 458–459.

Canadas, K., Baum, E., Lee, S., & Ostrower, S. T. (2010). Case report: Treatment failure using propanolol for treatment of focal subglottic hemangioma. *International Journal of Pediatric Otorhinolaryngology, 74*, 956–958.

Cavanaugh, F. (1955). Vocal palsies in children. *The Journal of Laryngology and Otology, 69*, 399–418.

Chan, Y. (2010). Nasal and sinus infections, pain, pressure. In K. J. Lee & Y. Chan (Eds.), *Health care reform through practical clinical guidelines ear nose throat* (pp. 201–207). San Diego, CA: Plural Publishing.

Chen, E., & Inglis, A. (2008). Bilateral vocal cord paralysis in children. *Otolaryngologic Clinics of North America, 41*(5), 889–901.

Christopher, K. L., & Morris, M. J. (2010). Vocal cord dysfunction, paradoxic vocal fold motion, or laryngomalacia? Our understanding requires and interdisciplinary approach. *Otolaryngoilogic Clinics of North America, 43*(1), 43–46.

Contensin, P., Gumpert, L., Gaudemar, I., Chaussain, M., & Dupont, C. (1997). Non-endoscopic techniques for the evaluation of the pediatric airway. *International Journal of Pediatric Otolaryngology, 41*, 347–352.

Cotton, R., & Willging, J. P. (1999). Subglottic stenosis in the pediatric patient. In A. Chinski & R. Eavy (Eds.), *II manual of pediatric otorhinolaryngology of the IAPO* (pp. 143–154). Buenos Aires: Interamerican Associationof Pediatric Otorhinolaryngology.

Daya, H., Hosni, A., Bejar-Solar, I., Evans, J., & Bailey, C. (2000). Pediatric vocal fold paralysis: A long-term retrospective study. *Archives of Otolaryngology— Head & Neck Surgery, 126*(1), 21–25.

de Jong, A. L., Kuppersmith, R. B., Sulek, M., & Friedman, E. M. (2000). Vocal cord paralysis in infants and children. *Otolaryngologic Clinics of North America, 33*, 131–149.

Derkay, C. S. (2001). Recurrent respiratory papillomatosis. *Laryngoscope, 111*(1), 57–69.

Desuter, G., Veyckemans, F., & Clement de Clety, S. (2004). Laryngeal web as a cause of upper airway obstruction in children. *Paediatric Anaesthesiology, 14*, 528–529.

Don, D. M., Yellon, R. F., Casselbrant, M. L., & Bluestone, C. D. (2001). Efficacy of a stepwise protocol that includes intravenous antibiotic therapy for the management of chronic sinusitis in children and adolescents. *Archives of Otolaryngology—Head & Neck Surgery, 127*, 1093–1098.

Doshi, D. R., & Weinberger, M. M. (2006). Long-term outcome of vocal cord dysfunction. *Annals of Allergy, Asthma & Immunology, 96*, 794–799.

Dyce, O., McDonald-McGinn, D., & Kirschner, R. (2002). Otolaryngologic manifestations of the 22q11.2 deletion syndrome. *Archives of Otolaryngology—Head & Neck Surgery, 128*(12), 1408–1412.

Dykewicz, M. S. (2003). Rhinitis and sinusitis. *Journal of Clinical Immunology, 111*(2), S520–S529.

Enjolras, O., Breviere, G., Roger, G., Tovi, M., Pellegrino, B., Varotti, E., et al. (2004). Vincristine treatment for function and life-threatening infantile hemangioma. *Archives Pediatrics, 11*, 99–107.

Frieden, I., Reese, V., & Cohen, D. (1996). PHACES syndrome: The association of posterior fossa brain malformations, hemangiomas, arterial anomalies, coarctation of the aorta and cardiac defects, and eye abnormalities. *Archives of Dermatology, 132*, 307–311.

Friedlander, S. (2010). Propranolol may benefit those with severe infantile hemangiomas. *Journal of Pediatrics, 156*(3), 506–507.

Gavin, L. A., Wamboldt, M., Brugman, S., et al. (1998). Psychological and family characteristics of adolescents with vocal cord dysfunction. *The Journal of Asthma, 35*, 409–417. Abstract.

Geelhoed, G. C., & Macdonald, W. B. (1995). Oral dexamethasone in the treatment of croup: 0.15 mg/kg versus 0.3 mg/kg versus 0.6 mg/kg. *Pediatric Pulmonology, 20*, 362–368. Abstract.

Giannoni, C., Sulek, M., Friedman, E., & Duncan, N. (1998). Gastroesophageal reflux associated with laryngomalacia: A prospective study. *International Journal of Pediatric Otolaryngology, 43*, 11–20.

Gorelick, M. H., & Baker, M. D. (1994). Epiglottitis in children, 1979 through 1992: Effects of *Haemophilus influenzae* type b immunization. *Archives of Pediatrics & Adolescent Medicine, 148*, 47–50.

Gupta, A. K., Mann, S. B., & Nagarkar, N. (1997). Surgical management of bilateral immobile vocal folds and long-term follow-up. *The Journal of Laryngology and Otology, 111*(5), 474–477. Abstract.

Hallden, C., & Majmudar, B. (1986). The relationship between juvenile laryngeal papillomatosis and maternal condylomata acuminata. *The Journal of Reproductive Medicine, 31*(9), 804–807.

Hartnick, C. J., Brigger, M. T., Willging, J. P., Cotton, R. T., & Myer, C. M. (2003). Surgery for pediatric vocal cord paralysis: A retrospective review. *The Annals of Otology, Rhinology, and Laryngology, 112*(1), 1–6. Abstract.

Healy, G. (1989). Subglottic stenosis. *The Otolaryngology Clinics of North America, 22*(3), 599–606.

Healy, G. (2000). Introduction to disorders of the upper airway. In R. Wetmore, H. Muntz, T. McGill, W. Potsic, G. Healy, & R. Lusk (Eds.), *Pediatric otolaryngology: Principles and practice pathways* (pp. 763–774). New York: Thieme.

Hengerer, A. S., & Klotz, D. A. (2003). Complications of nasal and sinus infections. In C. D. Bluestone, S. E. Stool, C. M. Alper, E. M. Arjmand, M. L. Casselbrant, J. E. Dohar, & R. F. Yellon (Eds.), *Pediatric otolaryngology* (4th ed., Vol. 2, pp. 1021–1031). Philadephia: W.B. Saunders.

Hicks, M., Brugman, S. M., & Katial, R. (2008). Vocal cord dysfunction/paradoxical vocal fold motion. *Primary Care: Clinics in Office Practice, 35*, 81–103.

Hollinger, L. D., Holinger, P. C., & Holinger, P. H. (1976). Etiology of bilateral abductor vocal cord paralysis in children 1 year of age and younger. *The Annals of Otology, Rhinology, and Laryngology, 85*, 428–436.

Hughes, C., & Dunham, M. (2000). Congenital anomalies of the larynx and trachea. In R. Wetmore, H. Muntz, T. McGill, W. Potsic, G. Healy, & R. Lusk (Eds.), *Pediatric otolaryngology: Principles and practice pathways* (pp. 775–786). New York: Thieme.

Inglis, A. F., Perkins, J. A., Manning, S. C., et al. (2003). Endoscopic posterior cricoid split and rib grafting in 10 children. *Laryngoscope, 113*(11), 2004–2009. Abstract.

Jephson, C., Manunza, F., Syed, S., Mills, N., Harper, J., & Hartley, B. (2009). Successful treatment of isolated subglottic haemangioma with propranolol alone. *International Journal of Pediatric Otorhinolaryngology, 73*, 1821–1823.

Karaman, E., Hacizade, Y., Isildak, H., & Kaytaz, A. (2008). Pott's puffy tumor. *Journal of Craniofacial Surgery, 19*(6), 1694–1697.

Karkos, P., Leong, S., Apostolidou, M., & Apostolidis, T. (2006). Laryngeal manifestations and pediatric laryngopharyngeal reflux. *American Journal of Otolaryngology—Head and Neck Medicine and Surgery, 27*, 200–203.

Klassen, T. P. (1997). Recent advances in the treatment of bronchiolitis and laryngitis. *Pediatric Clinics of North America, 44*, 249–261.

Klassen, T. P., Craig, W. R., Moher, D., Osmond, M. H., Pasterkamp, H., Sutcliffe, T. et al. (1998). Nebulized budesonide and oral dexamethasone for treatment of croup: A randomized controlled trial. *JAMA, 279*, 1629–1632. Abstract.

Knutson, D., & Aring, A. (2004). Viral croup. *American Family Physicians, 69*(3), 535–540.

Koempel, J., & Cotton, R. (2008). History of pediatric laryngotracheal reconstruction. *Otolaryngology Clinics of North America, 41*, 825–835.

Lacy, T. J., & McManis, S. E. (2004). Psychogenic stridor. *General Hospital Psychiatry, 16*, 213–223.

Lasley, M. V. (2000). Allergic and nonallergic rhinitides. In L. C. Altman, J. W. Becker, & P. V. Williams (Eds.), *Allergy in primary care* (pp. 109–119). Philadelphia: W.B. Saunders.

Lawley, L., Siegfried, E., & Todd, J. (2009). Propranolol treatment for hemangioma of infancy: Risks and recommendations. *Pediatric Dermatology, 26*(5), 610–614.

Leaute-Labreze, C., de la Roque, E., Hubiche, T., & Boralevi, F. (2008). Propranolol for severe hemangiomas of infancy. *New England Journal of Medicine, 358*, 2649–2651.

Lee, K. J. (2003). Pediatric otolaryngology. In K. J. Lee (Ed.), *Essential otolaryngology head and neck surgery* (8th ed., pp. 811–861). New York: McGraw-Hill.

Luong, A., & Roland, P. S. (2008). The link between allergic rhinitis and chronic otitis media with effusion in atopic patients. *Otolaryngologic Clinics of North America, 41*, 311–323.

Lusk, R. P. (2010). Pediatric chronic sinusitis. In R. S. Gaertner, R. Halpine, & P. W. Flint (Eds.), *Cummings otolaryngology: Head & neck surgery* (5th ed.). Chapter 195. Philadelphia: Mosby.

Mahboubi, S., Harty, M. P., Hubbard, A. M., & Meyer, J. S. (1996). Innominate artery compression of the trachea in infants. *International Journal of Pediatric Otolaryngology, 35*, 197–205.

Mandell, G. L., Bennett, J. W., & Dolin, R. (2010). Sinusitis. In G. L. Mandell, J. E. Bennett, & R. Dolin (Eds.), *Mandell, Douglas, and Bennett's principles and practice of infectious diseases* (7th ed.). Chapter 58. Philadelphia: Churchill Livingston.

Mathur, N. N., Kumar, S., & Bothra, R. (2004). Simple method of vocal cord lateralization in bilateral abductor cord paralysis in pediatric patients. *International Journal of Pediatric Otorhinolaryngology, 68*(1), 15–20. Abstract.

McDonald-McGinn, D., Zachai, E., & Goldmuntz, E. (2002). Chromosomal and cardiovascular anomalies associated with congenital laryngeal web. *International Journal of Pediatric Otolaryngology, 66*, 23–27.

McFadden, E. R., & Zawadski, D. K. (1996). Vocal cord dysfunction masquerading as exercise-induced asthma: A physiologic cause for "choking" during athletic activities. *American Journal of Respiratory and Critical Care Medicine, 153*, 942–947.

McGarvey, J., & Pollack, C. (2008). Heliox in airway management. *Emergency Medicine Clinics of North America, 26*(4), 905–920.

Miller, R., Gray, S., Cotton, R., Myer, C., & Netterville, J. (1990). Subglottic stenosis and Down Syndrome. *American Journal of Otolaryngology—Head and Neck Medicine and Surgery, 11*, 274–277.

Morris, M. J., Deal, L. E., Bean, D. R., et al. (1999). Vocal cord dysfunction in patients with exertional dyspnea. *Chest, 116*(6), 1676–1682.

Morris, M. J., Perkins, P. J., & Allan, P. F. (2006). Vocal cord dysfunction: Etiologies and treatment. *Clinical Pulmonary Medicine, 13*, 73–86.

Murty, G. E., Shinkwin, C., & Gibbin, K. P. (1994). Bilateral vocal fold paralysis in infants: Tracheostomy or not? *The Journal of Laryngology and Otology, 108*, 329–331.

Myer, C. M., O'Connor, D. M., & Cotton, R. T. (1994). Proposed grading system for subglottic stenosis based on endotracheal tube sizes. *Annals of Otol Rhinol Laryngology, 103*, 319.

Nicollas, R., & Triglia, J. (2008). The anterior laryngeal webs. *Otolaryngology Clinics of North America, 41*, 877–888.

O'Donnell, S., Murphy, J., Bew, S., & Knight, L. (2007). Aryepiglottoplasty for laryngomalacia: Results and recommendations following a case series of 84. *International Journal of Pediatric Otolaryngology, 71*, 1271–1275.

O-Lee, T., & Messner, A. (2008). Subglottic hemangioma. *Otolaryngology Clinics of North America, 41*, 903–911.

Orlow, S., Isakoff, M., & Blei, F. (1997). Increased risk of symptomatic hemangiomas of the airway in association with cutaneous hemangiomas in a "beard" distribution. *Journal of Pediatrics, 131*, 643–646.

Papsin, B., Abel, S., & Leighton, S. (1999). Diagnostic value of infantile stridor: A perceptual test. *International Journal of Pediatric Otolaryngology, 51*, 33–39.

Parikh, S. (2004). Pediatric unilateral vocal fold immobility. *Otolaryngologic Clinics of North America, 37*(1), 203–215.

Pereira, K. D., Mitchell, R. B., Younis, R. T., & Lazar, R. H. (1997). Management of medial subperiosteal abscess of the orbit in children-a 5 year experience. *International Journal of Pediatric Otorhinolaryngology, 38,* 247–254.

Phipps, C. D., Wood, W. E., Gibson, W. S., & Cochran, W. J. (2000). Gastroesophageal reflux contributing to chronic sinus disease in children. *Archives of Otolaryngology—Head & Neck Surgery, 126,* 831–836.

Pratter, M. R. (2006). Chronic upper airway cough syndrome secondary to rhinosinus diseases (previously referred to as postnasal drip syndrome) ACCP evidence-based clinical practice guidelines. *Chest, 129*(1), 1–12.

Quick, C. A., Watts, S. L., Krzyzek, R. A., & Faras, A. J. (1980). Relationship between condylomata and laryngeal papillomata. Clinical and molecular virological evidence. *The Annals of Otology, Rhinology, and Laryngology, 89*(5, Pt 1), 467–471.

Rafei, K., & Lichenstein, R. (2006). Airway infectious disease emergencies. *Pediatric Clinics of North America, 53*(2), 215–242.

Ramadan, H. H. (1999). Adenoidectomy vs endoscopic sinus surgery for the treatment of pediatric sinusitis. *Archives of Otolaryngology—Head & Neck Surgery, 125,* 1208–1211.

Richter, G., & Thompson, D. (2008). The surgical management of laryngomalacia. *Otolaryngology Clinics of North America, 41,* 837–864.

Rittichier, K. K., & Ledwith, C. A. (2000). Outpatient treatment of moderate croup with dexamehasone: Intramuscular versus oral dosing. *Pediatrics, 106,* 1344–1348. Abstract.

Roger, G., Denoyelle, F., & Triglia, J. (1995). Severe laryngolmalacia: Surgical indications and results in 115 patients. *Laryngoscope, 105,* 1111–1117.

Roosevelt, G. E. (2007). Acute inflammatory upper airway obstruction. In R. K. Kliegman & R. Behrman (Eds.), *Nelson textbook of pediatrics* (18th edition, pp. 1762–1766). Philadelphia: Saunders.

Rubin, A., & Sataloff, R. (2007). Vocal fold paresis and paralysis. *Otolaryngology Clinics of North America, 40,* 1109–1131.

Ruckenstein, M. J. (2001). Hearing loss, tinnitis, and otalgia. In G. E. Woodson (Ed.), *Ear, nose and throat disorders in primary care* (pp. 31–51). Philadelphia: W.B. Saunders.

Schild, J. A., & Holinger, L. D. (1980). Peroral endoscopy in neonates. *International Journal of Pediatric Otorhinolaryngology, 2,* 133–138. Abstract.

Scolnik, D., Coates, A. L., Stephens, D., Da Silva, Z., Lavine, E., & Schuh, S. (2006). Controlled delivery of high vs. low humidity vs. mist therapy for croup in emergency departments: A randomized controlled trial. *JAMA, 295,* 1274–1280.

Seear, M., Wensley, D. W., & West, N. (2005). How accurate is the diagnosis of exercise-induced asthma among Vancouver schoolchildren? *Archives of Disease in Childhood, 90*(9), 898–902.

Senbil, N., Yavuz Gurer, Y. K., Uner, C., & Barut, Y. (2008). Sinusitis in children and adolescents with chronic ore recurrent headache: A case-control study. *Journal of Headache Pain, 9,* 33–36.

Shah, R., Mora, B., Bacha, E., Sena, L. K., Buonomo, C., Del Nido, P., & Rahbar, R. (2007). The presentation and management of vascular rings: An otolaryngology perspective. *International Journal of Pediatric Otolaryngology, 71,* 57–62.

Shah, R. K. (2010). Epiglottitis in the United States: National trends, variances, prognosis and management. *Laryngoscope, 120*(6), 1256–1262.

Sinclair, C. F., & Berkowitz, R. G. (2007). Prior antibiotic therapy for acute sinusitis in children and the development of subperiosteal orbital abscess. *International Journal of Pediatric Otorhinolaryngology, 71*, 1003–1006.

Sobol, S., & Zapata, S. (2008). Epiglottitis and croup. *Otolaryngologic Clinics of North America, 41*(3), 551–566.

Wald, E. R. (2003). Rhinitis and acute and chronic sinusitis. In C. D. Bluestone, S. E. Stool, C. M. Alper, E. M. Arjmand, M. L. Casselbrant, J. E. Dohar, & R. D. Yellon (Eds.), *Pediatric otolaryngology* (4th ed., Vol. 2, pp. 995–1031). Philadelphia: Saunders.

Wald, E. R. (2008). Sinusitis. In S. S. Long, L. K. Pickering, & C. G. Prober (Eds.), *Principles and practice of pediatric infectious diseases* (3rd ed.). Chapter 34. New York: Churchill Livingston.

Weber, R. W. (2008). Allergic rhinitis. *Primary Care: Clinics in Office Practice, 35*, 1–10.

Zawin, J. (2000). Radiologic evaluation of the upper airway. In R. Wetmore, H. Muntz, T. McGill, W. Potsic, G. Healy, & R. Lusk (Eds.), *Pediatric otolaryngology: Principles and practice pathways* (pp. 689–736). New York: Thieme.

Zoumalan, R., Maddalozzo, J., & Holinger, L. (2007). Etiology of stridor in infants. *Annals of Otolaryngology Rhinology and Laryngology, 116*, 329–334.

Webliography

http://www.mahalo.com/montelukast

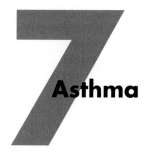

Asthma

Concettina Tolomeo, DNP, APRN, FNP-BC, AE-C,
Dawn Baker, MSN, CPNP, CCRC, and
Pnina Weiss, MD

ASTHMA

Asthma is an inflammatory disease characterized by obstruction and hyperresponsiveness of the airways. In the late 1980s, the National Heart, Lung, and Blood Institute established the National Asthma Education and Prevention Program (NAEPP) to educate clinicians, patients, and the public about asthma diagnosis and care. Its panel of experts created recommendations called the Expert Panel Report (EPR) to help guide health-care providers in the diagnosis and treatment of asthma. The EPR is updated on a regular basis. The last complete revision (Expert Panel Report 3 [EPR3]) was released in 2007. Since the initial recommendations were published in 1991, the number of deaths due to asthma has declined (National Heart Lung and Blood Institute [NHLBI], 2007).

The EPR3 is comprised of four components of asthma care and management. They include

- measures of asthma assessment and monitoring,
- education for a partnership in asthma care,
- control of environmental factors and comorbid conditions that affect asthma, and
- medications (NHLBI, 2007).

Nursing Care in Pediatric Respiratory Disease, First Edition. Edited by Concettina (Tina) Tolomeo.
© 2012 John Wiley & Sons, Inc. Published 2012 by John Wiley & Sons, Inc.

The diagnostic and management strategies discussed in this chapter are based on the EPR3.

EPIDEMIOLOGY

Asthma is considered one of the leading chronic childhood diseases currently affecting over 7 million children in the United States. Prevalence is estimated at 9% with the highest rates seen in school-age children. Although prevalence nearly doubled in the 1980s, it has since leveled off (Centers for Disease Control [CDC], n.d.,b). In young children, boys have higher rates than girls. However, girls have higher rates after puberty. In addition, prevalence rates are higher in non-Hispanic black and Puerto Rican children than in non-Hispanic white children (Akinbami, 2006). Childhood asthma prevalence rates are lowest in Asian children (Akinbami, Moorman, Garbe, & Sondik, 2009).

Nearly 60% of children currently diagnosed with asthma had one or more exacerbation in the previous year (Akinbami et al., 2009). In 2004, the mortality rate for asthma for children was 2.5 per 1 million (Centers for Disease Control [CDC], n.d.,b). Risk factors for asthma death include previous severe exacerbation, two or more hospitalizations in the past year, three or more emergency department (ED) visits in the past year, hospitalization or ED visit in the past month, use of greater than two canisters of a short-acting bronchodilator per month, difficulty perceiving asthma symptoms, poor socioeconomic status, and psychosocial stressors (NHLBI, 2007).

Non-Hispanic black children have higher ED visit rates and higher mortality rates than non-Hispanic white children (Akinbami, 2006). Morbidity and mortality rates are higher in the inner city population (Apter et al., 2001; Shapiro & Stout, 2002; Smith et al., 2004). It has been documented that poor children are 40% more likely to be hospitalized, and they experience more clinical and social dysfunction due to asthma than children who are not poor (Shapiro & Stout, 2002). There is also evidence that steroid resistance may be greater in African Americans (Celano et al., 2010). Furthermore, treatment disparities exist in minority populations (Akinbami et al., 2009).

Asthma is one of the most common causes of missed school days and is associated with high health-care costs. According to Kamble and Bharma (2009), asthma health-care costs (direct and indirect costs) in the United States are greater than $30 billion a year. Health-care costs for those with asthma are double those without asthma (Birnbaum et al., 2002).

Epidemiological studies have helped to provide an understanding of the natural history of asthma and the influence of heredity, gender, smoke, and environmental exposure on the development of asthma. Findings have revealed that maternal smoking is associated with decreased airway function, which may lead to bronchial hyperresponsiveness (BHR) (Dezateux et al., 2004). Furthermore, prenatal use of antibiotics and C-section delivery has been associated with an increased rate of atopy and asthma (Subbarao, Mandhane, & Sears, 2009). Prenatal nutrition has been inconsistent in its effect on asthma rates. In a birth cohort, 8-year longitudinal study, maternal consumption of peanuts was the only strong correlate between nutrition and asthma development (Willers et al., 2008). A protective effect of breast-feeding on the development of allergy and asthma has also been postulated but not consistently supported in studies. And finally, a large family size is thought to be protective against developing asthma.

The hygiene hypothesis proposes that exposure to early infections and bacterial serotypes influences the immune system to the nonasthma phe-notype, most likely by stimulating a preponderance of T-helper cell 1 (T_H1)-type responses (Schaub, Lauener, & Mutius, 2006). Factors such as rural living—particularly farm environment, having older siblings, and early exposure to infections—have been demonstrated to be protective (Liu, 2007; Von Mitius, 2010).

The Tucson Children's Respiratory Study evaluated the natural history of asthma through a longitudinal study of over 1,000 children followed from birth until adulthood. There were three distinct asthma phenotypes: (1) transient wheezers who have wheezing episodes that resolve by 3 years of age and have lower levels of lung function at birth; (2) nonatopic wheezers who continue wheezing after 3 years of age, but in general resolve by the age of 13 years; and (3) atopic wheezers who are sensitized to aeroallergens and go on to develop persistent asthma (Stern, Morgan, Halonen, Wright, & Martinez, 2008). Early-onset wheeze is typically related to decreased airway caliber and irritant exposure, while late-onset and persistent wheeze is attributed to genetic and environmental factors.

Genetics

Asthma has been described as a complex genetic disorder that does not follow the classic Mendelian pattern. Several genes have been discovered that are associated with the development of asthma, although the specific action of these genes is not fully understood. Genetic factors are felt to contribute not only to the asthma phenotype but also to its clinical course.

Candidate gene studies have identified an excess of 100 genes associated with allergy and asthma. Genome-wide association studies (GWAS) help find polymorphisms by looking at markers along the human genome called single-nucleotide polymorphisms. Frequency occurrence is studied to determine if a candidate gene is involved in a disease process. Unfor-tunately, other variables preclude such a generalization. Additionally, many of the genes originally found by GWAS have not been replicated consistently (Rogers et al., 2009). Genotypic characteristics have been sug-gested in the beta-adrenergic receptor pathway that could predict response to therapy. Individuals with polymorphisms in the $beta_2$ antagonist recep-tor ($β_2AR$) gene may have a variable response to short-acting beta agonists

(SABAs). African Americans have a greater predisposition to the development of asthma or to polymorphism in the β_2AR gene. Recently, patients with the Arg/Arg16 genotype have been shown to have an impaired response to long-acting beta agonists (LABAs) (Finkelstein, Bournissen, Hutson, & Shannon, 2009). Both genetic predisposition and gene–environment interactions help describe the allergic asthma phenotype.

Environment

A recent report highlighted the discovery of two independent loss-of-function genetic variants (R510X and 2282del14) in a key protein called filaggrin that was associated with an increase in the prevalence of asthma and atopic dermatitis (Palmer et al., 2006). The highest asthma and allergy burden is found in Westernized countries where a combination of lifestyle factors including diet, allergen exposure, urban life, air pollution, and widespread antibiotic use may contribute to asthma development. Early exposures to day care, older siblings, and farm environments are felt to be protective.

PATHOPHYSIOLOGY

One of the major hallmarks of asthma is inflammation that leads to airway obstruction and hyperresponsiveness. Airway obstruction is caused by bronchoconstriction, mucus hypersecretion, and edema. Inflammation occurs through the accumulation and interaction of a variety of cell types. Inflammatory mediators work by activating cell-specific surface receptors, which in turn begin a cascade of signaling events (NHLBI, 2007). These processes are complex and dynamic and are described next (Mason, Broaddus, Murray, & Nadel, 2000).

Inflammatory cells

Inhaled allergens trigger mast cells and T_H2 cells to release inflammatory mediators such as histamine and cysteinyl leukotrienes and cytokines such as interleukin-4 (IL-4) and interleukin-5 (IL-5). Cytokine production leads to activation of endothelial cells, release of collagen and matrix proteins, and eventual airway remodeling (Fitzgerald, Boulet, & O'Byrne, 2001).

Lymphocytes

Lymphocytes are involved in the regulation of airway inflammation through T_H1 and T_H2. The T_H1 phenotype has been described as being protective as it will produce IL-4 and interferon-y (IFN-y), which are known cellular defense mechanisms. Alternatively, the T_H2 cells release cytokines (IL-4,-5,-6,-9, and -13), which mediate allergic inflammation. An imbalance between T_H1 and T_H2 lymphocytes contributes to a chronic inflammatory cascade. In asthma, there is a predilection toward a T_H2-driven, immunoglobulin E (IgE)-predominant, eosinophilic response (Mason et al., 2000).

Eosinophils

Many children with asthma have an increased number of eosinophils in their airways. These cells contain inflammatory enzymes and a variety of proinflammatory cytokines. A higher eosinophilic burden has been associated with more severe asthma (NHLBI, 2007).

Neutrophils and dendritic cells

Neutrophils are found in both acute and chronic asthma, those with nocturnal symptoms, and in individuals who smoke. Their role is still not completely understood. They may contribute to a lack of steroid responsiveness.

Dendritic cells are the key antigen-presenting cells that interact with allergens on the airway surface and contribute to T_H2 cell differentiation (Mason et al., 2000).

Mast cells

Mediator release from mast cells is important in the pathogenesis of asthma. Mast cell degranulation can be activated by the allergen-induced pathway as well as by mechanical or thermal stimulation. Mast cells are also seen in smooth muscle airways, exercise-induced bronchoconstriction, and airway inflammation. Inhaled corticosteroids (ICSs) decrease the number of mast cells (Clark et al. 2000).

Macrophages

An increase in immature macrophages is seen in individuals with asthma. This may result in proinflammatory mediator release and tissue damage (Poston et al. 1992).

Inflammatory mediators

The production of mediators has been cited in the pathogenesis of asthma and may contribute to BHR. Both cytokine and chemokine cellular recruitment contributes to the activation of asthma.

Cytokines

Cytokines are produced from a number of cell types including previously described lymphocytes, eosinophils, and mast cells. They directly modify the inflammatory response in asthma and in turn determine asthma severity. Key cytokines include IL-1B and tumor necrosis factor-α (TNF-α), which exacerbates the inflammatory response and granulocyte-macrophage colony-stimulating factor (GM-CSF) (Clark et al. 2000). GM-CSF plays a key role in prolonging eosinophil survival. ICSs affect the balance of anti-inflammatory and proinflammatory cytokine expression.

Chemokines

Chemokines play a role in the recruitment of proinflammatory cells into the airways. One of the more studied is RANTES (regulated upon activation, normal T-cell expressed and secreted), which is a potent chemoattractant for T cells, eosinophils, basophils, macrophages, and mast cells. It induces recruitment of eosinophils in the airways of individuals with asthma (Fang, Wang, & Zhao, 2010).

IgE

IgE is important to the pathogenesis of allergic disease; it is the antibody responsible for the activation of the allergic response and causes acute bronchospasm and mucosal inflammation (Clark et al. 2000). Mast cells are known to have many IgE receptors and release inflammatory mediators such as histamines, tryptase, leukotrienes, prostaglandins, and other eicosanoids.

Novel therapies that target chemokines and other inflammatory cells are being studied. For example, monoclonal antibodies against IgE have been found to be effective in asthma treatment.

Histologically, one of the major features of asthma is the thickening of the bronchial subepithelial basement membrane. This process begins early and is seen even in mild disease. It is theorized that this reticular basement membrane thickening begins even before the diagnosis of asthma.

Ventilation and perfusion

In children with asthma, the airways are narrowed and there is increased resistance to airflow. Airways collapse on expiration and there is air trapping. Lung compliance is decreased, and it requires more work to move air through the airways. Hypoxemia or low oxygen levels may result because of atelectasis. Alveolar ventilation is decreased with subsequent carbon dioxide retention, acidosis, and, if untreated, respiratory failure. In some individuals, continued changes over time in airway structure can occur with fibrosis, mucous hypersecretion, epithelial cell injury, smooth muscle hypertrophy, and angiogenesis. Hyperplasia of the airways can make treatment difficult. Permanent changes can occur in the airway, leading to a progressive loss of lung function (Clark et al., 2000).

Phenotype

General triggers of asthma can vary with age. Respiratory infections (typically viral) predominate in infancy and in early childhood; in later life, inhalants, irritants, exercise, and cold exposure emerge as important triggers. For children under the age of 3 years, wheeze is often caused by a decrease in lung function and airway caliber. Presentation after 3 years is predominately related to elevated IgE and a parental history of asthma. Children tend to have more episodic events and more peripheral airway involvement than adults.

Exercise-induced bronchoconstriction is described as a transient airway narrowing typically 5–10 minutes following exercise, which usually resolves in 20–30 minutes. The proposed mechanism is that high ventilation associated with training irritates the airway lining and causes mediator release and injury to the airway. Cooling and drying of the airway epithelium is a trigger for bronchoconstriction. Exercise-induced asthma (EIA) occurs in up to 90% of individuals with asthma and is also seen in elite athletes (Milgrom & Taussig, 1999).

SIGNS AND SYMPTOMS

History

Clinical symptoms of asthma typically include cough, dyspnea, and wheeze. If the patient is old enough, he/she may complain of chest tightness. The symptoms may be intermittent or persistent. A complete history from the parent is imperative. Including older children in the discussion is also important as their perception may aid in the diagnosis (Watts, 2008).

An asthma cough can be hacking and nonproductive; it is often worse at night. Mucus hypersecretion may make the cough sound wet or productive. There may also be shortness of breath with activity. If only exercise-induced symptoms are present, it is important to ascertain when the cough occurs in relation to the activity and the physical condition of the child. Wheezing may or may not be present.

Certain history or symptoms may point to an alternative diagnosis or a comorbid condition. Foreign body aspiration may present with symptoms after a choking episode; toddlers are particularly at risk. Gastroesophageal reflux disease (GERD) can cause recurrent bouts of coughing or recurrent aspiration and should be suspected in children with a history of prematurity, feeding difficulties, or neurological deficit. Vocal cord dysfunction presents with wheezing and shortness of breath due to paradoxical adduction of the vocal cords during inspiration. Generally, it is more common in the adolescent and young adult population and does not respond to typical asthma therapy (Hill & Wood, 2009). With a history of frequent antibiotic use or recurrent pneumonia, an immune deficiency should be suspected.

A family history is also important when evaluating the child with asthma symptoms. A history of asthma, allergy, eczema, shortness of breath, or cough should be assessed. Wheeze and atopy are strong predictors of asthma (Schonberger et al., 2004). Review of the past medical history can reveal comorbid conditions, while a social history can elicit pet, smoking, or other allergen exposure. A comprehensive history can help establish the diagnosis of asthma and the severity of the presentation.

Physical examination

If the child is not experiencing current asthma symptoms, the physical examination may be completely normal. When examining the child, the nurse should look for allergic features, such as allergic shiners, boggy nasal turbinates, a nasal crease, and eczema. If the child is experiencing an exacerbation, observation of the chest may reveal accessory muscle use and hyperexpansion of the chest. Supraclavicular, suprasternal, subcostal, intercostal, and substernal retractions may be particularly noticeable in infants. Along with nasal flaring, these symptoms are indicative of respiratory distress.

The physical examination may also reveal a prolonged inspiratory-to-expiratory ratio. During an exacerbation, wheezing may be present. Furthermore, if the obstruction is severe enough, breath sounds may be significantly diminished. Clubbing of the fingers should raise the possibility of a chronic obstructive pulmonary disease such as cystic fibrosis (CF), primary ciliary dyskinesia, or immunodeficiency.

Assessment of oxygenation is frequently performed by pulse oximetry. However, there may be impending respiratory failure even if oxygen saturations are near normal. Because a clinical picture of tissue hypoxia is a late indicator of asthma severity, history and physical exam are critically important (Rebuck & Chapman, 1987).

DIAGNOSIS

Making an accurate diagnosis and determination of asthma severity is imperative because this information will ultimately guide therapy. An inaccurate diagnosis can result in inadequate treatment, which in turn can lead to increased morbidity and mortality. Thus, the diagnostic approach should be comprehensive and systematic in order to help ensure correct diagnosis and treatment.

One of the hallmarks of asthma is airflow obstruction that is at least partially reversible (NHLBI, 2007). This factor is important when establishing the diagnosis of asthma. Another factor that is necessary to establish the diagnosis of asthma is the presence of recurrent symptoms of airflow obstruction or airway hyperresponsiveness. Moreover, the diagnosis should only be made after other conditions that may present with similar symptoms (cough, wheeze, or dyspnea) are ruled out. Such conditions include sinusitis, allergies, CF, primary ciliary dyskinesia, heart disease, foreign body obstruction, vascular rings, tracheomalacia, tracheal stenosis or lesion, vocal cord dysfunction, and laryngeal web.

To diagnose asthma, the health-care provider should obtain a detailed medical history; this includes an environmental history to determine exposure to allergens, as well as a social history (number of missed school/work days due to asthma, insurance status, etc.) to determine the impact of asthma on quality of life, and barriers to care. The health-care provider should also perform a thorough physical examination; this includes a skin exam to assess for atopic dermatitis. If the child is old enough, spirometry should be obtained to confirm the diagnosis. Spirometry is used to assess the degree of airway obstruction and to determine the reversibility of airflow obstruction. Once the diagnosis of asthma is made, spirometry results are also used to classify disease severity and to monitor asthma control (NHLBI, 2007).

Children can generally start to perform spirometry around the age of 5. Spirometry is performed through a handheld device connected to a computer. A trained technician is crucial for coaching the child through the maneuver. For the young child or the child who is performing spirometry for the first time, incentive programs (such as a birthday cake with candles) are available and should be utilized when appropriate.

The American Thoracic Society (ATS) has standardized the performance and interpretation of spirometry and emphasized the importance of not extrapolating adult data for use in children. An accurate age, race, height, and weight should be obtained prior to testing so that results can be compared to reference values. Ideally, the child should exhale for 6 seconds; however, this may be difficult for young children. Therefore, for children less than 10 years of age, 3 seconds is considered acceptable (Miller et al., 2005). A minimum of three and a maximum of eight maneuvers should be completed to meet ATS criteria.

The two largest forced vital capacity (FVC) and forced expiratory volume in 1 second (FEV_1) values must be within 0.150 L of each other. For children with an FVC of ≤1.0 L, the two largest values should be within 0.100 L of each other (Miller et al., 2005). The FVC is the volume of air exhaled after the child takes a maximal breath. The FEV_1 is the volume of air exhaled in the first second of the FVC (Hyatt, Scanlon, & Nakamura, 1997).

If a child is undergoing reversibility testing (which is recommended for children suspected of having asthma), the postbronchodilator test should be performed 10–15 minutes after the administration of a SABA. Postbronchodilator FEV_1 values that increase ≥12% and 200 mL compared to baseline suggest a significant response (American Thoracic Society, 2005).

Spirometric categories and cutoffs for determining the severity of lung disease are arbitrary. In children, a lower limit of 80% predicted may be acceptable (American Thoracic Society, 2005). Normal spirometry is generally defined as an FEV_1 greater than 80% predicted; mild obstruction is an FEV_1 between 60 and 80% predicted; moderate obstruction is an FEV_1 between 40 and 60% predicted; and severe obstruction is less than 40% predicted. However, these same values do not apply when determining asthma severity and level of control. Severity and control spirometry cutoff values are listed in Tables 7.1 and 7.2.

In addition to performing spirometry upon initial evaluation to help determine asthma severity, spirometry should also be performed on a regular basis to assess the level of control. The EPR3 recommends performing spirometry at the initial assessment, after treatment is initiated and symptoms and peak expiratory flow rates (PEFRs) have stabilized, during periods of poor asthma control, and at least every 1–2 years (NHLBI, 2007).

Other tests that should be obtained as needed to rule out alternative diagnoses include chest X-ray, additional pulmonary function tests, bronchoprovocation studies, allergy/immunology testing, and biomarkers of inflammation.

Chest X-ray

A chest X-ray should be ordered if not previously obtained to rule out other diagnoses such as foreign body obstruction. Radiographic findings of the child with asthma may be normal or may reveal hyperinflation or peribronchial cuffing. If there is mucus retention, atelectasis may be present (Novelline, 2004).

Additional pulmonary function tests

Lung volumes may be obtained. An elevated total lung capacity (TLC) is consistent with asthma and airway obstruction. A decreased TLC is diagnostic of restrictive lung disease and alternative diagnoses should be considered. Inspiratory loops may be useful when considering the diagnosis of vocal cord dysfunction.

Bronchoprovocation studies

Bronchoprovocation or challenge studies may be helpful when children have symptoms consistent with asthma but have normal spirometry results. Two well-known bronchoprovocation tests include exercise and methacholine challenge testing (MCT). An exercise challenge test is indicated when symptoms occur with exercise. It can be performed in children greater than age 6. It involves obtaining baseline spirometry and heart rate followed by 4–6 minutes of maximal exercise (80–90% maximal heart rate for age) on a treadmill or bicycle ergometer. After the cessation of exercise, serial spirometry measurements are obtained. If there is a greater than 10% drop in FEV_1, it is a positive finding (American Thoracic Society, 1999). For

Table 7.1 Asthma severity classification and step therapy.

Severity measures		Age	Intermittent[a]	Persistent — Mild[a]	Persistent — Moderate[a]	Persistent — Severe[a]
Impairment	Symptoms[b]	0–4 5–11 >12	≤2 days/week	>2 days/week but not daily	Daily	Multiple times per day
	Nighttime symptoms[b]	0–4 5–11 >12	0 ≤2× per month	1–2× per month 3–4× per month	3–4× per month >1× per week but not every night	>1× per week Often 7×/week
	Activity limitation[b]	0–4 5–11 >12	None	Minor	Some	Extremely
	SABA use[b]	0–4 5–11 >12	≤2 days/week	>2 days/week but not daily >2 days/week but not >1× day	Daily	Several times per day
	Lung function FEV_1 FEV_1/FVC	0–4	N/A			
		5–11	Normal FEV_1 between exacerbations $FEV_1 > 80\%$ predicted $FEV_1/FVC > 85\%$ predicted	$FEV_1 > 80\%$ predicted $FEV_1/FVC > 80\%$ predicted	FEV_1 60–80% predicted FEV_1/FVC 75–80% predicted	$FEV_1 < 60\%$ predicted $FEV_1/FVC < 75\%$ predicted
		>12	Normal FEV_1 between exacerbations $FEV_1 > 80\%$ predicted FEV_1/FVC normal	$FEV_1 > 80\%$ predicted FEV_1/FVC normal	FEV_1 60–80% predicted FEV_1/FVC reduced by 5%	$FEV_1 < 60\%$ predicted FEV_1/FVC reduced by >5%

Normal FEV_1/FVC:
8–19 years old—85%
20–39 years old—80%
40–59 years old—75%
60–80 years old—70%

Risk	Exacerbation Requiring oral steroids	0–4	0–1 per year		
		5–11	≥2 in 6 months requiring steroids, or ≥4 wheezing episodes in 1 year lasting more than 1 day and affected sleep plus risk factors[c]		
		>12	≥2 per year		
Step therapy		0–4	1	2	3 and consider short course of oral steroids	
		5–11	1	2	3—medium-dose ICS option and consider short course of oral steroids	3—medium-dose ICS option or 4 and consider short course of oral steroids
		>12	1	2	3 and consider short course of oral steroids	3 or 4 and consider short course of oral steroids

Adapted from the National Asthma Education and Prevention Program (NAEPP) Expert Panel Report 3 (EPR3).

[a] Assign severity based on the most severe category in which any feature occurs.

[b] Based on recall over a 2- to 4-week period.

[c] Risk factors: either one of the following: physician-diagnosed atopy, parental history of asthma, evidence of sensitization to aeroallergens, or two of the following: evidence of sensitization to foods, eosinophilia (≥4%), or wheezing apart from colds.

SABA, short-acting beta agonist; FEV_1, forced expiratory volume in 1 second; FEV_1/FVC, forced expiratory volume in 1 second/forced vital capacity ratio; ICS, inhaled corticosteroid; N/A, not applicable.

Table 7.2 Asthma control and therapy adjustment.

Control measures		Age	Asthma control classification		
			Well controlled	Not well controlled	Very poorly controlled
Impairment	Symptoms[a]	0–4	≤2 days/week	>2 days/week	Multiple times per day
		5–11			
		>12			
	Nighttime symptoms[a]	0–4	≤1×/month	>1×/month	>1× per week
		5–11		≥2×/month	≥2×/week
		>12	≤2× per month	1–3×/week	≥4×/week
	Activity limitation[a]	0–4	None	Some	Extremely
		5–11			
		>12			
	SABA use[a]	0–4	≤2 days/week	>2 days/week	Several times per day
		5–11			
		>12			
	N/A	0–4	N/A		
	FEV_1 or peak flow	5–11	>80% predicted/personal best	60–80% predicted/personal best	<60% predicted/personal best
	FEV_1/FVC		>80%	75–80%	<75%
	FEV_1 or peak flow	>12	>80% predicted/personal best	60–80% predicted/personal best	<60% predicted/personal best
	ATAQ		0	1–2	3–4
	ACQ		≤0.75	≥1.5	N/A
	ACT		≥20	16–19	≤15

		0–4	5–11	>12
Risk	Exacerbation Requiring oral steroids	0–1 per year	2–3/year, ≥2 per year	>3/year
	Treatment-related side effects	Can vary from none to very troublesome. The level of intensity does not correlate to specific levels of control but should be a risk consideration.		
	Reduction in lung growth	N/A	Requires long-term follow-up	
	Progressive loss of lung function			(>12)
Action		0–4[b] Maintain current treatment; Follow-up every 1–6 months; Consider step down if well controlled × 3 months	5–11 Step up one step; Reevaluate in 2–6 weeks; For side effects, consider alternative option	>12 Consider short course of oral steroids; Step up one to two steps; Reevaluate in 2 weeks; For side effects, consider alternative option

Adapted from the National Asthma Education and Prevention Program (NAEPP) Expert Panel Report 3 (EPR3).

[a] Based on recall over a 2- to 4-week period.

[b] If not well controlled or very poorly controlled and there is no clear benefit in 4–6 weeks, consider an alternative diagnosis or adjusting therapy.

SABA, short-acting beta agonist; ATAQ, Asthma Therapy Assessment Questionnaire©; ACQ, Asthma Control Questionnaire©; ACT, Asthma Control Test™; FEV₁, forced expiratory volume in 1 second; FEV₁/FVC, forced expiratory volume in 1 second/forced vital capacity ratio.

MCT, baseline spirometry is again obtained. Methacholine (a chemical that increases parasympathetic tone in bronchial smooth muscles) is then administered via inhalation in varying concentrations. Spirometry is obtained after each dose of methacholine. A positive test is defined as a 20% decrease in FEV_1 from baseline or after the last dose of methacholine. This measure is known as the provocative concentration or PC20% (American Thoracic Society, 1999). MCT has a higher sensitivity than exercise challenge testing. Because bronchospasm may be induced with testing, the facility should be properly equipped with emergency medications and supplies such as albuterol, epinephrine, and supplemental oxygen. A newer bronchoprovocation study using mannitol is also available.

Allergy and immunology testing

If allergies are being considered in the differential diagnosis, testing should be performed by blood sampling (radioallergosorbent test [RAST]) or skin prick testing. These tests can be used to determine if the child is allergic to common indoor and outdoor allergens. An IgE level and complete blood count (CBC) should also be ordered. If an immune disorder is being considered, basic quantitative immunoglobulins should be obtained.

Biomarkers of inflammation

Biomarkers of inflammation such as sputum eosinophils and fractional concentration of nitric oxide (fraction of exhaled nitric oxide [FeNO]) are being utilized in some practices. However, according the EPR3, they require further evaluation before they can be recommended as a clinical tool for asthma management (NHLBI, 2007).

Determining severity

Once all other conditions have been ruled out and the child meets the diagnostic criteria for asthma, the health-care provider should classify the child's level of asthma severity. Severity is defined as the intrinsic intensity of the disease process (NHLBI, 2007). To obtain the most accurate assessment of severity, it is best to assess the child before he/she initiates long-term control therapy. However, because this is not always possible, severity can be inferred from the least amount of medication therapy necessary to maintain control (NHLBI, 2007).

Severity should be based on the domains of current impairment and future risk. Impairment is defined as the frequency and intensity of symptoms and functional limitations the child is currently experiencing or has recently experienced (NHLBI, 2007). Determining a child's current impairment requires an assessment of symptoms, nighttime awakenings, use of SABA for symptoms, exercise limitation, and lung function. Studies have demonstrated that the FEV_1/FVC ratio appears to be a more sensitive measure of severity in the impairment domain (NHLBI, 2007). Risk is defined as the likelihood of either asthma exacerbations, progressive decline in lung function or reduced lung growth, or risk of adverse effects from medications (NHLBI, 2007). An assessment of future risk includes an evaluation of the frequency of asthma exacerbations requiring oral systemic corticosteroids. Studies have revealed that the FEV_1 appears to be a useful measure for indicating risk for exacerbations (NHLBI, 2007).

The EPR3 lists four classifications of asthma severity: intermittent, mild persistent, moderate persistent, and severe persistent. Table 7.1 provides a chart to assist the health-care provider in determining asthma severity.

COMPLICATIONS

Asthma is associated with impaired quality of life, frequent utilization of acute care facilities, increased health costs, and missed school and work days (Guilbert et al., 2010). Inadequately treated asthma leads to impaired growth and weight gain and failure to thrive. Children with asthma have a higher incidence of psychological disorders including poor self-esteem, anxiety, and depression (Mrazek, 1992).

Asthma is associated with deterioration in lung function over time, which is exacerbated by smoking. This decrease in lung function may occur before the age of 2 years (Guilbert et al., 2004). Pathology has revealed evidence of remodeling in the airway wall with fibrosis and collagen deposition. There may be a link between asthma and the development of chronic obstructive pulmonary disease in adults (Martinez, 2009).

Asthma, along with most chronic pulmonary diseases, increases the prevalence of GERD (Berquist et al., 1981). Asthma may worsen obstructive sleep apnea. It leads to an increase in postsurgical complications (Kalra, Buncher, & Amin, 2005). Asthma is associated with increased morbidity from viral infections, such as influenza (Gaglani, 2002), sickle cell disease (Sylvester et al., 2007), and cardiac disease.

Asthma medications may cause side effects. Corticosteroids, both inhaled and oral, are associated with a decrease in linear growth and adrenal suppression in a dose-dependent manner. Corticosteroids cause oral thrush. Daily use of oral corticosteroids may cause immunosuppression and an increased susceptibility to infection (Leone, Fish, Szefler, & West, 2003).

Asthma exacerbations may lead to death. Fatalities have been associated with one or more life-threatening events, poor symptom control, frequent emergency room visits, the use of oral corticosteroids, impaired perception of the severity of obstruction, poor socioeconomic status, and psychiatric disease (NHLBI, 2007). An asthma attack may precipitate dissection of air along tissue planes. Air can dissect into subcutaneous tissue (subcutaneous emphysema), pleural space (pneumothorax), mediastinum (pneumomediastinum), around the heart (pneumopericardium), and, rarely, into the spinal cord (pneumorrhachis). A pneumothorax or pneumopericardium can result in inadequate ventilation and oxygenation and decreased cardiac output and shock.

MANAGEMENT

The overall goals of asthma management are to reduce impairment and risk. This includes preventing chronic symptoms, limiting the use of SABA, maintaining normal or near-normal lung function and activity levels, meeting the patient's/family's expectations of care, preventing exacerbations, minimizing the need for ED visits and hospitalizations, preventing loss of lung function, preventing reduced lung growth (in children), and experiencing little to no side effects from therapy (NHLBI, 2007).

Allergen avoidance and pharmacotherapy are utilized in combination to control and prevent asthma symptoms. Both require an individualized approach. Two other fundamental components of asthma management are education (discussed in the section "Nursing Care of the Child and Family") and the ongoing assessment of asthma control.

Allergen avoidance

Dermatophagoides pteronyssinus, also known as the dust mite (DM) is a common allergen and trigger of asthma symptoms. DMs thrive in humid environments and depend on human dander for their existence. Because there are high levels of DMs in mattresses, pillows, and bed covers, the child's bed is the major focus of DM control (NHLBI, 2007). Washing linens weekly can help control DMs (Arlian, Vyszenski-Moher, & Morgan, 2003). Linens should be washed in hot water (>130°F). In addition, the mattress and pillows should be encased in allergen-impermeable covers (NHLBI, 2007). Other actions that can be instituted to control DMs include keeping indoor humidity between 30 and 50%, removing carpets, eliminating and/ or minimizing stuffed toys, washing stuffed toys weekly, and avoiding lying on upholstered furniture (NHLBI, 2007).

Pet dander can also be an allergen and trigger for children with asthma. Recommendations for controlling animal antigens include bathing the pet regularly, keeping the pet out of the child's bedroom, keeping the child's bedroom door closed, and keeping the pet off of upholstered furniture. Of course, the ideal method of avoidance is to remove the pet from the home.

Outdoor allergens (tree, grass, and weed pollen, and mold such as *Alternaria*) can also trigger asthma symptoms. Avoidance measures include staying indoors with the windows closed and the air conditioner on during pollen season (NHLBI, 2007). Parents should be instructed to monitor pollen counts in their area. Other control measures include not hanging clothes outside on the line and having the child take a shower before going to bed if he/she was playing outdoors.

Smoking exposure is a common irritant and trigger of asthma symptoms (Gilliland et al., 2006). Reducing exposure is vital. Smoking should not be allowed in the car or at home.

Cockroach exposure is common in inner city areas and can be troublesome for children with asthma. Parents and children should be instructed to not leave food or garbage uncovered. To eliminate cockroaches, traps or boric acid are preferred. If chemical agents are necessary, the home should be well ventilated and the child should not return home until the odor has disappeared (NHLBI, 2007).

Pharmacotherapy

The primary goal of pharmacotherapy is to use an effective medication at the lowest dose possible to achieve control of symptoms and to reduce exacerbations. By doing so, one minimizes side effects and costs.

Asthma medications are divided into two categories: long-term control medications and quick-relief medications. Long-term control medications are used to achieve and maintain asthma control. They include the following drug classes: corticosteorids (ICSs and oral corticosteroids), cromolyn sodium, immunomodulators, leukotriene modifiers, LABAs, and methylxanthines. Quick-relief medications are used to treat acute symptoms and exacerbations. Quick-relief medications include anticholinergics, SABAs, and systemic corticosteroids (NHLBI, 2007). Specific medication classes, mechanisms of action, side effects, and names are discussed in Chapter 3. However, the following provides some general considerations for asthma pharmacotherapy. First, every child with asthma should be prescribed a SABA for rescue therapy to relieve symptoms of airflow obstruction. Second, a daily ICS is preferred for initiating therapy in infants and in young children (NHLBI, 2007). Findings have demonstrated the effectiveness of ICS in improving symptoms and in reducing exacerbations in infants and in children with asthma (Guilbert et al., 2006). The biggest concern that parents generally express is the potential effect on growth, which is temporary (Rottier & Duiverman, 2009). Parents should be reassured that in long-term studies with conventional dosing, the final growth was not affected (Agertoft & Pedersen 1994; Visser et al., 2004). Finally, omalizumab (anti-IgE antibody) therapy can be costly (Hendeles & Sorkness, 2007). Therefore, insurance and patient assistance programs should be investigated.

A stepwise approach to medication therapy is recommended to manage asthma (NHLBI, 2007). Table 7.1 provides a listing of the different steps and associated severity levels. The EPR 3 stepwise approach includes six steps and three different age groups (0- to 4-year-olds, 5- to 11-year-olds, and ≥12-year-olds). In all age groups, step 1 consists of as-needed use of a SABA to manage intermittent asthma. Steps 2–6 are used to manage persistent asthma and vary according to the age group and asthma severity level as outlined next:

- For children 0–4 years:
  - *Step 2.* Low-dose ICS is preferred. Cromolyn or montelukast is an alternative.
  - *Step 3.* Medium-dose ICS is preferred.

○ *Step 4.* Medium-dose ICS plus either a LABA or montelukast are preferred.
○ *Step 5.* High-dose ICS plus either a LABA or montelukast are preferred.
○ *Step 6.* High-dose ICS plus either a LABA or montelukast and oral corticosteroids are preferred.
● For children 5–11 years:
○ *Step 2.* Low-dose ICS is preferred. Cromolyn, leukotriene receptor antagonist, nedocromil, or theophylline is an alternative.
○ *Step 3.* Either low-dose ICS plus LABA, leukotriene receptor antagonist, or theophylline or medium-dose ICS is preferred.
○ *Step 4.* Medium-dose ICS plus a LABA are preferred. Medium-dose ICS plus either leukotriene receptor antagonist or theophylline are alternatives.
○ *Step 5.* High-dose ICS plus LABA are preferred. High-dose ICS plus either a leukotriene receptor antagonist or theophylline are alternatives.
○ *Step 6.* High-dose ICS plus LABA plus oral corticosteroid are preferred. High-dose ICS plus either a leukotriene receptor antagonist or theopylline plus oral corticosteroid are alternatives.
● For children ≥12 years:
○ *Step 2.* Low-dose ICS is preferred. Cromolyn, leukotriene receptor antagonist, nedocromil, or theophylline is an alternative.
○ *Step 3.* Either a low-dose ICS plus LABA or a medium-dose ICS is preferred. Low-dose ICS plus either leukotriene receptor antagonist, theophylline, or zileuton are alternatives.
○ *Step 4.* Medium-dose ICS plus LABA are preferred. Medium-dose ICS plus either leukotriene receptor antagonist, theophylline, or zileuton are alternatives.
○ *Step 5.* High-dose ICS plus LABA and consideration of omalizumab for patients with allergies are preferred.
○ *Step 6.* High-dose ICS plus LABA and oral corticosteroids and consideration of omalizumab for patients with allergies are preferred (NHLBI, 2007).

As health-care providers, it is important to remember that guidelines are not intended to replace clinical decision making. The stepwise approach is a fluid process that requires adjustment in treatment as necessary. The health-care provider should attempt to step down therapy if the child's asthma is well controlled for at least 3 months (NHLBI, 2007). If the child's asthma is not well controlled, a step-up in therapy may be necessary.

Not all symptoms are due to ineffective medication therapy. Other factors such as inhalation technique, adherence, allergen exposure, and comorbid conditions can play a significant role in the manifestation of symptoms. Therefore, before stepping up therapy, the health-care provider must assess inhaler technique as well as adherence to medications (pharmacy refill history and patient report are two methods that can be used to assess adherence). Furthermore, the environment should always be considered as a potential key factor. Parents should be asked if there have been any changes to their environment (i.e., new home/location, installation of carpeting, addition of pet, flooding, and presence of a live evergreen tree) recently or since the last visit. Information regarding changes to the environment may not be voluntarily reported by the parents or the child because such changes are part of normal everyday life and may not appear to them to be related to asthma. However, they can trigger asthma symptoms and should be assessed. Furthermore, identifying and treating comorbid conditions such as allergies, GERD, or sinusitis can positively influence asthma symptoms and eliminate the need for a step-up in therapy. A final consideration is the potential for aspirin sensitivity. Although more common in individuals of Eastern European and Japanese descent and rare in children, aspirin sensitivity can also worsen symptoms (Farooque & Lee, 2009). Generally, symptoms include profound rhinorrhea, tearing, and severe bronchospasm occurring within 1 hour of exposure. After confirmatory testing, these medications should be avoided.

Monitoring control

In addition to allergen avoidance and pharmacotherapy, assessment of asthma control is an important component of asthma management. The level of control will dictate changes in medication therapy. Control is defined as the degree to which manifestations of asthma are minimized and goals are met (NHLBI, 2007). Like severity, control is also determined based on the domains of current impairment and future risk. Specific areas of assessment include symptoms, lung function, quality of life, history of exacerbations, adherence to and side effects caused by medications, patient–provider communication and satisfaction, and biomarkers of inflammation. Evaluation of these areas is based on parent/child recall over the past 2–4 weeks. Control is described as well controlled, not well controlled, and very poorly controlled. Table 7.2 provides the asthma control chart and recommendations for adjustment in therapy.

The EPR3 recommends that all children with asthma receive follow-up care every 2–6 weeks initially and when making adjustments in therapy. Once control is achieved, follow-up care should occur every 1–6 months to determine whether or not goals of therapy are being met (NHLBI, 2007).

Assessment of asthma control should also occur at home. Parents (and the child if old enough) should be instructed on how to monitor their asthma. In addition to assessing symptoms, children with moderate or severe persistent asthma, children with a history of severe exacerbations, and children who have difficulty perceiving airflow obstruction and worsening asthma may benefit from the use of a peak flow meter to assess asthma control at home (NHLBI, 2007). A peak flow meter is a handheld device used to measure the PEFR or the maximum flow rate than can be generated during a forced expiratory maneuver. The PEFR is a measure of the large airways (Yoos & McMullen, 1999). To use a peak flow meter, the child should be instructed to

- place the indicator at "0,"
- stand or sit up straight and tall,
- take a deep breath,
- place the mouthpiece in the mouth (behind teeth) with lips wrapped tightly around the mouthpiece, and
- blow fast and hard in a single breath.

The above steps will cause the indicator to move up the peak flow meter barrel. The corresponding number is the actual peak flow. The steps should be repeated for a total of three times. The highest of the three readings is the PEFR that should be recorded.

The PEFR readings are compared against the child's peak flow zones and are used to self-manage asthma and to assess control in the home setting. The child's peak flow zones should be based on his/her personal best or the predicted, whichever is higher. The personal best is the highest PEFR that the child can achieve over a 2- to 3-week period of time when his/her asthma is well controlled. The predicted is based on a chart of normal PEFRs and is based on height and sex. The peak flow zone system can be explained to parents and children using the traffic light analogy. The green zone (>80% of personal best or predicted) indicates that asthma is well controlled on current therapy. The yellow zone (50–80% of personal best or predicted) indicates that asthma is not well controlled and requires assessment and intervention such as the use of a SABA. The red zone (<50% of personal best or predicted) is considered the "danger zone" and requires immediate medical attention.

The peak flow meter is an effort-dependent device. Therefore, before taking action based on a single reading, the parents should assure that proper technique was used during the measurement. If the lips are not tightly placed around the mouthpiece, the values may be falsely low. Alternatively, if the child coughs or spits into the device, the values may be falsely high.

Managing exacerbations

Although preventing exacerbations is a goal of asthma management, exacerbations continue to occur. In 2005, approximately 3.8 million children experienced an asthma exacerbation in the previous year (Akinbami, n.d.).

Exacerbations are also classified according to level of severity: mild-moderate (PEFR or $FEV_1 \geq 40\%$ predicted) or severe (<40% predicted). It is important to recognize that severe exacerbations can occur at any level of asthma severity; in other words, even those with intermittent asthma can have a severe exacerbation. Exacerbations are managed either at home or in the hospital, depending on their level of severity.

The focus of home asthma exacerbation management is early intervention (NHLBI, 2007). This focus further underscores the importance of teaching parents and children how to self-manage asthma. General home management includes knowing how to use an asthma action plan, recognizing early signs of an exacerbation, and removing allergens from the environment. During an exacerbation, the parent/child should promptly initiate SABA therapy, monitor response to therapy, and stay in contact with a primary care provider (PCP).

Initial home therapy includes the use of a SABA, up to two treatments (nebulizer or two to six puffs of the metered-dose inhaler [MDI] formulation), 20 minutes apart. If the child responds well to the SABA (no wheezing or dyspnea and PEFR in the green zone), the parents should contact the health-care provider for additional instructions. The child can use the SABA every 3–4 hours for 24–48 hours. In addition, the health-care provider may want to consider a short course of oral corticosteroids at this time. If the response to the initial SABA is incomplete (persistent wheezing or PEFR in the yellow zone), the parent should contact the health-care provider immediately so that oral steroids can be initiated. If the response to the initial SABA is poor (marked wheezing, dyspnea, or PEFR in the red zone), the child needs urgent evaluation. The health-care provider should be contacted immediately, the SABA should be repeated, and an oral steroid should be initiated. If the child is in distress, he/she should go directly to the ED or call 911 (NHLBI, 2007).

A severe exacerbation associated with a PEFR or FEV_1 less than 40% predicted usually requires an emergency room visit and possible hospitalization. Children with severe status asthmaticus are at risk for sudden deterioration and respiratory arrest. They must be sequentially and frequently assessed by physical exam, FEV_1 or PEFR if possible, and oxygen saturation by pulse oximetry (SpO_2). Supplemental oxygen should be given, if necessary, to keep oxygen saturation ≥90%. Most providers keep oxygen saturation ≥95% in order to give the patient as much reserve as possible. High-dose inhaled SABA is given with ipratropium with MDI plus valved holding chamber every 20 minutes or via nebulization continuously for 1 hour. Oral corticosteroids should be given if the patient has not already received them. If there is no improvement after continued therapy and the PEFR or FEV_1 remains under 70% predicted, then the patient should be admitted to the hospital. In-hospital therapy consists of supplemental oxygen, continued use of SABA, and corticosteroids. Intravenous hydration may be necessary if the patient has been unable to drink or eat. A PEFR or FEV_1 less than 40% despite aggressive treatment will likely require admission to an intensive care unit. Signs of impending or actual respiratory failure include drowsiness, confusion, severe respiratory distress, and arterial carbon dioxide level (PCO_2) ≥42 mm Hg. Adjunct therapies such as intravenous magnesium or heliox-driven albuterol nebulization may be considered. Intubation and mechanical ventilation may be necessary.

If the child is experiencing frequent exacerbations or is not meeting goals of therapy, the health-care provider should consider a referral to an asthma specialist. Other reasons to consider a referral to an asthma specialist are if the child is exhibiting atypical signs and symptoms, if there are problems with the differential diagnosis, or if additional testing is required (NHLBI, 2007).

NURSING CARE OF THE CHILD AND FAMILY

The primary role of the nurse is to provide education to the child and family so that they are able to self-manage the asthma. Education for the child with asthma and his/her family is an integral component of asthma management and the EPR3. National certification for asthma educators has been available since 2002 from the National Asthma Educator Certification Board (National Asthma Educator Certification Board, n.d.). Asthma self-management education programs have been proven effective. In a published meta-analysis, Coffman and colleagues revealed that providing asthma education in the pediatric setting decreases the mean number of ED visits and hospitalizations and the odds of an ED visit (Coffman, Cabana, Halpin, & Yelin, 2008). Other pediatric asthma education studies have also demonstrated an increase in asthma knowledge, self-efficacy, adherence, and quality of life, and a decrease in ED visits, hospitalizations, and costs when children and their parents participate in asthma self-management education programs (Butz et al., 2005; Greineder, Loane, & Parks, 1999; Kelly et al., 2000; Newcomb, 2006).

After the diagnosis of asthma is established, care should be given to the child and family to ensure that they have a basic understanding of asthma and how it is managed. The educational process should be comprehensive and ongoing. It should include all members of the health-care team and should occur across various settings.

Additionally, the nurse should develop a partnership with the parents and the child. This partnership includes the development of mutually agreed-upon treatment goals. The child should be involved as much as possible in establishing goals of therapy. The nurse must create an environment that encourages open communication. Such a relationship will allow the nurse to effectively assess barriers to care as well as adherence to treatment.

All patients should receive basic education regarding asthma in a culturally competent manner. The essential components of an educational program include basic facts about asthma, how to assess the level of control, how asthma is treated (this includes information about medications and allergen avoidance), how to use prescribed devices, how to respond to signs and symptoms of worsening asthma, and when and where to seek medical attention.

The educational plan should be individualized to meet the needs of the parents and child and should include the provision of an asthma action plan. Prior to providing the education, the nurse should make an assessment of what the parents and child already know about asthma. This evaluation provides the nurse with the opportunity to reinforce accurate messages and to correct inaccurate ones. The nurse should also determine how much information to provide at each setting so as not to overwhelm the parents and the child.

Basic facts

When providing information about the basic facts, the nurse must emphasize the role inflammation plays in asthma. This will help the parents and child understand the purpose of the medications prescribed. The use of pictures or models is helpful.

Allergen/trigger avoidance

The parents and the child should receive individualized instruction and advice regarding environmental control measures (specific measures were discussed earlier in this chapter). Unfortunately, environmental control measures such as carpet removal or professional extermination services can be costly and are not covered by insurance companies. In such situations, the nurse should work with the family and refer them to resources that are available in the community. When discussing environmental control measures, the nurse should remember to include an assessment of the daycare and school environment as the child spends a great deal of time in those locations.

Respiratory viruses are a common trigger for asthma symptoms. In addition to practicing good hand washing, the parents should be encouraged to have their child (if not allergic to the vaccine or eggs) vaccinated with the influenza vaccine. The CDC recommends that children 6 months of age and older receive the influenza vaccine. Depending on the age of the child, either one or two doses may be required (Centers for Disease Control [CDC], n.d.,a). A recent univariate analysis found that the influenza vaccine reduced ED visits and use of oral steroids (Ong, Forester, & Fallot, 2009).

Medications and delivery devices

When providing information about medications, the nurse should include the name of the medication, the dose, the dosing interval, and the side effects. Because oral candidiasis is a potential side effect of ICSs, the parents and child should be instructed to have the child rinse his/her mouth after the ICS is administered. Another important fact to reinforce in regard to medications is the difference between long-term control medications and quick-relief medications.

Because most asthma medications are administered via inhalation, the nurse must ensure that the parents and child know and follow the correct technique and priming recommendations. This starts by making sure the most appropriate delivery device is selected for the child. The nurse plays an integral role in determining the most suitable device. Factors to consider when choosing a device include the child's ability to use the device correctly, the preferences of the child for the device, the availability of the drug/device combination, the compatibility between the drug and the delivery device, convenience, durability, the cost of the device, and the potential for reimbursement (Dolovich et al., 2005).

Parents often assume a nebulizer is a more effective form of medication delivery; however, the MDI used with or without spacer/holding chamber is appropriate for the delivery of ICSs and SABAs at home, in the hospital, and in the ED (Dolovich et al., 2005). Previous studies have demonstrated that MDIs are as effective as nebulizers in treating individuals with asthma. However, data in the treatment of those experiencing severe exacerbations are not as strong (Castro-Rodriguez & Rodrigo, 2004). If the child is prescribed a nebulizer, the "blow-by" technique should be discouraged. Furthermore, if the child is not old enough to use a mouthpiece (with a nebulizer or a holding chamber), the nurse should fit the child for an appropriate-sized mask.

Inspiratory flow rates are also important when selecting a medication delivery device. If the child does not take a deep breath, the medicine will not adequately reach the lower airways. With MDIs, if the inhalation is too fast, the medication may be deposited in the back of the throat rather than in the lower airways. Having the child inhale slowly and deeply over a count of 10 (for a younger child, have him/her count to 10 with the fingers of his/her other hand) is the proper technique for an MDI. With dry powder inhalers (DPIs), if the inspiratory effort is weak/slow, the device will not be activated properly; this will have a negative impact on deposition to the lower airways. DPIs are more effective when the child inhales rapidly (Dolovich et al., 2005). An assessment of the inhaler technique can be made with the use of the In-Check DIAL. The In-Check DIAL is a hand-held device used to measure inspiratory flow rate. This device and its use are described in Chapter 3.

Self-management

The parents and child should be instructed on how to self-manage asthma at home. This is best accomplished with the use of an asthma action plan (Bhogal, Zemek, & Ducharme, 2006). The child should be involved in the development of the asthma action plan, and it should be written in terms that are understood by the parent and older child. Studies have demonstrated that keeping teaching materials simple and concise improves health-care knowledge (Paasche-Orlow et al., 2005).

Key elements of an asthma action plan include what to do on a daily basis, when to step up therapy, and when to contact the health-care provider. The asthma action plan should also include environmental control measures and contact telephone numbers for the health-care provider (NHLBI, 2007).

In a Cochrane Review evaluating symptom versus peak flow-based asthma action plans, no significant differences in rates of exacerbations requiring oral steroids or admissions, lung function, symptom scores, and quality of life were noted. Findings did reveal that children using symptom-based asthma action plans experienced a lower risk of exacerbations requiring an acute care visit. Furthermore, children preferred symptom-based plans. However, data were insufficient to recommend using one method over the other (Bhogal et al., 2006). Thus, asthma action plans can be based on symptoms and/or PEFR. If the plan is based on PEFRs, the nurse must ensure that the parent/child knows how to use the peak flow meter and how to respond to the readings. If the child is experiencing symptoms or a decrease in PEFRs (yellow or red zone), he/she should take action by adding a SABA to the daily medications and by contacting the health-care provider if the SABA does not relieve symptoms.

Adherence and barriers to care

The nurse must work with the child to determine if there are any barriers to carrying out the agreed-upon asthma action plan. Adherence to therapy has a major impact on asthma control. There are many factors that contribute to nonadherence. They can be patient related, caregiver related, or disease related. Examples include patient/family psychological disorders, lack of insurance, long wait times for appointments, inconvenient office hours, lack of communication with the health-care provider, medication side effects, and the need for daily therapy (Adams, Dreyer, Dinakar, & Portnoy, 2004). Forgetfulness is the primary reason identified for nonadherence (Matsui, 2007). If medication administration is difficult at home (i.e., the child wakes up late or forgets to take his/her medication), the nurse can work with the family and the school nurse to make arrangements to have the medications administered at school if possible.

The best way to assess adherence is to use a nonjudgmental approach. The nurse must remember that there may be underlying issues that the parents have not shared with the health-care provider (i.e., fear of ICS side effects, not knowing how to recognize symptoms, inability to give the medicine twice a day, not recognizing the need for daily medications). By communicating with the parents/child and addressing the concerns, adherence will likely improve (Williams et al., 2007).

Anticipatory guidance

Anticipatory guidance is important for parents and children. Parents should be made aware that giving medications to infants, toddlers, and preschoolers can sometimes be difficult. For oral medications, the nurse should prepare the parents by informing them that the younger child may try to spit out the medication because of the taste. Some medications can be flavored by the pharmacy; parents should be instructed to check with their local pharmacy to determine if this option is available.

For inhaled medications, the nurse should provide the parents with developmentally appropriate methods (demonstrating medication administration on the child's favorite doll, allowing the child time to touch and explore the mask, holding chamber, etc., employing distractions such as singing to the child) to help ensure adequate medication delivery. The parent should be reassured that any difficulty with medication administration is related to developmental maturity level and will resolve as the child becomes accustomed to the device.

School-related issues also require attention. The nurse should encourage the parents to discuss the fact that their child has asthma with the school nurse and teachers. The nurse should also ensure that the school is provided with a copy of the written asthma action plan, a SABA plus a nebulizer or holding chamber (often called spacer), and an authorization for medication administration. If the child is old enough, the nurse should work with the family and other health-care providers to allow the child the ability to carry his/her own SABA while in school. If this is allowed by the school system, written instructions for the school, along with parental permission to carry the SABA, are necessary. Easy access is key to early intervention. The NAEPP has partnered with various organizations to ensure that children are allowed to carry their own medications. Legislation has been enacted by a number of states to allow for self-administration (NHLBI, 2007).

Physical activity at home and in school should be promoted. Parents sometimes limit their child's activities because they are afraid the exercise will exacerbate their child's asthma. However, parents should be made aware that children with asthma can and should exercise. The child himself/herself should also be encouraged to participate in physical activities. If needed, treatment with a SABA before exercise can be prescribed to prevent symptoms of exercise-induced bronchoconstriction.

Finally, there are a number of organizations that provide educational materials to people with asthma as well as health-care providers. Parents should be informed about the existence of these organizations and should be provided with their contact information. Helpful resources include

- Allergy & Asthma Network Mothers of Asthmatics
  1-800-878-4403
  http://www.breatherville.org

- American Academy of Allergy, Asthma and Immunology
  1-414-272-6071
  http://www.aaaai.org
- American College of Allergy, Asthma & Immunology
  1-847-427-1200
  http://www.acaai.org
- Association of Asthma Educators
  1-888-988-7747
  http://www.asthmaeducators.org
- Asthma and Allergy Foundation of America
  1-800-727-8462
  http://www.aafa.org
- National Heart, Lung, and Blood Institute
  1-301-592-8573
  http://www.nhlbi.gov

Follow-up care

At each follow-up visit, the nurse should reinforce previous educational messages and provide new information as needed. During each visit, the nurse should focus on expectations of the visit, asthma control, parents' and child's goals and preferences, medications, and quality of life (NHLBI, 2007). Device technique and appropriateness should be evaluated at each visit because as the child grows, he/she may need a bigger size mask or may be able to switch from the mask to the mouthpiece.

When reviewing technique, the nurse can begin by asking who administers the medication. The nurse can then give a demonstrator to the parents or child and ask them to "show me how you take your medicine at home." After assessing the technique, the nurse should first provide encouragement and praise the steps that were performed correctly. Next, the nurse should correct any errors that were noted. Common mistakes include not forming a tight seal with the mask or mouthpiece and poor inspiratory effort. In addition to evaluating technique, the holding chamber should be assessed for cracks and loss of valve function. Finally, the written asthma action plan should be reviewed and revised as needed.

It is important to remember that follow-up education should not be limited to the office setting. Every encounter with the parents and child should be viewed as an opportunity to reinforce teaching (Szpiro, Harrison, VanDenKerkjof, & Lougheed, 2009); this includes ED visits and hospitalizations.

REFERENCES

Adams, C. D., Dreyer, M. L., Dinakar, C., & Portnoy, J. M. (2004). Pediatric asthma: A look at adherence from the patient and family perspective. *Current Allergy and Asthma Reports, 4*, 425–432.

Agertoft, L., & Pedersen, S. (1994). Effects of long-term treatment with an inhaled corticosteroid on growth and pulmonary function in asthmatic children. *Respiratory Medicine, 88*(5), 373–381.

Akinbami, L. J. (2006). The State Of Childhood Asthma, United States, 1980-2005.. Retrieved from http://www.cdc.gov/nchs/data/ad/ad381.pdf.

Akinbami, L. J. (n.d.). Asthma prevalence, health care use and mortality: United States, 2003–2005. Retrieved from http://www.cdc.gov/nchs/data/hestat/asthma03-05/asthma03-05.htm.

Akinbami, L. J., Moorman, J. E., Garbe, P. L., & Sondik, E. J. (2009). Status of childhood asthma in the United States. *Pediatrics, 123*, S135–S145.

American Thoracic Society. Guidelines for methacholine and exercise challenge testing. (1999). Retrieved from http://www.thoracic.org/statements/resources/pfet/methacholine1-21.pdf.

American Thoracic Society. (2005). Interpretative strategies for lung function tests. Retrieved from http://www.thoracic.org/statements/resources/pfet/pft5.pdf.

Apter, AJ, Van Hoof, TJ, Sherwin, TE, Casey, BA, Petrillo, MK, & Meehan, TP (2001). Assessing the quality of asthma care provided to Medicaid patients enrolled in managed care organizations in Connecticut. *Annals of Allergy, Asthma, & Immunology, 86*(2), 211–218.

Arlian, L. H., Vyszenski-Moher, D. L., & Morgan, M. S. (2003). Mite and mite allergen removal during machine-washing of laundry. *Journal of Allergy and Clinical Immunology, 111*(6), 269–273.

Berquist, W. E., Rachelefsky, G. S., Kadden, M., Siegel, S. C., Katz, R. M., Fonkalsrud, E. W., et al. (1981). Gastroesophageal reflux-associated recurrent pneumonia and chronic asthma in children. *Pediatrics, 68*(1), 29–35.

Bhogal, S., Zemek, R., & Ducharme, F. M. (2006). Written action plans for asthma in children. *Cochrane Database of Systematic Reviews*, (3), CD005306.

Birnbaum, H. G., Berger, W. E., Greenberg, P. E., Holland, M., Auerbach, R., Atkins, K. M., et al. (2002). Direct and indirect costs of asthma to an employer. *The Journal of Allergy and Clinical Immunology, 109*(2), 264–270.

Butz, A., Pham, L., Lewis, L., Lewis, C., Hill, K., Walker, J., et al. (2005). Rural children with asthma: Impact of a parent and child asthma education program. *The Journal of Asthma, 42*, 813–821.

Castro-Rodriguez, J. A., & Rodrigo, G. J. (2004). B-agonists through metered-dose inhaler with valved holding chamber versus nebulizer for acute exacerbation of wheezing or asthma in children under 5 years of age: A systematic review with meta-analysis. *The Journal of Pediatrics, 145*(2), 172–177.

Celano, M. P., Linzer, J. F., Demi, A., Bakeman, R., Oyeshiku Smith, C., et al. (2010). Treatment adherence among low-income, african american children with persistent asthma. *The Journal of Asthma, 47*, 317–322.

Centers for Disease Control (CDC). (n.d.,a). Influenza vaccination: A summary for clinicians. Retrieved from http://www.cdc.gov/flu/professionals/vaccination/vax-summary.htmhttp://www.cdc.gov/flu/professionals/vaccination/vax-summary.htm.

Centers for Disease Control (CDC). (n.d.,b). The state of childhood asthma, United States, 1980–2005. Retrieved from http://www.cdc.gov/asthma/.

Clark, T. J. H et al. (2000). *Asthma* (4th ed.). New York: Oxford University Press.

Coffman, J. M., Cabana, M. D., Halpin, H. A., & Yelin, E. H. (2008). Effects of asthma education on children's use of acute care services: A meta-analysis. *Pediatrics, 121,* 575–586.

Dezateux, C., Lum, S., Hoo, A., Hawdon, J., Costeloe, K., & Stocks, J. (2004). Low birth weight for gestation and airway function in infancy: Exploring the fetal origins hypothesis. *Thorax, 59*(1), 60–66.

Dolovich, M. B., Ahrens, R. C., Hess, D. R., Anderson, P., Dhand, R., Rau, J. L., et al. (2005). Device selection and outcomes of aerosol tehrapy: Evidence-based guildenes. *Chest, 127*(1), 335–371.

Fang, Q., Wang, F., & Zhao, D. (2010). Association between regulated upon activation, normal T cells expressed and secreted (RANTES) -28C/G polymorphism and asthma risk—A meta-analysis. *International Journal of Medical Sciences, 7*(1), 55–61.

Farooque, S. P., & Lee, T. H. (2009). Aspirin-sensitive respiratory disease. *Annual Review of Physiology, 71,* 465–487.

Finkelstein, Y., Bournissen, F. G., Hutson, J. R., & Shannon, M. (2009). Polymorphism of the ADRB2 gene and response to inhaled beta-agonists in children with asthma: A meta-analysis. *The Journal of Asthma, 46*(9), 900–905.

Fitzgerald, J. M., Boulet, E. P., & O'Byrne, P. M. (2001). *Evidenced based asthma management* (Vol. 3). Ontario: BC Decker.

Gaglani, M. J. (2002). Rationale and approach to target children with asthma for annual influenza immunization. *Seminars in Pediatric Infectious Diseases, 13*(2), 97–103.

Gilliland, F. D., Islam, T., Berhane, K., Gauderman, W. J., McConnell, R., Avol, E., et al. (2006). Regular smoking and asthma incidence in adolescents. *American Journal of Respiratory and Critical Care Medicine, 174,* 1094–1100.

Greineder, D. K., Loane, K. C., & Parks, P. (1999). A randomized controlled trial of a pediatric asthma outreach program. *The Journal of Allergy & Clinical Immunology, 103*(3), 436–440.

Guilbert, T. W., Garris, C., Jhingran, P., Bonafede, M., Tomaszewski, K. J., & Bonus, T. (2011). Asthma that is not well-controlled is associated with increased healthcare utilization and decreased quality of life. *The Journal of Asthma, 48*(2), 126–132.

Guilbert, T. W., Morgan, W. J., Krawiec, M., Lemanske, R. F., Jr., Sorkness, C., Szefler, S. J., et al. (2004). The prevention of early asthma in kids study: Design, rationale and methods for the Childhood Asthma Research and Education network. *Controlled Clinical Trials, 25*(3), 286–310.

Guilbert, T. W., Morgan, W. J., Zeriger, R. S., Mauger, D. T., Boehmer, S. J., Szefler, S. J., et al. (2006). Long-term inhaled corticosteroids in preschool children at high risk for asthma. *New England Journal of Medicine, 354,* 1985–1997.

Hendeles, L., & Sorkness, C. A. (2007). Anti-immunoglobulin E therapy with Omalizumab for asthma. *The Annals of Pharmacotherapy, 41*(9), 1397–1410.

Hill, V. L., & Wood, P. R. (2009). Asthma epidemiology, pathophysiology, and initial evaluation. *Pediatrics in Review,* (30), 331–336.

Hyatt, R. E., Scanlon, P. D., & Nakamura, M. (Eds.) (1997). *Interpretation of pulmonary function tests, a practical guide*. Philadelphia: Lippincott William & Wilkinsm.

Kalra, M, Buncher, R, & Amin, RS (2005). Asthma as a risk factor for respiratory complications after adenotonsillectomy in children with obstructive breathing during sleep. *Annals of Allergy, Asthma & Immunology, 94*(5), 549–552.

Kamble, S., & Bharma, M. (2009). Incremental direct expenditure of treating asthma in the United States. *The Journal of Asthma, 46*(1), 73–80.

Kelly, C. S., Morrow, A. L., Shults, J., Nakas, N., Strope, G. L., & Adelman, R. D. (2000). Outcomes evaluation of a comprehensive intervention program for asthmatic children enrolled in Medicaid. *Pediatrics, 105*(5), 1029–1035.

Leone, F. T., Fish, J. E., Szefler, S. J., & West, S. L. (2003). Systematic review of the evidence regarding potential complications of inhaled corticosteroid use in asthma: Collaboration of American College of Chest Physicians, American Academy of Allergy, Asthma, and Immunology, and American College of Allergy, Asthma, and Immunology. *Chest, 124*(6), 2329–2340.

Liu, A. H. (2007). Hygiene theory and allergy and asthma prevention. *Paediatric and Perinatal Epidemiology, 21*, 2–7.

Martinez, F. D. (2009). The origins of asthma and chronic obstructive pulmonary disease in early life. *Proceedings of the American Thoracic Society, 6*(3), 272–277.

Mason, R. J., Broaddus, V. C., Murray, J. H., & Nadel, J. A. (2000). *Murray and Nadel's textbook of respiratory medicine* (3rd ed.). New York: WB Saunders.

Matsui, D. (2007). Current issues in pediatric medication adherence. *Pediatric Drugs, 9*(5), 283–288.

Milgrom, H., & Taussig, L. M. (1999). Keeping children with exercise-induced asthma active. *Pediatrics, 104*(3), 1–7.

Miller, M. R., Hankinson, J., Brusasco, V., Burgos, F., Casaburi, R., Coates, A., et al. (2005). Standardisation of spirometry. *European Respiratory Journal, 26*, 319–338.

Mrazek, D. A. (1992). Psychiatric complications of pediatric asthma. *Annals of Allergy, 69*(4), 285–290.

National Asthma Educator Certification Board. (n.d.). Promoting excellence in Asthma education, history. Retrieved from http://www.naecb.org/about/history.htm.

National Heart Lung and Blood Institute (NHLBI). (2007). Guidelines for diagnosis and management of Asthma (EPR-3). Retrieved from http://www.nhlbi.nih.gov/guidelines/asthma/.

Newcomb, P (2006). Results of an asthma disease management program in an urban pediatric community clinic. *Journal for Specialists in Pediatric Nursing, 11*(3), 178–188.

Novelline, R. A. (2004). *Fundamentals of radiology* (6th ed.). Cambridge, MA: Harvard University Press.

Ong, B. A., Forester, J., & Fallot, A. (2009). Does influenza vaccination improve pediatric asthma outcomes? *The Journal of Asthma, 46*(9), 477–480.

Paasche-Orlow, M. K., Riekert, K. A., Bilderback, A., Chanmugam, A., Hill, P., Rand, C. S., et al. (2005). Tailored education may reduce health literacy disparities in asthma self-management. *American Journal of Respiratory and Critical Care Medicine, 172,* 980–986.

Palmer, C., Irvin, A. D., Terron-Kwiatkowski, A., Zhao, Y., Liao, H., Lee, S. P., et al. (2006). Common loss-of-function variants of the epidermal barrier protein filaggrin are a major predisposing factor for atopic dermatitis. *Nature Genetics, 38,* 441–446.

Poston, R. N., Chanez, P., Lacoste, J. Y., Litchfield, T., Lee, T. H., & Bousquet, J. (1992). Immunohistochemical characterization of the cellular infiltration in asthmatic bronchi. *The American Review of Respiratory Disease, 145*(4), 918–921.

Rebuck, A. S., & Chapman, K. R. (1987). Asthma: 1. Pathophysiologic features and evaluation of severity. *Canadian Medical Association Journal, 136,* 351–354.

Rogers, A. J., Raby, B. A., Lasky-Su, J. A., Murphy, A., Lazarus, R., Klanderman, B. J., et al. (2009). Assessing the reproducibility of asthma candidate gene associations, using genome-wide data. *American Journal of Respiratory and Critical Care Medicine, 179*(12), 1084–1090.

Rottier, B. L., & Duiverman, E. J. (2009). Anti-inflammatory drug therapy in asthma. *Paediatric Respiratory Reviews, 10*(4), 214–219.

Schaub, B., Lauener, R., & von Mutius, E. (2006). The many faces of the hygiene hypothesis. *The Journal of Allergy and Clinical Immunology, 117*(5), 969–977.

Schonberger, H., van Schayck, O., Muris, J., Bor, H., vanden Hoogen, H., Knottnerus, A., et al. (2004). Towards improving the accuracy of diagnosing asthma in early childhood. *European Journal of General Practice, 10*(4), 18–145.

Shapiro, G. G., & Stout, J. W. (2002). Childhood Asthma in the United States: Urban issues. *Pediatric Pulmonology, 33,* 47–55.

Smith, S. R., Jaffe, D. M., Fisher, E. B., Trinkaus, K. M., Highstein, G., & Strunk, R. C. (2004). Improving follow-up for children with asthma after an acute emergency department visit. *Journal of Pediatrics, 145*(6), 772–777.

Stern, D. A., Morgan, W. J., Halonen, M., Wright, A. L., & Martinez, F. D. (2008). Wheezing and bronchial hyper-responsiveness in early childhood as predictors of newly diagnosed asthma in early adulthood: A longitudinal birth-cohort study. *Lancet, 372*(96), 1058–1064.

Subbarao, P., Mandhane, P. J., & Sears, M. R. (2009). Asthma: Epidemiology, etiology and risk factors. *Canadian Medical Association Journal, 181,* 181–190.

Sylvester, K. P., Patey, R. A., Broughton, S., Rafferty, G. F., Rees, D., Thein, S. L., et al. (2007). Temporal relationship of asthma to acute chest syndrome in sickle cell disease. *Pediatric Pulmonology, 42*(2), 103–106.

Szpiro, K. A., Harrison, M. B., VanDenKerkjof, E. G., & Lougheed, M. D. (2009). Asthma education delivered in an emergency department and an asthma education center. A feasibility study. *Advanced Emergency Nursing Journal, 31*(1), 73–85.

Visser, M. J., van der Veer, E., Postma, D. S., Arends, L. R., de Vries, T. W., Brand, P. L., et al. (2004). Side-effects of fluticasone in asthmatic children: No effects after dose reduction. *The European Respiratory Journal, 24*(3), 420–425.

Von Mitius, E. (2010). 99th Dahlem conference on infection, inflammation and inflammatory disorders: Farm lifestyles and the hygiene hypothesis. *Clinical and Experimental Immunology, 160*, 130–135.

Watts, B. (2008). Outpatient management of asthma in children age 5–11 years: Guidelines for practice. *Journal of the American of Academy of Nurse Practitioners, 21*, 261–269.

Willers, S. M., Wijga, A. H., Brunekreef, B., Kerkhof, M., Gerritsen, J., Hoekstra, M. O., et al. (2008). Maternal food consumption during pregnancy and the longitudinal development of childhood asthma. *American Journal of Respiratory and Critical Care Medicine, 178*(2), 124–131.

Williams, L. K., Joseph, C. L., Peterson, E. L., Ells, K., Wang, M., Chowdhry, V. K., et al. (2007). Patients with asthma who do not fill their inhaled corticosteroids: A study of primary nonadherence. *Journal of Allergy and Clinical Immunology, 120*(5), 1153–1159.

Yoos, H. L., & McMullen, A. (1999). Symptom monitoring in childhood asthma: How to use a peak flow meter. *Pediatric Annals, 28*(1), 31–39.

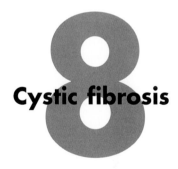

Cystic fibrosis

Antoinette Gardner, RN, MEd, CCRC, AE-C, and
Kimberly Jones, MD

EPIDEMIOLOGY

Cystic fibrosis (CF) is a chronic, life-shortening, multisystem disease affecting approximately 30,000 individual in the United States. It is the most common autosomal recessive disorder in the Caucasian population, affecting approximately 2,500–3,500 live births. The incidence is lower in other ethnic groups; specifically, 1:9,000 Hispanics, 1:15,000 African Americans, and 1:30,000 Asian Americans are affected (Hamosh et al., 1998). According to the Cystic Fibrosis Foundation (CFF) Registry (Cystic Fibrosis Foundation [CFF], 2010a), the median age at diagnosis is 5 months, with a median predicted survival of 37.42 years. This median predicted age of survival is up from 32 years in 2000. In fact, survival over the past 20 years has been significantly improved; this is in part due to earlier diagnosis by newborn screening as well as to new and emerging therapies to stabilize and/or improve lung function and nutritional state. The steady rise of the median predicted age of survival suggests how improvements in treatment and care are advancing the lives of those with CF (CFF, 2010d).

PATHOPHYSIOLOGY

The gene for CF was first isolated to the long arm of chromosome 7 in 1989 (Kerem et al., 1989). Since that time, more than 1,800 different mutations

Nursing Care in Pediatric Respiratory Disease, First Edition. Edited by Concettina (Tina) Tolomeo.
© 2012 John Wiley & Sons, Inc. Published 2012 by John Wiley & Sons, Inc.

have been identified (Cystic Fibrosis Centre at the Hospital for Sick Children in Toronto, 2010). The basic defect is the cystic fibrosis transmembrane conductance regulator (CFTR), a transmembrane protein responsible for moving sodium and chloride across the epithelial cell surface. The CFTR protein is located on the cell membrane of epithelial surfaces. A defect in this protein causes secretions within the respiratory tract as well as the gastrointestinal and reproductive tracts to become thick and sticky, leading to impaired clearance of secretions and obstruction of the exocrine ducts and epithelial channels. The most common mutation, ΔF508, is a single deletion of the amino acid, phenylalanine, and is associated with defective production and trafficking of the CFTR protein.

There are five different classes of mutations identified. Class I mutations are associated with a defect in protein production secondary to a nonsense mutation, frameshift mutation, or splice-site mutation that results in essentially no production of protein. Class II mutations result in defective trafficking of the protein so that little to no CFTR protein reaches the cell surface (e.g., ΔF508). Class III mutations are associated with defective regulation of the CFTR so that there is diminished ion channel activity. Class IV mutations result in diminished ion flow with conduction defects. Class V mutations result in decreased production of the CFTR protein (Rowe, Miller, & Sorscher, 2005).

There is enormous variability between the genotype and phenotypic features seen in patients with CF. Recent work has demonstrated that this may be in part due to genetic modifiers. Approximately 20% of patients with CF have variants in one or both of the following: (1) transforming growth factor beta (TGF-beta) 1 gene and (2) mannose-binding lectin (MBL). Polymorphisms in the TGF-beta 1 gene, which is a suppressor of T cell activation and cytokine production, are associated with more severe manifestations of lung disease (Drumm et al., 2005). In patients with CF carrying variant MBL alleles, reduction in lung function, increased risk of chronic *Burkholderia* and *Pseudomonas* infections, and early death have been seen (Garred et al., 1999). These effects are more pronounced in patients carrying variant alleles in both TGF-beta 1 and MBL.

The predominant morbidity occurs in the respiratory tract where thick, inspissated secretions cause progressive airway obstruction. Over time, the secretions within the airway become colonized with a variety of bacteria, the most common being *Pseudomonas aeruginosa* (found in 55% of the CF population in 2007). Recruitment of inflammatory cells to fight the bacteria results in the release of mediators that damage airway walls, leading to bronchiectasis and fibrosis.

SIGNS AND SYMPTOMS

Based on the 2008 National CF Registry data (Cystic Fibrosis Foundation, 2009), 44% of all patients diagnosed with CF presented with respiratory symptoms. Chronic or recurrent cough, wheeze, recurrent pneumonia, or bronchitis can be seen related to thickened secretions and progressive airway obstruction. These findings can be associated with persistent radiographic changes that fail to clear with treatment. Upper airway disease, such as chronic sinusitis and nasal polyps, occurs frequently in this population and may be the only presenting symptoms in older patients.

Gastrointestinal manifestations are often the most common early and initial presentation. Meconium ileus is seen in 20% of patients; approximately 10% of these patients ultimately require corrective surgery. In older infants, steatorrhea, failure to thrive, and voracious appetites can be seen. In such cases, infants typically consume large amounts of formula/food, but, despite excessive caloric intake, they fail to gain weight. This picture is associated with greasy, foul-smelling, and frequently bulky stools (steatorrhea) that are characteristic of fat malabsorption.

The same thick secretions seen within the airways are seen within the gastrointestinal tract. In the pancreas, there are exocrine glands that secrete digestive enzymes that pass through a ductal system and lead to the small intestine to facilitate absorption of carbohydrates, proteins, and fats. Thickened secretions lead to plugging of the exocrine ducts of the pancreas, causing an autodegradation of the pancreas and ultimately a fatty-replaced pancreas that is nonfunctional. Pancreatic insufficiency results in the inability to absorb fats and fat-soluble vitamins from the diet. This leads to malnutrition and failure to thrive. Studies such as fecal elastase enable clinicians to make the diagnosis of pancreatic insufficiency and to initiate treatment.

Ninety-eight to ninety-nine percent of postpubertal males with CF have obstructive azoospermia secondary to an absent or rudimentary vas deferens. The abnormality with the vas deferens occurs during the embryological development. During this time, thickened secretions prevent the canaliculization of the developing vas deferens. There are reports of a subset of patients with congenital bilateral absence of the vas deferens (CBAVD) without respiratory or pancreatic abnormalities; these patients are not classified as having CF unless they also have phenotypic features of respiratory or gastrointestinal manifestations consistent with CF (Chillon et al., 1995).

Other less common presentations include skin rash due to fatty acid vitamin deficiency as well as other manifestations of fat-soluble vitamin deficiency. Vitamin A deficiency is associated with an increased risk for the development of respiratory and diarrheal infection, a decrease in growth rate, and slowing of bone development (Michel et al., 2009). Late findings associated with vitamin A deficiency include bulging fontanel secondary to increased intracranial pressure, conjunctival xerosis, and night blindness. Symptoms of vitamin D deficiency include rickets, although this is rarely seen in the present day due to adequate amounts of vitamin D in most infant formulas. Vitamin E deficiency can be associated with hemolytic disease in infancy, diminished deep tendon reflexes (DTRs), and muscle weakness. Vitamin K deficiency can cause easy bruising and, rarely, severe bleeding.

Older patients may come to medical attention with atypical presentations. Examples of such presentations include diabetes, cirrhosis, chronic or recurrent pancreatitis, rectal prolapse, focal biliary cirrhosis, appendicitis, or gallbladder disease.

DIAGNOSIS

The diagnosis of CF (excluding newborn screening) can be made when the patient has the following (Boyle, 2003):

(a) The presence of one or more phenotypic characteristics
(b) A history of CF in a sibling along with elevated sweat chloride concentrations on two separate occasions
(c) The identification of two known disease-causing CF mutations
(d) *In vivo* demonstration of the characteristic abnormalities in ion transport across the nasal epithelium seen in CF patients

The only acceptable method for sweat chloride testing is the quantitative pilocarpine iontophoresis sweat test. This test is performed at experienced centers following standard guidelines (CFF, 2010a).

For people over the age of 6 months:

●   Chloride levels at or above 60 mmol/L are consistent with CF.
●   Chloride levels between 40 and 59 mmol/L are borderline.
●   Chloride levels below 40 mmol/L are negative for CF.

The sweat chloride test must be repeated on two separate occasions as there can be occasional false positives or negatives.

DNA testing is performed (1) when the sweat chloride test is inconclusive (intermediate), (2) as part of the newborn screening process in certain states, and (3) in some centers even in patients with positive sweat chloride tests for research and for epidemiological or prognostic purposes. However, as new therapies targeted toward the specific classes of mutations emerge, DNA testing may be needed for identifying which patients will respond to such therapies.

Molecular analysis has become quite complex and often is performed as a two-tiered process. Initial analysis often examines the most common 80–85% of all mutations. However, further analysis can be performed if a second mutation is not identified with the initial testing or to detect deletions, duplications, or sequence variations. DNA testing is most commonly performed from a blood sample but can also be performed from a buccal smear or saliva.

Nasal potential difference (PD) is another test that can help make the diagnosis. The respiratory epithelia, including the nasal epithelia, regulate the composition of fluids on airway surfaces by the transport of ions such as sodium and chloride. The active transport of ions generates a transepithelial electrical PD that can be measured *in vivo*. Abnormalities of ion transport in CF patients result in a different pattern than people without CF. This pattern can be distinguished by the following:

(a) Higher basal PD
(b) Larger inhibition of PD after perfusion of nasal epithelia by amiloride, a sodium channel inhibitor
(c) Little or no change in PD after nasal profusion with isoproterenol (due to the absence of CFTR-mediated chloride secretion) (Rosenstein & Cutting, 1998)

Newborn screening is now being performed in all 50 states and in the District of Columbia. Each state has its own screening program, but all screens are based on the use of immunoreactive trypsinogen (IRT) as a first-line screen. The IRT can be performed on a dried blood sample from a heel stick obtained at the same time as the phenylketonuria (PKU) test. If the IRT is elevated, the state refers the patients for a repeat IRT or mutational analysis. If the test is abnormal, the patient is then referred for sweat chloride testing, preferably when the infant is at least 2 weeks of age or >2 kg if asymptomatic. Sweat test cutoff values are slightly different for infants less than 6 months of age (Farrell et al., 2008):

For children who are less than 6 months old:

* Chloride levels at or above 60 mmol/L are consistent with CF.
* Chloride levels between 30 and 59 mmol/L are borderline and need to be interpreted on a case-by-case basis.
* Chloride levels below 30 mmol/L are negative for CF.

New guidelines published in 2009 for the management of infants diagnosed by newborn screening have been developed in an attempt to standardize the care of these patients across the different centers. Recommendations for timing of follow-up, age at which nutritional testing should be performed, and so on, have been recommended (Borowitz et al., 2009b). For those patients with an intermediate or negative sweat test and one or two CFTR mutations, but one mutation is designated as nondisease causing, a new designation has been proposed. These patients are given the diagnosis of CFTR-related metabolic syndrome and are followed by a CF specialist closely during the first 2 years of life for any signs or symptoms suggestive of disease consistent with CF (Borowitz et al., 2009a).

COMPLICATIONS

The pulmonary manifestations of CF may be complicated by numerous factors, including types of infection (atypical mycobacterium, *Burkholderia cepacia*, etc.), bronchiectasis, and progressive respiratory dysfunction. The most common bacteria identified within the airways of patients with CF during the first few years of life include *Staphylococcus aureus* and *Haemophilus influenzae*. Over time, *P. aeruginosa* becomes the predominant organism occurring in up to 80% of the adult population. Recent studies have noted a change in the epidemiology of these organisms with a trend toward a lower incidence of *Pseudomonas* and an increasing incidence of *S. aureus* (particularly methicillin-resistant *S. aureus*), as well as other organisms such as *Stenotrophomonas maltophilia* and *Achromobacter xylosoxidans* (LiPuma, 2010). This may be a result of improved infection control within CF centers or may be related to the recent introduction of eradication protocols targeting first acquisition of *Pseudomonas*.

Less common organisms such as atypical mycobacteria (*Mycobacterium avium* complex or *Mycobacterium abscessus*) can also colonize airways of these patients, leading to rapid decline in lung function. *B. cepacia*, a gram-negative bacterium found in water and soil, is another organism that can be associated with rapid decline in lung function, although the incidence of this organism has remained stable at 3–4% of the population. Fungal infections may also pose a problem in this population with the most common fungus recovered being *Aspergillus*. *Aspergillus* rarely causes invasive infection; rather, it most commonly results in an allergic reaction to the fungus. This is known as allergic bronchopulmonary aspergillosis (ABPA). ABPA is manifested by an elevated total IgE, a positive skin test for *Aspergillus* or a demonstration of serum-specific IgE to *Aspergillus*, and the demonstration of clinical deterioration not responsive to conventional therapy with antibacterial treatment.

Additional pulmonary complications can include hyperreponsive airways, with asthma-like symptoms of wheezing and chest tightness. This is more commonly seen in the younger population, and most of these children are responsive to bronchodilators. Hemoptysis may also occur in the CF population, occurring in approximately 1 in 115 patients per year. Massive hemoptysis, defined as >240 cc in a 24-hour period, occurs in 4.1% of the population. The incidence of pneumothorax is approximately 3.4%. Hemopytsis and pneumothorax are both more commonly seen in older patients with more advanced disease (Flume et al., 2010).

Numerous complications involving the gastrointestinal system can also arise. In infants, prolonged neonatal jaundice can result secondary to inspissated bile within the liver and may be the presenting manifestation. Distal intestinal obstructive syndrome (DIOS), previously known as meconium ileus equivalent, is characterized by recurrent episodes of partial or complete small bowel obstruction. DIOS can occur with regular frequency in patients over 5 years of age and most commonly in patients over 20 years of age. DIOS is also often seen in those patients with a history of meconium ileus. In 2008, DIOS occurred in almost 4% of the population (Cystic Fibrosis Foundation, 2009).

Hepatic disease can be mild (e.g., elevated serum levels of hepatic enzymes) or severe, such as biliary cirrhosis with or without portal hypertension. In the liver, inspissated secretions within the bile duct along with impaired secretion of mucins from submucosal glands cause increased concentration and impaired movement of bile acids. Intrahepatic biliary ducts then become blocked with abnormal secretions, leading to biliary cirrhosis and portal hypertension marked by splenomegaly and esophageal varices. Hepatic disease is present in approximately 15% of the population. Cystic fibrosis liver disease (CFLD) was the primary cause of death in 9% of the population in 2008 (Cystic Fibrosis Foundation, 2009). CFTR mutations have been linked to liver disease; the vast majority (>95%) of CFLD occurs in patients with two "severe" (pancreatic insufficient) CFTR alleles. Furthermore, males are more likely than females (2:1) to experience CFLD (Knowles et al., 2010).

As the CF population ages, it is increasingly recognized that those patients with pancreatic exocrine insufficiency are at risk for the development of endocrine pancreatic insufficiency and subsequent development of cystic fibrosis-related diabetes mellitus (CFRD). Certain risk factors make the development of CFRD more likely such as chronic oral steroid use, female gender, and advancing age. Yearly screening of random blood glucose is recommended for all patients.

Osteopenia/osteoporosis is another complication recognized in the adolescent and adult population (10% of population affected in 2008) (Cystic Fibrosis Foundation, 2009). Risk factors include poor nutritional state, delayed puberty, malabsorption of fat-soluble vitamins specifically vitamins K and D, reduced muscle mass and weight-bearing activity, hepatobiliary disease, and, in some patients, chronic oral steroid use. In addition, chronic inflammation alters remodeling by increasing osteoclastic activity while the bone-rebuilding osteoblasts are understimulated leading to bone loss. Because of this potential complication, bone density evaluation is recommended beginning at age 18 (if not performed earlier) and, if normal, is repeated every 5 years.

MANAGEMENT

Pulmonary management

The goal of management in CF is to prevent or slow the progression of disease. Therapies are aimed at thinning the mucus, improving airway clearance of secretions, and decreasing bacterial burden within the airways. Frequent courses of antibiotics are often needed with exacerbations.

Bronchodilators

Airflow obstruction is central to this disease process and can be caused by secretions within the airway, inflammation of the airway walls, or airway destruction. A subgroup of patients also has a component of bronchoconstriction secondary to airway hyperreactivity. Short-acting beta agonists (such as albuterol) have been recommended for routine use (Flume et al., 2007) prior to airway clearance, prior to administration of other inhaled therapies to improve deposition of these medications, and/or prior to exercise in those with a component of airway hyperreactivity (Konig et al., 1995).

Dornase alfa

Neutrophils are recruited into the airways to fight bacteria that are colonizing the airways. As neutrophils die, they leave behind DNA strands that contribute to the overall viscosity of the sputum. Dornase alfa thins secretions within the airways of CF patients by cleaving DNA strands from degenerating neutrophils. Based on the recommendations of the CFF, dornase alfa should be offered to all patients over 6 years of age regardless of bacterial colonization, pulmonary signs and symptoms, or lung function. It has also been suggested for use in patients younger than 6 years of age with associated pulmonary signs and symptoms (Fuchs et al., 1994).

Hypertonic saline

Due to altered chloride transport, the periciliary fluid layer within the airways is relatively dehydrated. This reduction impairs ciliary transport of mucus and debris from the airways. Several studies have demonstrated that the inhalation of 7% hypertonic saline increases the height of the periciliary fluid layer by osmotically driven forces, rehydrating that fluid layer. This translates to an improvement in airway clearance of secretions, as well as improved lung function. The CFF Consensus Committee recommends the use of hypertonic saline in patients 6 years of age or older regardless of pulmonary signs or symptoms after pretreatment with a bronchodilator (Donaldson et al., 2006; Flume et al., 2009a).

Inhaled antibiotics

Several antibiotics with activity against *Pseudomonas* are now available in a nebulized form for use with CF. Inhaled tobramycin nebulized twice daily has been shown to decrease bacterial burden, improve pulmonary function (forced expiratory volume in 1 second [FEV_1]), and reduce exacerbations. The guidelines recommend the use of tobramycin by nebulization for patients 6 years of age and older with chronic *Pseudomonas* colonization. Inhaled tobramycin has also been incorporated into several eradication strategies to eradicate *Pseudomonas* with first acquisition on deep throat or sputum culture.

Fewer studies have been performed with inhaled colistin. Colistin has activity against *Pseudomonas* even in those strains that are multidrug resistant. It has been found that colistin forms toxic breakdown products once it has been mixed in a solution that can be damaging to the lungs. It is recommended that this product be reconstituted in sterile water just prior to nebulization. Due to the paucity of studies with this drug, the CFF Guidelines Committee was unable to make any formal recommendations regarding the use of this drug.

In early 2010, the Food and Drug Administration (FDA) approved inhaled aztreonam for use in CF. A small portable nebulizer that increases convenience for the patient administers this drug. Studies with this formulation have shown improvement in respiratory symptoms in patients over 7 years of age, with an FEV_1 between 25 and 75% of predicted, and chronic *Pseudomonas* or *B. cepacia* colonization (Cayston: Indications and Usage, 2010).

Macrolide therapy

Macrolide therapy was initially used in panbronchiolitis, a disease with lung findings similar to CF (McArdle & Talwalkar, 2007; Tamaoki, Kadota, & Takizawa, 2004). Macrolide therapy clinical trials in patients with CF have shown improved lung function and reduced pulmonary exacerbations (Adams & Congelton, 2008; Friedlander & Albert, 2010). Azithromycin was chosen for these trials due to the low incidence of gastrointestinal side effects. In patients with chronic *P. aeruginosa*, this oral antibiotic improved lung function and weight gain and decreased hospitalization rate. Follow-up studies are in progress (Flume et al., 2009a). The CFF Guidelines Committee recommends the use of macrolide therapy for patients 6 years and older with chronic *Pseudomonas* colonization. Cultures should be obtained prior to initiating this therapy to look for atypical mycobacteria. If patients are positive for atypical mycobacteria, macrolide therapy should be discontinued to prevent induction of macrolide resistance (Saiman et al., 2003; Wagner & Burns, 2007).

Inhaled corticosteroids and anti-inflammatory medications

Inhaled steroids and anti-inflammatory medications are important to control airway inflammation. The recurrent infections that are present in CF contribute to narrowing of the airways and decreased airflow. These medications help control airway edema and thus over time can assist in preserving lung function.

Airway clearance

Airway clearance has been the cornerstone of respiratory care in CF for decades. Despite this, there remain few studies that can conclusively demonstrate sustained or short-term benefits from this therapy. The CFF Pulmonary Guidelines Committee has evaluated the evidence that is available and has made four recommendations. The first is that airway clearance should be recommended for all patients with CF regardless of age or degree of pulmonary impairment. It is felt that there is sufficient evidence to demonstrate that airway clearance improves sputum clearance, helps to maintain lung function, and can improve quality of life. The second and third recommendations state that although no form of airway clearance has been proven to work better than another, for each individual, one method may work better than another. Therefore, when prescribing airway clearance for patients, therapy should be individualized based on age, patient preference, and so on. The final recommendation is that aerobic exercise should be encouraged for patients with CF as an adjunct therapy for airway clearance (Flume et al., 2009b).

Airway clearance therapy should be performed prior to eating or at least 1 hour after eating to avoid stomach upset and emesis that may occur with coughing. Bronchodilators and/or mucolytics should be administered prior to or during the therapy, depending on the method used. To allow maximum penetration into the airways, inhaled antibiotics and inhaled corticosteroids should always been administered after airway clearance.

Chest physical therapy (postural drainage and percussion)

Traditional manual chest percussion with postural drainage has been the standard by which all airway clearance techniques are measured. Five components are utilized in this technique including percussion, postural drainage, vibration, deep breathing, and cough. This technique includes placing the child in different positions to drain secretions from the various lung segments utilizing gravity to move the secretions from smaller to larger airways. Clapping and vibrating the chest is accomplished by using a cupped hand or device, such as a palm cup with infants, to loosen secretions and to allow the child to cough mucus out.

Some infants, toddlers, children, and adults may experience worsened heartburn and vomiting in certain postural drainage positions. This most frequently occurs when lying in the Trendelenburg position, wherein the head is down lower than the feet. Positions should be modified in those experiencing complications.

A cough called the "huff" cough is often effective in moving mucus up the airways. The huff cough involves taking a deep breath, holding for 2–3 seconds, followed by a forced exhalation with an open mouthed (much like "steaming up a window or mirror") (Flume et al., 2009b). The huff cough can be used with most airway clearance techniques.

Positive expiratory pressure therapy

Positive expiratory pressure (PEP) therapy delivers pressure through a face mask and resistor. This therapy utilizes an expiratory resistor designed to create positive pressure during exhalation and to lengthen the expiratory phase. The accumulated pressure allows the airways to stay open during exhalation to allow air to get behind mucus to assist in its removal. The huff cough is also utilized in this technique. Furthermore, bronchodilator deposition can be enhanced when administered with PEP therapy (Flume et al., 2009b; Saiman & Siegel, 2003).

Airway oscillating devices

There are different types of oscillating PEP devices that assist in the vibration of the large and small airways to move and loosen mucus for expectoration. Deep breathing and forced exhalation are important for airway clearance using this technique. These devices require exhaling into them numerous times to create the positive pressure vibration. They are typically followed by a series of huff and cough maneuvers (Flume et al., 2009b). Examples of oscillating PEP devices include the Acapella® and the Flutter®.

High-frequency chest compression

High-frequency chest compression (HFCC) is a technique of giving chest percussion by an electric device. This device has a vest that fits over the child's trunk that connects to a generator by hoses. The machine delivers chest percussion at varying rates/frequencies during inflation. Airflow is created within the lung by the inflation and deflation of the vest causing pulses of pressure that vibrate the airways. These vibrations cause the airflow to increase at low volume resulting in an increased mobilization of sputum (Hansen & Warwick, 1990). The pressure of the delivered percussion is adjustable and the health-care provider (physician, nurse practitioner, physician assistant) chooses the settings and the frequency of therapy which is individualized to optimize sputum production. It is important that deep breathing and coughing be encouraged periodically while using this method to help mobilize secretions.

Active cycle of breathing technique and autogenic drainage

Active cycle of breathing technique (ACBT) is a set of breathing maneuvers that involves short gentle breaths followed by deep breaths with three-second breath holds to build up pressure behind the mucus and finally adding the huff cough to remove mucus. It utilizes breath control or normal gentle breathing, thoracic expansion exercises, and forced expiratory technique. This technique can begin to be taught at 3–4 years of age but will likely require assistance until 8–10 years of age.

The autogenic drainage (AD) technique involves breathing at different lung volumes to dislodge mucus, collect, and then clear it. It is a difficult technique to learn and is not recommended in children under 12 years old. Huff cough and breathing techniques are critical for either of these airway clearance techniques (Flume et al., 2009b; Saiman & Siegel, 2003).

Exercise

Although it is not an airway clearance method, regular aerobic exercise is encouraged as an adjunctive therapy to other airway clearance techniques (Flume et al., 2009b).

Oral or intravenous antibiotics

Despite the numerous therapies mentioned earlier, patients with CF have acute exacerbations requiring the use of oral or intravenous antibiotics. While there is no clear consensus on defining an exacerbation, most agree that increased cough and/or sputum from baseline, decline in pulmonary function and/or oxygen saturation, weight loss, or increased fatigue necessitates the use of antibiotics. Antibiotics are chosen based on bacteria found on the most recent culture from the respiratory tract. Oral antibiotics are generally chosen if the exacerbation is mild and treatment is generally for 14–21 days.

Intravenous antibiotics are chosen when an exacerbation is moderate to severe or if there has been a failure to respond to oral antibiotic therapy. With intravenous therapy, two antibiotics are generally chosen based on susceptibility profiles to cover any gram-negative organisms. The most commonly chosen antibiotics include aminoglycosides (such as tobramycin or amikacin), in combination with an extended spectrum pencillin (e.g., piperacillin), an extended third- or fourth-generation cephalosporin (ceftazadime or cefepime), carbapenems (meropenem or imipenem), or a monobactam (aztreonam). Additional organisms commonly seen such as *S. aureus* (methicillin sensitive or methicillin resistant) may require the use of a third intravenous antibiotic. Treatment time with intravenous antibiotics varies from 10 days to 3 weeks depending on clinical response (Gibson, Burns, & Ramsey, 2003; Flume et al., 2009a).

Gastrointestinal management

Pancreatic enzymes

The majority of patients with CF are pancreatic insufficient and require the use of supplemental enzymes or pancreatic enzyme replacement therapy (PERT) for the breakdown and adequate absorption of their food. Pancreatic enzymes are dosed based on the weight of the patient and the amount of lipase per capsule. The number of enzymes will increase as the child grows, generally maintaining a range of 1,000–2,500 lipase units/kg/meal. Patients should not exceed 10,000 lipase units/kg/day (Michel et al., 2009). Enzymes are taken immediately before meals and snacks containing fats and remain active for up to 30 minutes.

Fat-soluble vitamins

In addition to standard vitamin supplementation, CF patients who are pancreatic insufficient also require additional doses of the fat-soluble vitamins (vitamins A, E, D, and K). Special CF-specific formulations of vitamins (fat soluble in water-miscible form) have been created to ensure adequate absorption and subsequent amounts of the fat-soluble vitamins. The CFF recommends yearly monitoring of serum levels.

H2 antagonists or proton pump inhibitors

Drugs that decrease gastric acidity such as H2 antagonists or proton pump inhibitors may improve pancreatic enzyme function. Unfortunately, pancreatic enzymes are often not completely effective due to the low pH of the intestinal tract (Davis, 2006). Steps to increase gastric pH such as the addition of H2 antagonists or proton pump inhibitors may improve pancreatic enzyme function and may lead to enhanced absorption (Davis, 2006). Unlike their symptomatic use in gastroesophageal reflux disease, these medications should be taken daily if they are being used to enhance pancreatic enzyme activity.

Nutritional supplementation

Some patients have higher caloric needs due to increased energy requirements. Often oral high-calorie supplements are initiated as a first step. In those patients unable to consume enough calories orally to support continued growth or maintenance of an adequate body mass index (BMI) percentile, a gastrostomy will be placed, and enteral feedings administered overnight may be used to supplement any oral intake.

Insulin

CFRD occurs in 15–20% of the population. The prevalence is 2% in children, 19% in adolescents, 40% in young adults, and 45–50% in those over 30 years of age (Stecenko & Moran, 2010). The development of CFRD is associated with worsening nutritional status and decline in pulmonary function. Annual screening is recommended by the CFF for children over 10 years of age during a clinically stable period. If diabetes is confirmed, the standard therapy is subcutaneous insulin or the use of an insulin pump. CF patients are to continue a high-calorie, high-protein diet despite the diagnosis of diabetes. The only dietary restriction made is to limit the intake of simple sugars (Stecenko & Moran, 2010).

Emerging therapies

Alternative chloride channel agonists

Denufosol, a P2Y(2) agonist currently in phase III testing, is an example of an alternate chloride channel activator designed to correct the ion transport defect in CF. This activation results in an increase in airway surface hydration, which results in improved airway clearance. Denufosol is delivered by nebulization three times daily (Jones & Helm, 2009; Kellerman et al., 2008).

Sodium channel blockers

In the CF airway, decreased chloride secretion and increased salt absorption is observed. The decreased chloride secretion appears to be a direct consequence of defective CFTR; however, the increased salt absorption is believed to result from the failure of CFTR to restrict salt absorption through a sodium channel named the epithelial Na^+ channel, ENaC (Berdiev, Qadri, & Benos, 2009). This contributes to the overall dehydrated state of the airway surface liquid seen in CF. Drugs that would block ENaC and hence sodium resorption could potentially improve airway surface liquid depth and therefore improve mucociliary clearance. Studies with amiloride, a short-acting sodium channel blocker, have shown conflicting results. Second-generation amiloride analogues that are more potent are being studied (Zeitlin, 2010).

Osmotic agents

As discussed earlier, the inhalation of 7% hypertonic saline increases the height of the periciliary fluid layer by osmotically driven forces, rehydrating that fluid layer. Other therapies utilizing this same concept are currently being studied. One such drug is inhaled mannitol. Mannitol has been studied as a dry powder inhalation delivered twice daily. It is currently in phase III testing (Jones & Helm, 2009; Zeitlin, 2010).

CFTR modulation

Class I mutations are associated with a defect in protein production because of a nonsense mutation, frameshift mutation, or splice-site mutation that results in premature termination of DNA translation. This is known as a premature stop codon (PTC). One area of modulation under investigation is the use of agents that allow transcription through the PTC during mRNA translation, producing functional full-length CFTR. One such agent under investigation is PTC124 (ataluren). This oral agent has shown promise in improved nasal PD measurements in phase II trials and is currently in phase III testing (Clancy, 2010; Mogayzel & Flume, 2010).

Class II mutations (e.g., Delta F508) are associated with abnormal folding of the CFTR protein, so it is retained in the endoplasmic reticulum where it is sent for degradation. VX809 is an oral agent in development, known as a corrector, which helps move the defective CFTR protein to the proper place in the airway cell membrane and improves its function as a chloride channel, although it is still not fully active. The use of a potentiator (described next) in combination with VX809 could potentially restore CFTR function in the most common mutation for CF (Clancy, 2010; Mogayzel & Flume, 2010). A phase IIa trial was completed in 2009. A trial of VX809 plus VX-770 is planned.

In class III mutations, the protein is made, but the gating properties of the channel are diminished, not allowing normal transport of ions. VX770, an oral agent known as a potentiator, may act on the CFTR protein and may help open the chloride channel in CF cells (Clancy, 2010; Mogayzel & Flume, 2010). Phase I dosing has been completed in healthy volunteers and

CF patients. A phase II trial in CF patients with at least one copy of the G551D mutation in their CF gene demonstrated improvements in biological measures of CFTR function (nasal PD and sweat chloride) and clinical measures of pulmonary health (FEV_1). Two phase III studies (one for pediatric and one for adolescent/adult patients) completed enrollment in the summer of 2010 (CFF, 2010c).

Gene therapy

The gene defect in CF was discovered in 1989 and since that time, attempts to replace the defective CF gene with wild-type CFTR have been attempted. Although gene transfer has been accomplished, long-lasting effects have not been achieved. Two vectors currently under study by the UK Gene Therapy Consortium include liposomes and retroviruses. Liposomes have a low toxicity to the cell but are not efficient at gene transfer. Retroviruses are highly efficient at entering the nucleus to transfer DNA, but due to high immunogenicity, they usually result in the DNA being silenced. Continued work in this area is ongoing (Jones & Helm, 2009).

NURSING CARE OF THE CHILD AND FAMILY

With current technological and medication advances, taking care of a child with CF can be quite overwhelming. Helping a patient and family to manage the care associated with CF takes coordination by a variety of health team members. Nurses, whether a licensed practical nurse (LPN), a registered nurse (RN), or a nurse practitioner (NP), are an integral part of this team. In many CF care centers, a nurse is the overall coordinator of care (or CF coordinator). However, even when another team member functions in this role, the nurse often oversees the overall plan of care and acts as a liaison between the various team members. The CF coordinator and nurse play an important role in case management; education; adherence issues; empowering patients and families toward self-care; dealing with psychosocial challenges; and advocating for the family with schools, employers, insurance companies, other family members, and other care providers.

In both the inpatient and outpatient settings, the nurse obtains a health history and performs a physical examination. Questions regarding interval respiratory health history should include

- changes in frequency or severity of cough;
- changes in sputum production, color, consistency, or amount;
- presence of wheezing;
- presence and description of dyspnea or any increase in work of breathing;
- changes in activity tolerance;

- presence of hemoptysis and description to include amount and frequency; and
- increased need for pulmonary medications.

Other important items to include in the history are changes in appetite, weight loss, abdominal pain, stool frequency and description, headaches, as well as any symptoms related to sinus disease.

The nurse will generally utilize inspection and auscultation as part of the routine pulmonary physical examination. During inspection, it is important to observe the patient's general appearance and color. The nasal passages should be observed for obstruction and polyps. The nurse should note the respiratory rate, work of breathing, any use of accessory muscles, presence of retractions, shape of the chest (barrel chest, in which the anterior–posterior diameter approximates transverse diameter), digital clubbing, and color of skin and nail beds. During auscultation, it is important to listen in all segments and to describe any adventitial sounds present. If crackles or wheezing are present, the description should include the segmental location—whether anterior or posterior, if the sounds are fine or coarse, intermittent or persistent, and if the breath sounds are decreased or diminished. The nurse is often the first health-care provider to see the patient and must be able to identify signs of distress and to communicate the appropriate findings to the other health-care providers.

Infection control while attending clinics and while hospitalized is an ongoing concern for patients with CF. The nurse as part of the CF care team has an important role in enforcing guidelines in these areas and in helping patients and families understand the reasons for implementing infection control guidelines. Infection control has become increasingly important, as many different organisms have been found to spread between patients. Guidelines have been established by the CFF for standard and transmission-based precautions, hand hygiene for health-care workers, cleaning of equipment, and education of patients.

Evidenced-based recommendations from the CFF (Saiman & Siegel, 2003) for decreasing transmission of organisms include the following:

(1) Hand washing
   (a) Use of antibacterial soap and water when hands are soiled with body fluids or have visible secretions
   (b) Use of antibacterial soap and water after direct contact with an object soiled by secretions
   (c) Use of alcohol-based gel or antibacterial soap and water if there is no visible dirt/residue
(2) Encouraging patients to
   (a) clean their hands often, especially after coughing, sneezing, or blowing their nose
   (b) avoid spas and hot tubs without enough chlorine to kill *P. aeruginosa*

    (c)   not attend events sponsored by the CFF, for example, Great Strides, if colonized with *B. cepacia*

    (d)   only attend camps that are not CF specific

(3) Patients who do not live in the same household should be encouraged to

    (a)   avoid activities such as hand shaking, hugging, or kissing, and

    (b)   keep at least 3 ft between themselves and other CF patients

Education on infection control for patients and families includes cleaning and disinfection of equipment, safe handling of secretions, hand washing, and maintaining a distance of 3 ft or more from other CF patients. Education about the care of respiratory equipment is particularly important. Recommendations from the CFF Consensus Guidelines on Infection Control for cleaning and disinfecting respiratory equipment include the following:

(1) Cleaning immediately with soap and water and

(2) Disinfecting using one of the following (refer to the manufacturer's instructions for the type of nebulizer being used):

    (a)   Boil in water for 5 minutes.

    (b)   Microwave (in water) for 5 minutes.

    (c)   Place in dishwasher, if the water is hotter than 158°F and maintained for 30 minutes.

    (d)   Soak in a solution of 1 part household bleach and 50 parts water for 3 minutes.

    (e)   Soak in 70% isopropyl alcohol for 5 minutes.

    (f)   Soak in 3% hydrogen peroxide for 30 minutes.

(3) If using any of the last three options; rinse with sterile water.

(4) Air dry (Saiman & Siegel, 2003).

Preventative care is time-consuming and at times can be overwhelming for the patient and/or the family. The nurse can assist in setting up a routine for day-to-day living with CF. Keeping lines of communication open is essential for this process. The goals of the patient and family must be considered and incorporated into the overall plan of care recommended by the provider. The plan must be reevaluated on a regular basis, recognizing and respecting the patient's and family's changing needs over time.

The daily management plan should include medications, airway clearance techniques, and a nutritional plan for adequate and appropriate calorie intake and daily nutritional requirements. Education should include verbal and written materials appropriate for the child and family. The education plan should also include a discussion about outcome measures and guidelines recommended by the CFF for routine health maintenance. The nurse can play a critical role in encouraging routine health maintenance at the CF care center.

Recommended health maintenance for CF patients includes

- four visits to an accredited CF center clinic;
- four respiratory cultures, either by throat swab or sputum;
- two pulmonary function tests (PFTs) if physically able;
- an influenza (flu) vaccine if >6 months of age;
- vitamin A, D, and E levels, and prothrombin time measured annually;
- an oral glucose tolerance test (OGTT) to screen for CF-related diabetes in people with CF aged 10 years and older; and
- an annual test to measure liver enzymes (Cystic Fibrosis Foundation, 2009).

Other suggested testings include a chest X-ray—every 2–4 years if clinical status is stable, annually if frequent respiratory infections or declining lung function is present. Additionally, a serum IgE is recommended for screening for ABPA annually for patients 6 years of age and older.

Routine visits with the interdisciplinary team are critical for improved care of CF patients. These visits should include the following team members: physician, respiratory/physical therapist, nutritionist, social worker, and nurse at minimum. At some CF centers, appointments will include visits to psychologists/psychiatrists, child life specialists, geneticists, or physicians from other specialty care areas.

Unfortunately, the cost of routine care and management is high, and referrals to appropriate agencies for assistance are often necessary for families to meet the needs of the CF child. The nurse can help make these referrals. The emotional cost for the patient and caregivers should not be overlooked. Referrals to support groups or contact information for other parents can provide needed resources to families. The CFF has local chapters throughout the United States. It also has social/educational support documents located on its Web site, which can be found at http://www.cff.org.

Due to infection control concerns, it has become more difficult for children and adolescents with CF to obtain peer-to-peer support. Face-to-face contact is discouraged, and it is recommended that all CF patients limit contact with other people with CF or stay at least 3 ft from others with CF. Electronic and online communication has been increasingly observed.

Adherence to routine health maintenance and the plan of care is often an issue for people living with a chronic illness such as CF. Nurses should be cognizant of the potential for nonadherence so that they can anticipate and address it.

Factors that negatively influence adherence include inadequate knowledge and skills, lack of communication with the health-care team, and not identifying barriers. Inadequate knowledge and skills may involve misunderstandings or confusion about the disease or treatments, skills not taught or reinforced, and forgetting to provide reeducation or updates as the child gets older. Lack of communication may include lack of time to educate or for the learner to ask questions, not assessing the actual knowledge of the child or the caregiver, the caregiver's anxiety about asking questions or admitting lack of knowledge; and lack of documentation of education (Quittner, 2007).

Strategies to promote adherence include

- assessment of how education is provided and documented by the care team, followed by strategies to target the education;
- administering a written knowledge assessment of the patient and caregivers at least annually, followed by reeducation at the next visit; and
- using a collaborative approach with the family to build trust and a positive relationship (Quittner, 2007).

Education is one of the most important functions of the nurse when working with children with CF and their families. Education must begin at the time of diagnosis and must be reinforced at every visit. Education should include the parents and/or other caregivers (including extended family if appropriate), patient and siblings at appropriate developmental stages, daycare providers, and school personnel. Others may need education in specific situations.

Education is provided and reinforced by several members of the care team and takes place in a variety of settings, including the outpatient and inpatient settings and in many CF care centers during family education programs. Topics for ongoing CF education should include CF disease-specific topics such as pulmonary issues (e.g., PFTs, lung health, and sinus disease); growth and nutrition; potential complications of CF and prescribed therapies; basic understanding of the pathophysiology of CF; reproductive issues; transplantation; hospitalization/home care; and end-of-life care. Topics relating to living with CF should also be addressed and should include an individualized plan of care, with a focus on incorporating it into daily life, family life—parents/siblings, school/work issues, finances/insurance, stressors/coping, adherence issues, and self-management of the disease. Documentation of interdisciplinary education and achievement of goals and objectives is imperative to provide all healthcare team members with an up-to-date picture of the needs of each child and family.

It is also important for the care team to help prepare the child and family for transition at a variety of developmental stages. There are different educational goals and expectations for the child as he/she becomes older. As children with CF transition to subsequent developmental stages, they should be provided with more information about CF and should be expected to assume more responsibility for their own care. Self-management is the goal and, with thoughtful preparation and coordination by the pediatric care team, CF patients will be better able to have a smooth transition into independent ongoing care in an adult environment. Table 8.1 provides

Table 8.1 Cystic fibrosis (CF) education plan with developmental transitions.

	Date	Team member
Stage I: diagnosis to age 6		
Discuss CF impact on the child/family		
Purpose/consent for CF registry		
CF basic education—discuss genetics of cystic fibrosis		
Respiratory		
Chronic pulmonary therapy		
Airway clearance		
Infection control measures		
Gastrointestinal		
Nutrition—diet		
Pancreatic enzymes		
Growth and development		
Role of the primary care provider		
Immunization management		
Healthy coping strategies		
Utilizing community resources		
Discuss transition into stage II		
Stage II: ages 6–10		
Discuss CF impact on the child/family		
Child begins participation in medical history		
Importance of following plan of care		
Performing PFTs		
Discuss the importance of airway clearance		
Discuss the importance of enzyme use		
Discuss increased salt intake during summer		
Management of CF in a school setting		
Effective communication with family/health-care team		
Discuss stage III		
Stage III: ages 10–12		
Discuss CF impact on the child/family		
Child primary provider of medical history		
Child masters names and reason for all therapies		
Discuss airway clearance and changes needed		
Identify barriers and potential solutions to barriers		
Effective communication with family/health-care team		
Discuss stage IV		

an example of a checklist that can be used to plan for the age/development-based educational needs from birth to 12 years old.

In 2010, the Cystic Fibrosis Foundation Patient Education Committee approved a set of performance objectives developed by the Baylor College of Medicine, Texas Children's Hospital. The "CF Core Self-Management Performance Objectives for Patients and Families—2010" (CFF, 2010b) is a set of behaviors that provide a method for CF centers to plan and evaluate systematic health education and care interventions to enhance CF self-management. The behaviors identified (divided into eight major categories) relate to gastrointestinal, respiratory, and psychosocial goals. Each goal includes its own specific skill set. The following provides a sample (the broad goals for the two respiratory measures and one of the psychosocial measures) of the performance objectives.

Respiratory health performance objectives (CFF, 2010b)

Measure I: patient/family manages lower and upper respiratory tract infection

(a) Takes preventive measures for contagious respiratory infections and respiratory irritants
(b) Monitors change in symptoms, suggesting respiratory infection
(c) Treats lower respiratory infection
(d) Monitors response and improvement in respiratory infection
(e) Uses inhaled antibiotic for chronic *P. aeruginosa* infection
(f) Manages upper respiratory tract infection

Measure II: Manages airway obstruction

(a) Monitors for symptoms and signs of airway obstruction
(b) Performs airway clearance maneuvers agreed on with CF clinician
(c) Uses inhaled medication to facilitate clearance of secretions
(d) Manages airway inflammation and hyperreactivity
(e) Monitors lung status with CF clinician using objective studies
(f) Engages in developmentally appropriate activities

Measure VII: Utilizes health-care services for maintenance of health and management of problems

(a) Establishes a mutually trusting relationship with members of the CF health-care team
(b) Feels confident in knowing how and when to contact each health-care provider if/when needed, that is, primary care provider (PCP), CF health care.
(c) Makes and keeps routine CF health maintenance appointments (quarterly visits)
(d) Seeks timely medical assistance for complications of CF
(e) Follows through on referrals for information and services
(f) Recognizes the need for ancillary services (i.e., dietary, counseling, and pulmonary physical rehab)
(g) Makes and keeps appointments for referrals

(h) Seeks assistance in overcoming obstacles that prevent the patient from receiving treatments (i.e., medication side effects, refills, and no chest physical therapy [CPT] partner)

(i) Attends to age-specific general health maintenance (i.e., vaccinations and dental and vision checkups)

The nurse and the health-care team can use the specific skills identified for the goals associated with each health performance objective to develop an individualized education plan and tracking tool for documentation purposes in a specific CF care center or hospital setting. The specific skills listed in the document can provide objective measures for evaluating the patient and family's achievement of each performance objectives. This form could also be used to document the comprehensive education plan for the patient. Table 8.2 provides an example of how Measure I-a could

Table 8.2 Sample individualized tracking form.

Respiratory health performance objective tracking	What was taught, date, and who taught	Achieved, demonstrated, or stated objective
I. Management of lower respiratory infection—takes preventive measures for contagious respiratory infections and respiratory irritants		
1. Gets flu shot annually	August 1, 2010—reinforced the importance of getting an influenza shot from a PCP or a health unit this fall—KJ, MD	October 5, 2008—copy of influenza immunization record printed from state database, placed in chart
2. Immunizations are up-to-date for age	April 5, 2008—discussed the importance of getting immunizations as recommended, gave "Respiratory: Stopping the Spread of Germs" handout—KJ, MD	October 5, 2009—immunization record printed from state database and all are up-to-date, placed in chart
3. Avoids others who have respiratory infections—child now in day care	January 28, 2009—reeducated about why it is important to avoid people with respiratory infections—SQ, RN	
4. Effectively cleans hands with soap and water	January 28, 2009—demonstrated hand washing techniques, gave "Respiratory: Stopping the Spread of Germs"—SQ, RN	May 30, 2009—both parent and child were able to demonstrate good hand washing techniques
5. Effectively cleans hands with alcohol-based hand sanitizer		August 1, 2010— redemonstrated good technique, postreview— parent and child
6. States when to clean hands	August 1, 2010—review of hand washing—SQ, RN	

Adapted from the Cystic Fibrosis Family Education Program ©Baylor College of Medicine (CFF, 2010b).

be evaluated and documented (adapted from the "CF Core Self-Management Performance Objectives for Patients and Families—2010"; CFF, 2010b).

As it has become increasingly important to involve the child and the family in the self-management of CF, there has been an increased expectation that patients and families become an integral part of the CF care team. The CFF has encouraged people with CF and their families to become active participants in care and to become partners of their CF care centers. This participation is expected to help improve the quality of care for patients and ultimately to improve the care center.

The CF Foundation has suggested a framework for various levels of participation by patients and families. Individual CF centers have varying degrees of involvement, and since these levels build upon each other, increased participation can be implemented in gradual stages. The levels of patient and/or family involvement in a CF care center include

- patients or families as participants, wherein they may respond to surveys and questionnaires and/or be members of a focus group;
- patients or families as advisory board members, in which they may be involved as members of CF center committees or a specific center task force and/or may serve on advisory boards for the quality improvement team within the CF center;
- patients or families as active advisors or consultants, wherein they are active task force/committee members, faculty for staff education, participants at collaborative meetings/conferences, mentors for others (patients, families, or staff), trainers for other patients and families, and providers for staff orientation and/or work closely with the quality improvement team; and
- patients and families as coleaders, in which they may serve as facilitators, content experts, evaluators of the team, authors, and/or be members of the team as hospital/clinic employees (Cystic Fibrosis Foundation, 2006).

The nurse as a team member with direct contact with the entire family can play a vital role in identifying patients or family members to assist in the CF quality improvement activities. On the CFF's Web site section about living with CF, it states "research has shown that if a person is more involved in their healthcare, they can get better results and feel more satisfied with that care" (CFF, 2010e). By working together as partners, CF care teams and patients can provide quality care that will help to make life better and longer for people with CF.

REFERENCES

Adams, N. P., & Congelton, J. (2008). Diffuse panbronchiolitis. *European Respiratory Journal, 32*(1), 237–238.

Berdiev, B. K., Qadri, Y. J., & Benos, D. J. (2009). Assessment of the CFTR and ENaC association. *Molecular BioSystems, 5*(2), 123–127.

Borowitz, D., Parad, R. B., Sharp, J. K., et al. (2009a). Cystic Fibrosis Foundation practice guidelines for the management of infants with cystic fibrosis transmembrane conductance regulator-related metabolic syndrome during the first two years of life and beyond. *Journal of Pediatrics, 155,* s106–s116.

Borowitz, D., Robinson, K. A., Rosenfeld, M., et al. (2009b). Cystic Fibrosis Foundation evidence-based guidelines for management of infants with cystic fibrosis. *Journal of Pediatrics, 155*(Suppl. 6), S73–S93.

Boyle, M. (2003). Nonclassic cystic fibrosis and CFTR-related diseases. *Current Opinion in Pulmonary Medicine, 9*(6), 498–503.

Cayston: Indications and usage (2010). Retrieved from http://www.cayston.com.

Chillon, M, Casaid, B, Mercier, B, et al. (1995). Mutations in the cystic fibrosis gene in patients with congenital absence of the vas deferens. *New England Journal of Medicine, 332*(22), 1475–1480.

Clancy, J. P. (2010). Ongoing research into CFTR modulation. *Advanced Studies in Medicine, 10*(1), 14–18.

Cystic Fibrosis Centre at the Hospital for Sick Children in Toronto. (2010). Cystic Fibrosis Mutation Database. Retrieved from Cystic Fibrosis Mutation Database: http://www.genet.sickkids.on.ca/cftr/app.

Cystic Fibrosis Foundation (CFF). (2006). Action guide for accelerating improvement in Cystic Fibrosis Care. Retrieved from http://clinicalmicrosystem.org/materials/workbooks/cystic_fibrosis_action_guide.pdf.

Cystic Fibrosis Foundation (CFF). (2009). Cystic Fibrosis Foundation Registry 2008 Annual Report. Bethesda, MD: Cystic Fibrosis Foundation.

Cystic Fibrosis Foundation (CFF). (2010a). Cystic Fibrosis Foundation Registry 2009 Annual Report. Bethesda, MD: Cystic Fibrosis Foundation.

Cystic Fibrosis Foundation (CFF). (2010b). 2010 CF Core Self-Management Performance Objectives. Retrieved from https://portcf.outcome.com/.

Cystic Fibrosis Foundation (CFF). (2010c). Drug development pipeline. Retrieved from http://www.cff.org/research/DrugDevelopmentPipeline/#CFTR_MODULATION.

Cystic Fibrosis Foundation (CFF). (2010d). Frequently asked questions. Retrieved from http://www.cff.org/AboutCF/Faqs/#What_is_the_life_expectancy_for_people_who_have_CF_(in_the_United_States)?.

Cystic Fibrosis Foundation (CFF). (2010e). Living with CF. Retrieved from http://www.cff.org/LivingWithCF/QualityImprovement/WhatYouCanDo/.

Davis, P. B. (2006). Cystic fibrosis since 1938. *American Journal of Respiratory and Critical Care Medicine, 173*(5), 475–482.

Donaldson, SH, Bennett, WD, Zeman, KL, et al. (2006). Mucus clearance and lung function in cystic fibrosis with hypertonic saline. *New England Journal of Medicine, 354,* 241–250.

Drumm, M. L., Konstan, M. W., Schluchter, M. D., et al. (2005). Genetic modifiers of lung disease in cystic fibrosis. *New England Journal of Medicine, 353*(14), 1443–1453.

Farrell, P. M., Rosenstein, B. J., White, T. B., et al. (2008). Guidelines for diagnosis of cystic fibrosis in newborns through older adults: Cystic fibrosis Foundation consensus report. *Journal of Pediatrics, 153*(2), S4–S14.

Flume, P. A., Mogayzel, P., Robinson, K., et al. (2009a). Cystic fibrosis pulmonary guidelines: Treatment of pulmonary exacerbations. *American Journal of Respiratory and Critical Care Medicine, 180,* 802–809.

Flume, P. A., Mogayzel, P., Robinson, K., et al. (2010). Cystic fibrosis pulmonary guidelines: Pulmonary complications: Hemoptysis and pneumothorax. *American Journal of Respiratory and Critical Care Medicine, 182,* 298–306.

Flume, P. A., O'Sullivan, B. P., Robinson, K. A., et al. (2007). Cystic fibrosis pulmonary guidelines: Chronic medications for maintenance of lung health. *American Journal of Respiratory and Critical Care Medicine, 176,* 957–969.

Flume, P. A., Robinson, K. A., O'Sullivan, B. P., et al. (2009b). Cystic fibrosis pulmonary guidelines: Airway clearance therapies. *Respiratory Care, 54*(4), 522–537.

Friedlander, A. L., & Albert, R. K. (2010). Chronic macrolide therapy in inflammatory airways diseases. *Chest, 138*(5), 1202–1212.

Fuchs, H., Borowitz, D. S., Christiansen, D. et al. (1994). Effect of aerosolized recombinant human DNase on exacerbations of respiratory symptoms and on pulmonary function in patients with cystic fibrosis. *New England Journal of Medicine, 331,* 637–642.

Garred, P., Pressler, T., Madsen, H. O., et al. (1999). Association of mannose-binding lectin gene heterogeneity with severity of lung disease and survival in cystic fibrosis. *Journal of Clinical Investigation, 104*(4), 431–437.

Gibson, R. L., Burns, J. L., & Ramsey, B. W. (2003). Pathophysiology and management of pulmonary infections in cystic fibrosis. *American Journal of Respiratory and Critical Care Medicine, 168,* 918–951.

Hamosh, A., FitzSimmons, S. C., Macek, M., Jr., et al. (1998). Comparison of the clinical manifestations of cystic fibrosis in black and white patients. *Journal of Pediatrics, 132*(2), 255–259.

Hansen, L. G., & Warwick, W. J. (1990). High-frequency chest compression system to aid in clearance of mucus from the lung. *Biomedical Instrumentation & Technology, 24*(4), 289–294.

Jones, A. M., & Helm, J. M. (2009). Emerging treatments in cystic fibrosis. *Drugs, 69*(14), 1903–1910.

Kellerman, D., Evans, R., Mathews, D., et al. (2008). Denufosol: A review of studies with inhaled P2Y(2) agonists that led to phase 3. *Pulmonary Pharmacology and Therapeutics, 21*(4), 600–607.

Kerem, B. R., Rommens, J. M., Butchanan, J. A., et al. (1989). Identification of the cystic fibrosis gene: Genetic analysis. *Science, 245,* 1073–1080.

Knowles, M. C., Commander, D., Stonebraker, J. R., et al. (2010). Genetic modifiers and CF liver disease. The 24th Annual North American CF Conference. Supplement 33, 122–123. Baltimore: *Pediatric Pulmonology.*

Konig, P., Gayer, D., Barbero, G. J., et al. (1995). Short-term and long-term effects of albuterol aerosol therapy in cystic fibrosis: A preliminary report. *Pediatric Pulmonology, 20,* 205–214.

LiPuma, J. (2010). The changing microbial epidemiology in cystic fibrosis. *Clinical Microbiology Reviews, 23*(2), 299–323.

McArdle, J. A. & Talwalkar, J. S. (2007). Macrolides in cystic fibrosis. *Clinics in Chest Medicine*, *28*(2), 347–360.

Michel, S. H., Magbool, A., Hanna, M. D., et al. (2009). Nutrition management of pediatric patients who have cystic fibrosis. *Pediatric Clinics of North America*, *56*, 1123–1141.

Mogayzel, P. J., & Flume, P. A. (2010). Update in cystic fibrosis 2009. *American Journal of Respiratory and Critical Care Medicine*, *181*, 539–544.

Quittner, A. Accelerating the rate of improvement in cystic fibrosis care: Presentation at Learning and Leadership Collaborative V, March 29, 2007, Baltimore.

Rosenstein, B., & Cutting, G. (1998). The diagnosis of cystic fibrosis: A consensus statement. *Journal of Pediatrics*, *132*(4), 589–595.

Rowe, S. M., Miller, S., & Sorscher, E. J. (2005). Mechanisms of disease: Cystic fibrosis. *New England Journal of Medicine*, *352*, 1992–2001.

Saiman, L., Marshall, B. C., Mayer-Hamblett, N., et al. (2003). Azithromycin in patients with cystic fibrosis chronically infected with *Pseudomonas aeruginosa*: A randomized controlled trial. *The Journal of the American Medical Association*, *290*, 1749–1756.

Saiman, L., & Siegel, J. (2003). Cystic Fibrosis Foundation: Infection control recommendations for patients with cystic fibrosis: Microbiology, important pathogens, and infection control practices to prevent patient to patient transmission. *Infection Control Hospital Epidemiology*, *24*(5), 52–56.

Stecenko, A. A., & Moran, A. (2010). Update on cystic fibrosis-related diabetes. *Current Opinion in Pulmonary Medicine*, *16*(6), 611–615.

Tamaoki, J., Kadota, J., & Takizawa, H. (2004). Clinical implications of the immunomodulatory effects of macrolides. *American Journal of Medicine*, *117*(Suppl. 9A), 5S–11S.

Wagner, T., & Burns, J. (2007). Anti-inflammatory properties of macrolides. *Pediatric Infectious Disease Journal*, *26*, 75–76.

Zeitlin, P. L. (2010). Ongoing research into other emerging therapies. *Advanced Studies in Medicine*, *10*(1), 19–23.

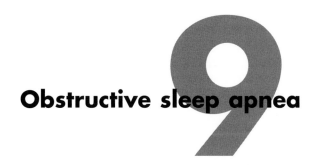

Obstructive sleep apnea

Linda Niemiec, MSN, RN, CPNP, and
Lewis J. Kass, MD

INTRODUCTION

Obstructive sleep apnea (OSA), which essentially is difficulty breathing
and sleeping at the same time, is a very common problem in the pediatric
population. Despite being so common, OSA is a frequently missed diagnosis. It is not clear why OSA is not considered sooner in the differential
diagnosis for a child who is experiencing snoring, irritability, hyperactivity,
restless sleep, and chronic respiratory problems. Perhaps it is due to the
relative infancy of the diagnosis of OSA. As recently as the early 1980s,
OSA in children was considered a rare diagnosis. However, no matter what
the reason, making an accurate and timely diagnosis is imperative because
if left untreated, OSA can be associated with cognitive, behavioral, cardiovascular, and metabolic consequences. We are likely to realize in the near
future and as outlined so exquisitely by Gozal et al. (Gozal & Kheirandish-
Gozal, 2010) that the morbidity associated with OSA in the form of neurocognitive, cardiovascular and metabolic manifestations are interrelated.
They are likely shaped by individual susceptibility, environment and lifestyle, and severity of OSA (Gozal & Kheirandish-Gozal, 2010). That places
the responsibility on us as caregivers to identify problems early and to treat
them accordingly.

Nursing Care in Pediatric Respiratory Disease, First Edition. Edited by Concettina (Tina) Tolomeo.
© 2012 John Wiley & Sons, Inc. Published 2012 by John Wiley & Sons, Inc.

It is therefore important that nurses and nurse practitioners receive adequate training and information regarding OSA. The knowledge gained from this training and information can help nurses and nurse practitioners identify symptoms of OSA in children. Identification of symptoms can ultimately lead to proper diagnosis and hopefully avoidance of complications associated with OSA.

EPIDEMIOLOGY

The diagnosis of OSA has steadily increased over the past decade, in large part due to increased awareness and screening, but also due to the number of centers that perform the diagnostic testing necessary to identify OSA. Current medical literature states OSA occurs in children of all ages, from toddlers to adolescents, with estimates of prevalence from 2 to 4% (Meltzer et al., 2010). The peak incidence of OSA is between the ages of 2 and 6 years, coinciding with the peak age of lymphoid hyperplasia, when the tonsils and adenoids reach their maximum size in relationship to the upper airway dimensions.

Habitual snoring occurs in up to 12% of the general pediatric population and in most children with OSA. However, a history of snoring is insufficient to diagnose OSA because not all children who snore have OSA (Perez & Davidson, 2008). OSA is equally common in boys and girls. However, following the onset of puberty, OSA is more common in males.

The incidence of pediatric OSA appears to be on the upswing. This is most likely due to the notable increase in child and adolescent obesity over the past decade. Recent studies have found that the risk of OSA among adolescents (age ≥ 12 years) increases 3.5-fold with each standard deviation increase in body mass. The risk of OSA was not significantly increased with increasing body mass in younger children (Kohler, 2009).

Among otherwise healthy children, adenotonsillar hypertrophy, obesity, and upper respiratory problems are conditions that predispose children to OSA (Lumeng & Chervin, 2008). Adenotonsillar hypertrophy is usually the result of multiple etiologies, the most common of which are proliferation of lymphoid tissue, recurrent upper respiratory infections, allergic irritants, chronic nasal obstruction, and pharyngeal edema from gastroesophageal reflux. These etiologies all have in common the feature of an anatomically or functionally narrowed upper airway. Other risk factors include respiratory problems such as sinusitis, chronic rhinitis, asthma, African American ethnicity, family history of OSA, and low socioeconomic status (Benninger & Walner, 2007).

Medical, neurological, or dental conditions that reduce airway size, affect the muscle control of the upper airway, or impact the collapsibility of the upper airway also place a child at an increased risk of OSA. Examples include the following:

- Cerebral palsy
- Down syndrome
- Craniofacial abnormalities (micrognathia, retrognathia, midface hypoplasia, Pierre–Robin syndrome)
- History of prematurity/low birth weight
- Muscular dystrophy
- Achondroplasia
- Orthodontic problems (high, narrow hard palate, malocclusions).

PATHOPHYSIOLOGY

OSA in children is a syndrome characterized by recurrent periods of elevated upper airway resistance with partial or complete intermittent airflow obstruction of the upper airway during sleep, and can be associated with snoring, episodic oxyhemoglobin desaturation, hypercapnia, and repeated arousals (Sheldon, Ferber, & Kryger, 2005). In order to understand the pathophysiology associated with disturbed nighttime sleep, one needs some understanding of normal nighttime sleep in children. There are expected norms for length of sleep time and sleep architecture based on age and development. An excellent review of such norms appears in Dr. Jodi Mindell's *Clinical Guide to Pediatric Sleep* (Mindell & Owens, 2003).

It is presumed that sleep serves a restorative purpose, especially during deep non-REM stage N3 sleep. REM sleep is frequently spoken of in lay circles as "the deepest sleep," but in fact the brain is as metabolically active during REM sleep as it is during wakefulness. Experts believe that REM serves a purpose of rehearsal and learning. For example, if in school we learn that $2 + 2 = 4$, it is during REM sleep that such information is rehearsed and put into our internal "hard drive." Accordingly, any disruption in the continuity, quality, or quantity of sleep can have major impacts on neurocognitive development (Gozal et al. 2007), learning and general well-being.

The most common cause for childhood OSA is adenotonsillar hypertrophy, but enlarged tonsils and adenoids alone do not account for the entire pathophysiological process. OSA is linked to a relationship between structural and neuromuscular variables within the upper airway. Though several studies show that children with OSA have enlarged tonsils and adenoids when compared to their age-matched cohorts, not every child with large tonsils has OSA, and some children have persistent OSA despite having a tonsillectomy and adenoidectomy. Thus, structural factors alone cannot be fully accountable for OSA (Au & Li, 2009). It is believed that OSA occurs in children because the size of their airway is small in relation to the size of their tonsils and adenoids. Furthermore, other issues such as neuromuscular tone, nasal airway anatomy, and mandibular and midface structure can all add to the effect that airway caliber has on OSA.

Airflow obstruction during sleep can be associated with hypoxemia and hypercarbia and the sequelae associated with these blood gas alterations. Much focus in recent years has been on the oxidative stress associated with intermittent hypoxemia as well as the vast hemodynamic changes that occur repetitively all night long secondary to arousals from sleep. The current thinking is that this pathophysiology sets the patient up for conditions of chronic inflammation such as asthma, metabolic dysfunction, and cardiovascular stress (Gozal & Kheirandish-Gozal, 2008).

Numerous studies have been published over the past 5 years describing the findings of increased levels of mediators of inflammation (Gozal et al., 2008; Gozal, 2009; Tauman, O'Brien, & Gozal, 2007). It is still not clear whether the inciting event for the inflammatory cascade is the arousal from sleep itself, independent of oxygenation, or whether the intermittent hypoxia is the trigger. No doubt this debate will continue for many years. Suffice to say, however, that there is a link connecting OSA, obesity, asthma, and cardiovascular disease (Gozal & Kheirandish, 2006; Gozal & Kheirandish-Gozal, 2008).

When it comes to arousals from sleep versus hypoxemia, it is unclear which of the two is more problematic. It is well described that children with OSA manifest poor school performance and other neurocognitive deficits (Kheirandish & Gozal, 2006). The question is whether the source of the problem is due to arousals from sleep or the effects of intermittent or persistent hypoxemia. It is likely a combination of both (Gozal & Kheirandish, 2006).

For years, it has been scrutinized as to whether snoring is an innocent sound or whether snoring in and of itself is problematic (O'Brien et al., 2004a). Studies have demonstrated that snoring, which is often described as "harmless" primary snoring (PS), is associated with elevated systemic blood pressures (Amin et al., 2004). In addition, PS is known to be associated with children scoring higher on scales of inattentiveness and impulsivity.

The presence of snoring may actually serve as a source of arousal from sleep, which the technology at hand may not yet to be able to pick up. The vibrations in the upper airway (which we call snoring) have been hypothesized to damage the neuromuscular end plate in the upper airway. This damage may then render the patient with diminished tone in the upper airway, which is one of the proposed mechanisms for OSA. At the very least, snoring indicates that there is an increase in upper airway resistance (Marshall, 2007) that begs further investigation. Thus, no degree of snoring should be considered normal.

SIGNS AND SYMPTOMS

OSA can masquerade as hyperactivity, poor school performance, exercise intolerance, asthma, and chronic cough. Therefore, snoring is not the only symptom associated with OSA. The following list outlines additional important symptoms that could be elicited during a sleep interview:

- Restless sleep
- Sweating
- Audible noisy breathing
- Mouth breathing
- Unusual sleeping positions
- Nightly awakenings
- Enuresis
- Early morning awakenings
- Difficulty waking up in the morning
- Late for school because of sleepiness in the morning
- Daytime sleepiness
- Poor focus in class
- Poor behavior in school or at home
- Hyperactivity
- Poorly responsive to attention deficit/hyperactivity disorder (ADHD) medications
- Poor school grades
- Daytime irritability
- Daytime napping (after the age of 5)
- Trouble falling asleep at night

It is clear to see that such a symptom list is extensive. However, any one of the above symptoms could be a clue toward identifying OSA. A number of the above symptoms deserve special attention. Restlessness, for example, may need to be elicited in a number of ways, especially if the child no longer spends any sleep time with the parent. For an older child, you can ask whether the sheets are all kicked off the bed by morning. For younger children who still spend some time (or a lot of time) sleeping with parents, you may hear parents make comments like

- I will never sleep with him again. He kicks me all night long.
- He circles the bed like a clock.
- We shared a bed in a hotel on vacation last week and he kept me up all night long.

In regard to sweating, parents can often be very dramatic about the amount of perspiration. They may describe children soaking the sheets with sweat, needing to change the sheets, or needing to change the pajamas. Sometimes, the history of sweating is masked by adaptations that the child has made over the years, such as sleeping without sheets or blankets, only sleeping in underwear, or sleeping with fans or air conditioners even during the wintertime.

Some unusual sleep positions that may need to specifically be asked about include sleeping with the neck hyperextended. In addition, sometimes toddlers and young children will sleep with knees under the chest and bottom up in the air. Raising or heaving of the shoulders and chest may also be described.

Enuresis is an important symptom. It is one of the most common problems seen in a pediatric primary care office and ranks near the top in terms of most troubling problems for a patient and family. While the exact mechanisms have not been identified, there is a strong link between nocturnal enuresis and OSA. Some proposed mechanisms include patients with OSA having increased levels of morning brain natriuretic peptide (Capdevila et al. 2008). Arousals, hypoxemia, and excessive sleepiness have also been suggested as potential causes. Regardless of the exact mechanism, for many patients, treatment for OSA has resulted in improvement or even complete elimination of nocturnal enuresis (Basha et al., 2005).

The following is a list of medical conditions that might be elicited by history and should raise concern about possible OSA:

- Poorly controlled asthma despite maximal medical therapy and appropriate environmental controls
- Obesity
- Insulin resistance
- Recurrent tonsillitis
- Gastroesophageal reflux
- Attention deficit disorder with or without hyperactivity
- Failure to sleep train despite appropriate efforts
- Unexplained nocturnal hypoxemia discovered during a hospitalization for asthma or other illness
- Persistent nocturnal enuresis despite all efforts at assessment and management
- Growth disturbance (unexplained by any other cause)
- Neurodevelopmental delays (unexplained by any other cause)

In addition to a detailed history, the physical exam can be very informative. Tonsils can be easily visualized and are often described as big or small. Tonsils can be scored on a scale of 1+ to 4+. Tonsils that are scored as 1+ and 2+ are frequently described as normal; 3+- and 4+-sized tonsils are described as enlarged. However, the following points should be kept in mind:

(1) Tonsil size is not always correlated with severity of OSA. Patients with small tonsils can still have significant OSA. Said alternatively, lack of intervention for OSA should not be based on tonsil size alone.

(2) The tonsillar tissue that you see may just be the "tip of the iceberg." When a patient goes to sleep or receives anesthesia and neuromuscular tone decreases, the full extent of the tonsils can be revealed as they

fall into the midline of the oropharynx, giving you a more realistic picture.

(3) There can be mobility to the tonsillar tissue that is even evident on physical exam. During swallowing, or during the respiratory cycle or during an elicited gag reflex, such mobility can become fairly obvious.

In addition to obtaining lateral head X-rays or performing direct visualization with nasal endoscopy, adenoidal hypertrophy can usually be assessed on physical exam by assessing the quality of the voice. One's voice becomes hyponasal (or termed *nasal* in lay speak) in quality when there is significant obstruction by the adenoids. In clinical practice, this can be assessed by asking the patient to say the name "Mickey Mouse" while pinching the nose and while not pinching the nose. If the adenoids are significantly enlarged, the Mickey Mouse phrase sounds the same, pinching or no pinching.

Enlarged adenoids can also lead to the typical "adenoid facies." Adenoid facies can comprise open-mouth breathing, audible mouth breathing, and blueness around the lips and under the eyes (allergic shiners).

The use of the Mallampati score has recently come into vogue as a tool to judge airway obstruction. The Mallampati classification is an anesthesia tool used to describe the degree of overlap between the soft palate and the base of the tongue. Anesthesiologists use the score as an aid in predicting the degree of difficulty of intubation. The score is correlated with the presence of OSA. It is a scale from 1 to 4, with 4 describing severe overlap of the soft palate over the tongue base. While the published reports on OSA and Mallampati score describe an adult population, assessing a Mallampati score in kids is yet another clue that can be used in one's assessment (Nuckton et al., 2006).

Visualization and auscultation of the chest can elicit clues to the diagnosis of OSA as well. If you look very carefully, one can oftentimes pick up a small pectus excavatum, which can suggest long-standing increased work of breathing during sleep. When a pectus excavatum is identified, one needs to determine if the patient was born with this chest wall deformity or whether it is acquired. When a pectus excavatum is present from birth and simply grows in parallel with the child's growth, it is clinically insignificant. However, if the parents cannot remember it from birth, then it may have been acquired over time and might be an insidious sign of increased work of breathing during sleep.

Auscultation can sometimes be noteworthy for diminished breath sounds. Adenotonsillar hypertrophy can obstruct normal breathing such that the breath sounds are rendered less loud than you might expect.

Sometimes the most important element to the physical exam comes from just observing the child from afar. Sleepiness can be assessed if the child yawns a lot, seems unexpectedly quiet or withdrawn, or even falls asleep. Hyperactivity and impulsivity can manifest as the child bouncing all over the room, getting into things, and being poorly focused and poorly behaved. Fidgeting, leg bouncing, irritability, and tantrums are all easily observable and important to note. While all of these behaviors can of course be associated with normal childhood growth and development, over time, the skilled and experienced practitioner can begin to determine behaviors suggestive of excessive daytime sleepiness that stand out as abnormal. Furthermore, since sleep disorders of any cause (i.e., not just OSA) can masquerade as depression, anxiety, hyperactivity, or impulsivity, such global observations are of paramount importance.

OSA can have a major impact on growth; therefore, tracking height, weight, and body mass index need to be part of every office visit (Bonuck, Freeman, & Henderson, 2009). OSA can effect growth on both ends of the spectrum. In more severe cases, it can be associated with failure to thrive. In addition, it can be associated with insulin resistance and subsequent obesity (Gozal & Kheirandish-Gozal, 2009; Kohler, 2009; Spruyt et al., 2008).

When OSA has become long-standing and has begun to affect the cardiovascular system, there can be additional physical findings that become more obvious. Blood pressure can be elevated, and aberrant second heart sounds related to right heart strain can become pronounced (Sheldon et al., 2005).

DIAGNOSIS

The diagnosis of OSA has evolved over the years. Even though polysomnography (the overnight sleep study) remains the gold standard (Sheldon et al., 2005) for diagnosis, utilization and interpretation remains a challenge. If after evaluation the child is suspected of having OSA, he/she should ideally be referred for a sleep study. However, even when a child is referred, challenges exist. For example, many sleep labs do not study children and even fewer sleep labs study very young children and babies. Furthermore, the various monitoring devices involved with a sleep study can be frightening to children. Thus, when possible, it is preferred that the child is studied in a pediatric sleep lab staffed by pediatric trained sleep technicians. These pediatric trained technicians have the experience needed to get a child into the room, feel comfortable, engaged, and as willing a participant as possible.

The electrode leads are used to provide a complete assessment of cardiorespiratory, brain, and muscular physiology during sleep. Electroencephalogram leads assess brain wave activity and are designed to differentiate sleep stages and arousals. Their primary purpose is not to pick up seizure activity, but when obvious, epileptic activity can be seen.

Muscle activity is assessed by electromyogram leads placed on the chin and limbs. Muscular tone in the chin is a correlate for tone in the whole body and therefore can serve as an aid in distinguishing between stages of sleep. For example, there is nearly absent muscular tone during REM sleep;

therefore, the chin lead will be silent during REM. The chin lead also becomes active during bruxism and lip-smacking.

Airflow can be assessed by an airflow pressure transducer at the nose and by oronasal thermistors at the nose and mouth. End tidal or transcutaneous CO_2 recording is often available and at times is invaluable in making the diagnosis of OSA.

Determination of chest and abdominal wall excursion allows one to gauge respiratory effort and to classify apneas as central or obstructive. Limb leads assess leg movements. Snore microphones assess snoring. Finally, real-time video is useful in observing sleep positions, restlessness, and seizures, and in verifying what may be unclear from the electrodes as seen on the computer monitor.

As extensive and cumbersome as this array of monitoring sounds and appears, it remains the gold standard for a variety of reasons. First of all, it has long been known that relying solely on history, audiotape or videotape, is insufficient for diagnosing OSA. Second, there are a variety of combinations and permutations using data from the full set of leads whereby a study can be judged positive and diagnostic for OSA. Additionally, OSA is frequently sleep stage specific (REM), and since REM is clustered in the latter half of the night, a full night's monitoring is required. If one only performs an abbreviated study or a nap study, a majority of obstructive events might be missed. Finally, since OSA is but one reason (albeit very common) for restless and disturbed nighttime sleep, full polysomnography is as necessary to rule OSA in, as it is to rule other entities out.

Utilization of the sleep lab is also an issue of debate. As previously mentioned, in an ideal world with unlimited medical and financial resources, every child suspected of having OSA would have a sleep study. This, of course, is not an ideal world, and resources are limited as are skilled and trained personnel. The general guidelines for recommending a sleep study are as follows:

(1) If the OSA diagnosis is in question
(2) If the parent requires the information in order to be comfortable with the idea of possible surgical intervention such as adenotonsillectomy
(3) If the ENT surgeon requests the study
(4) If the child is very young or medically fragile

Other reasons for ordering a sleep study include the following:

(5) If the diagnosis and treatment of ADHD is being considered (Chervin et al., 2006; Hoban, 2008)
(6) If a child is insulin resistant or obese (Gozal, Capdevila, & Kheirandish-Gozal, 2008; Kohler, 2009; Nakra et al., 2008)
(7) If a child has persistent nocturnal enuresis
(8) If a child has difficult-to-control asthma (Ramagopal et al., 2009).

In a recent study by Bhattacharjee et al. (2010), expanded use of sleep studies is also advocated both pre- and postadenotonsillectomy (Bhattacharjee et al., 2010). However, performing a sleep study following adenotonsillectomy is not routinely done since posttreatment, a parent's objective assessment is oftentimes suggestive enough to make one feel confident that OSA has resolved or at least improved.

COMPLICATIONS

The morbidity or pathological consequences of OSA in children are multi-faceted and potentially complex. If left untreated or unidentified, OSA may lead to substantial morbidity, affecting multiple organ systems that may not be completely reversed with appropriate treatment. The possible complications of OSA in children can be divided into three major categories: behavioral disturbances (Chervin et al., 2006)/learning deficits (Gozal et al. 2007), cardiovascular (Gozal & Kheirandish, 2006), and compromised somatic growth. Furthermore, these complications associated with OSA are the result of four categories of upper airway obstruction during sleep: increased work of breathing, intermittent hypoxemia, sleep fragmentation, and alveolar hypoventilation (O'Brien & Gozal, 2005).

Children with OSA may be obese or may exhibit poor growth (Bonuck et al., 2009). In infants, poor growth may manifest as failure to thrive. The mechanisms responsible for growth deceleration may be multifactorial but seem to be due in large part to the increased energy expenditure that is necessary to meet the demands of an elevated work of breathing during sleep. It is possible that decreased appetite (a result of reduced olfaction due to enlarged adenoids) and difficulty swallowing (secondary to tonsillar hypertrophy) may play a role in a minority of cases. However, the exact causes underlying the development of growth retardation in OSA are not fully defined. Current research suggests that nocturnal growth hormone secretion may be disrupted and decreased in children with increased upper airway resistance during sleep. This finding is particularly applicable to pediatric OSA because even in children who are classified as "snorers" and who do not fulfill the criteria for OSA, there is evidence of stunted growth. Hence, the evidence strongly suggests that children who suffer from disrupted sleep have altered growth hormone levels. Finally, growth disruption in pediatric OSA does not appear to be associated with increased daily energy requirements but involves a combination of increased nighttime energy expenditure caused by increased respiratory effort and, most importantly, disruption of the growth hormone pathway. While the exact pathophysiology underlying decreased circulation of growth hormone in children remains unclear, it is known that these hormone levels will recover and return to normal after adenotonsillectomy and that rebound or catch-up growth will occur. Indeed, improved growth and weight gain, whether desired or not, has been reported after surgical treatment of OSA (Kiris et al., 2010).

Because children have greater vascular compliance than adults, the severity of blood pressure elevation in pediatric patients with OSA is not as prominent as those described in adults. Nevertheless, alterations in blood pressure do occur and are manifested primarily as higher diastolic blood pressure during wakefulness. Frequent oxygen desaturations during sleep are common in children with OSA, and the resultant autonomic alterations are the by-product of both the episodic hypoxia that accompanies OSA and also the repeated nighttime arousals and carbon dioxide elevations that occur (Tauman et al., 2007). The intermittent hypoxia that occurs in children with OSA may cause elevations of pulmonary artery pressure and hence leads to right ventricular dysfunction (Kheirandish-Gozal et al., 2006). A recent study demonstrated that right ventricular mass index and wall thickness were greater in children with OSA and children with an apnea–hypopnea index (AHI) of 10 or greater had a right and left ventricular mass greater than the 95th percentile (Hoban, 2008). As a result of systemic circulatory effects, recurrent hypoxia and hypercapnia can have a deleterious effect on pulmonary circulation and can lead to pulmonary vascular hypertension. Hypoxia-induced pulmonary vasoconstriction and the resultant elevation of pulmonary artery pressure is a serious consequence of OSA in children and can lead to persistent pulmonary hypertension and cor pulmonale. The long-term consequences of the effects of pediatric OSA on cardiovascular morbidity have yet to be explored and researched further. A particularly revealing animal experiment exposed rodents to a model of OSA at an age corresponding to the peak prevalence of OSA in children. The results found that there was an increased attenuation of the baroreceptors that control blood pressure function lasting into late adulthood. The results of the study postulate that early childhood insults to the cardiovascular system may lead to lifelong consequences and that exposure to hypoxia during childhood may exacerbate the pulmonary vascular response to subsequent hypoxia in adulthood (Gozal, Daniel, & Dohanich, 2001). Therefore, early identification of children with pediatric OSA may lead to the detection of a population potentially at risk for the development of hypertension and heart disease.

In the early years of a child's development, parents may receive different opinions from professionals/adults who view their child in different settings. A kindergarten teacher who observes the child unable to sit quietly during story time may call him "inattentive." A coach who sees a child running rowdily and unable to follow directions may label him "wild." A pediatrician seeing the child for an office visit may diagnose him with "attention deficit disorder" and may prescribe stimulant medication. Finally, a sleep medicine specialist may consider that the aforementioned child may have an underlying sleep disorder. Indeed, some of the earliest descriptions of childhood OSA reported hyperactivity, inattention, and learning problems as frequently associated symptoms. Reports of decreased intellectual function in children with tonsillar and adenoidal hypertrophy date back to the 19th century when Hill reported on "the stupid lazy child who breathes through his mouth instead of his nose, snores, and is restless at night." School difficulties have been cited repeatedly in case studies of children with OSA (Gozal et al. 2007; Kheirandish & Gozal, 2006).

Researchers are also discovering that there are detrimental cognitive, developmental, and behavioral consequences of OSA in children (O'Brien et al., 2004b). Valid connections have been made between OSA and reduced verbal IQ, decreased cognitive function, lower Bailey developmental scores, and poor school performance. Contemporary studies have demonstrated that effective treatment of OSA is associated with at least partially reversible behavioral and learning deficits. One study discussed a large sample of first graders who were failing at school and who had a sixfold increase in the incidence of OSA when compared to the prevalence of OSA in the general pediatric population. However, 1 year after undergoing surgical removal of hypertrophic tonsils, the children's overall school performance was significantly improved (Gozal et al., 2007). This suggests that OSA may impose adverse and persistent cognitive outcomes and lowered academic achievement, particularly when it presents during critical phases of brain growth and development. Such findings clearly provide a strong argument for early identification and effective treatment to prevent long-lasting consequences (Hoban, 2008).

It has been estimated that up to 30% of children with habitual snoring or OSA have hyperactivity and inattention. OSA in children may cause daytime neurobehavioral symptoms that resemble or mimic those of ADHD. The impact of OSA on childhood development and behavior—specifically hyperactivity and inattention—has been well published. The ADHD symptoms that these children exhibit should not be confused with true ADHD, but rather a lack of behavioral inhibition secondary to repeated sleep arousals and hypoxic episodes that ultimately affect memory, motor control, and self-control. The exact pathophysiology by which OSA contributes to hyperactivity remains unknown. It has been surmised that both the sleep fragmentation and the hypoxia that characterizes OSA lead to changes resulting in the cognitive and behavioral dysfunction.

MANAGEMENT

The decision to initiate treatment should be made on a case-by-case basis once OSA is confirmed. This requires cautiously weighing the anticipated risks and benefits of treatment. Factors to consider are the child's age, polysomnographic abnormalities, and whether there are underlying medical issues or complications related to OSA.

It is widely accepted that adenotonsillectomy is considered the first-line treatment for childhood OSA (Suen, Arnold, & Brooks, 1995). Several studies have evaluated the success rate for adenotonsillectomy in children with OSA secondary to adenotonsillar hypertrophy, and all suggest that an overwhelming majority of patients have an improvement in both symptoms and polysomnographic findings postoperatively; resolution occurs in 75–90% of otherwise healthy patients. Even in children with relatively small tonsils, adenotonsillectomy is often successful (Goldberg et al., 2005). This can be attributed to the fact that relaxed muscle tone, especially during REM sleep, may result in otherwise small-appearing tonsils having a significant impact and ability to obstruct the airway. Most sleep specialists agree that both the tonsils and adenoids should be removed, regardless if one or the other appears more enlarged. This stems from the belief that OSA is the result of both structural and neuromotor abnormalities. Thus, widening the airway and decreasing resistance as much as possible improves airflow (Kuhle et al., 2009; Lipton & Gozal, 2003).

Regrowth of the adenoid tissue may occur, especially in young children. One study demonstrated lymphoid regrowth occupying up to 40% of the nasopharynx. It is important to keep in mind that if a child develops a recurrence of OSA symptoms after adenotonsillectomy, they should be evaluated by an ear, nose, and throat (ENT) specialist to determine whether the adenoids have regrown and whether revision adenoidectomy is warranted.

Potential complications of adenotonsillectomy include hemorrhage, anesthetic complications; immediate postoperative problems, such as pain and poor oral intake; and respiratory decompensation. In addition, patients with severe OSA may develop respiratory complications, such as pulmonary edema. The Academy of Pediatrics Clinical Practice Guideline recommends that high-risk patients be hospitalized overnight after adenotonsillectomy and be monitored continuously with pulse oximetry.

Adenotonsillectomy is a relatively simple procedure with a low complication rate; most patients with OSA have a complete resolution of symptoms. Therefore, it is the preferable choice of treatment when compared to long-term use of continuous positive airway pressure (CPAP), where adherence is often a problem. However, adenotonsillectomy should not be taken lightly. As with any surgery, there are inherent risks. For this reason, it is recommended that all children have polysomnographic proof of OSA prior to surgery (Wei, Barretto, & Gerber, 2005).

Many reviews of OSA in children demonstrate a relationship between sleep positioning and worsening sleep apnea (Cuhadaroglu et al, 2003). Apneas tend to be worse when a child sleeps on his/her back due to the effect of gravity. In the supine position, hypertrophic tonsils may partially or fully collapse and occupy a significant proportion of the upper airway. In addition, decreased airway muscle tone during sleep may cause the uvula and/or tongue to prolapse into the hypopharyngeal airway and against the soft palate, leading to airway obstruction. Children with OSA tend to breathe best (have a lower AHI) when in the left lateral decubitus position.

Most children sleep in a variety of positions throughout the night and are generally not able to avoid the supine position. A "tennis ball technique" can be employed to train children to avoid sleeping on their back.

The tennis ball is placed into a sock and safety pinned to the back of the patient's shirt. Elevating the head of the bed may also be helpful. Head elevation reduces swelling of the turbinates and may reduce vascular congestion in the neck, thereby improving the nasal airway and potentially enlarging the diameter of the pharyngeal airway. Additionally, one may try the use of sleeping on a foam wedge pillow. Bear in mind that most studies have shown that positional sleep therapy achieves only a slight improvement in the AHI and is generally not helpful in managing severe sleep apnea (Cuhadaroglu et al, 2003; Rich, 2003).

As tonsils and adenoids consist of lymphoid tissue, several studies have focused on the use of steroids to reduce the inflammation and thereby the size of the tissue. A number of clinical trials have shown a modest improvement in OSA, with an AHI reduction from 11 to 6 events/h following a 6-week course of intranasal corticosteroids. While the results demonstrated that treatment with intranasal corticosteroids resulted in a reduction in the number of apneas in most children, it did not result in complete cessation. Furthermore, the children continued to have sleep-related hypoxia of the same magnitude as before (Brouillete et al., 2001). It is possible that nasal decongestants or intranasal corticosteroids may be more effective in specific subsets of children, such as those whose symptoms of OSA seem to be due to allergic rhinitis, allergies, and/or asthma. In children with mild OSA, both intranasal corticosteroids and montelukast have been shown to reduce symptoms and the degree of obstruction; however, they can only be recommended for short-term use to ameliorate symptoms in children with OSA on the waiting list for adenotonsillectomy.

Systemic steroids will definitely shrink adenotonsillar tissue, but since long-term use of systemic steroids is not safe, this is not a practical treatment plan for OSA. Short (5 days) courses of oral steroids can be used in certain circumstances when there is an urgent need to shrink the tonsils transiently. However, it is important to note that there can be rebound following the course.

Rapid maxillary expansion (RME) is an orthodontic treatment used to separate or widen the maxilla and the maxillary dental arch and to improve the nasal airway (Pirelli, 2010). RME may serve as an intervention for some children with OSA who exhibit abnormalities in craniofacial morphology associated with nasal obstruction due to a narrow maxilla. RME involves the insertion of a dental appliance into the mouth. The appliance contacts the roof of the mouth and is held in place by anchoring the device to the child's molars. RME is also commonly referred to as a palate expander. The benefits of orthodontic expansion continue to be explored in pediatric sleep medicine literature. A recent study, albeit with a small sample size ($n = 31$), demonstrated that after 4 months of RME, the mean AHI had decreased from 12 to less than 1 event/h. This study was performed on a group of nonobese children who had OSA, a high arched palate and either no adenotonsillar hypertrophy or a prior adenotonsillectomy (Pirelli, 2010). For those children who do not have resolution of OSA symptoms postadenotonsillectomy, treatment with orthodontic expansion should be explored, especially in children who have difficulty accepting CPAP therapy.

Weight loss is recommended for all obese patients, especially those with OSA. The evidence for an association between obesity and OSA is well documented, with obesity shown to be a risk factor in both adults and children. However, weight reduction treatment for the obese child/adolescent can be extremely challenging and is notoriously difficult to achieve. Weight loss requires motivation on both the part of the child and the family. Even when weight loss does occur, progress happens slowly. Therefore, interim management is often required. Although adenotonsillectomy can be effective even in morbidly obese children, it is important to keep in mind that postoperative persistence of OSA is more frequent (Lipton & Gozal, 2003). In addition, CPAP can also be used pending surgery.

Recent studies in extremely obese adolescents indicate that significant weight loss after bariatric surgery was associated with either complete resolution of OSA in the majority of patients or a significant reduction in OSA severity (Kalra et al., 2005). Patients with significant obesity should have good follow-up care and should undergo postoperative polysomnography to determine whether further treatment, such as CPAP, is necessary.

For the nearly 15% of kids for whom adenotonsillectomy is ineffective or incompletely effective, CPAP becomes a very important second-line intervention. CPAP delivered by nasal mask, full face mask, or nasal pillow blows air gently through the upper airway in order to ease one's work of breathing. Since OSA is defined by increased resistance to airflow in the upper airway, CPAP's effectiveness occurs by helping to overcome the airway resistance regardless of location (Guilleminault et al., 1995; Marcus et al., 1995; Palombini, Pelayo, & Guilleminault, 2004). Adenotonsillectomy results in a cure when the greatest place of obstruction is at the nose or in the oropharynx. However, these are only two areas where there can be an increase in airway resistance. Other sources of resistance can occur due to dynamic defects such as pharyngomalacia, laryngomalacia, or tracheomalacia. Furthermore, obstruction can occur due to unique craniofacial features or neuromuscular conditions that render adenotonsillectomy ineffective. Finally, one must remember that the ability to achieve adequate inhalation assumes that the muscles of respiration are working properly and are not impeded by any comorbid conditions. Weak chest wall muscles in certain neuromuscular conditions (spinal muscle atrophy, muscular dystrophy, Down syndrome) may not generate enough force to overcome normal or even just slightly increased upper airway resistance and may result in OSA. Additionally, diaphragmatic function can be compromised due to the hyperinflation associated with asthma. This, too, may then result in an inability to overcome normal upper airway resistance.

Given all the myriad of places and conditions where upper airway resistance can exist, one cannot help but stand in amazement that adenotonsillectomy works as well as and as often as it does. However, in instances where surgery is not effective, CPAP can generally be the solution for any level of obstruction due to increased airway resistance. In fact, if surgery were not so overwhelmingly curative and if adherence was not an issue, CPAP could be considered first-line therapy for OSA in children, as it is for adults.

There are a number of advantages and benefits to CPAP therapy for pediatric OSA. First of all, it is a nonsurgical form of therapy and is therefore extremely attractive for families fearful of surgery. Second, CPAP can serve as a bridge to surgery in children who are either very young or for whom one cannot find an ENT surgeon willing to operate. CPAP has been found to be safe and effective in newborns through and beyond adolescence. Finally, in those for whom surgery is incompletely effective, CPAP can be utilized in an attempt to completely treat OSA.

One disadvantage to CPAP therapy is that it can be seen as cumbersome and labor-intensive. CPAP involves placing a mask over the child's face and securing it with headgear over the head or behind the head. For some young children, this can seem scary and therefore can be met with resistance. However, when carefully approached, children after the age of 2 can successfully utilize CPAP therapy. When parents are involved and dedicated, CPAP can usually be accomplished. It is useful to remind parents and children that even if CPAP is used for only a few hours of sleep, these few hours will be better than the night before when CPAP was not in use. These small successes and sensations of improved sleep quality oftentimes build on themselves, leading to more time spent on CPAP and less resistance.

Another disadvantage is that the use of CPAP requires another sleep study in order to titrate the appropriate air pressure. For some children, this then becomes their third sleep study. (Many children have a second diagnostic study to prove that OSA is still present and to what degree, thus making the CPAP study their third study overall.) However, with the increased use of autotitrating CPAP machines where air pressure delivered is changed automatically based on the child's need, there is less of a medical need for the study. There is, however, a practical requirement for the CPAP titration study. Such a study is oftentimes required in order for insurance companies to agree to pay for the device. The CPAP titration study, however, does serve a few other important "medical" purposes. First, it exposes the child to the device in a controlled setting. Second, it allows the technicians to fit the child with an appropriate mask. Finally, it also allows the parent to observe that "CPAP is not the worst thing in the world!" More often than not, children and parents report during office follow-up how the day following the CPAP titration study was a much better day. These small observable successes help the process to move forward with greater ease.

CPAP adherence can be monitored via a data card from the CPAP machine. Such a download of information can inform caregivers about the number of hours and days of CPAP use. It is important to note that insurance companies sometimes track usage data in order to justify continued payment of the device. Adherence can also be monitored clinically. If CPAP is in use and is working properly, it can result in greater daytime alertness, less restless sleep, decreased snoring, improved school grades, and improved behavior. There can even be improved metabolism in the form of less insulin resistance and weight loss. Furthermore, many parents and children who had been diagnosed as having ADHD find that with the use of CPAP, their hyperactivity diminishes as does their need for stimulant medication.

In circumstances where CPAP cannot be used because of displeasure or discomfort on the part of the child, the following options exist:

(a)   Wait another 6 months and try again.
(b)   Have a conversation with the ENT surgeon in order to see if, in fact, there is anything surgical that could be useful such as
    a.   uvulopalatopharyngoplasty,
    b.   tongue reduction,
    c.   turbinate surgery, and
    d.   pillar procedure.
(c)   Consider other treatment options as outlined earlier.

NURSING CARE OF THE CHILD AND FAMILY

The American Academy of Pediatrics recommends that parents/caregivers of children be asked about snoring during routine health-care visits. This recommendation reflects the observation that habitual snoring is often present in children who have OSA. Sleep disorders are common in children and adolescents; however, sleep-related issues are often not discussed during well child visits in part due to parents not raising the issue and providers not asking caregivers about symptoms of sleep problems. Indeed, several studies have found that sleep disorders, including OSA, may be underdiagnosed in pediatric practices. The standard review of systems covered in a well child visit often does not include a sleep assessment. Nurses who work in primary care practices can incorporate a simple question, "Does your child snore," in their patient assessment, and document it within the electronic medical record or have it included in the office questionnaire that parents are routinely asked to complete.

School nurses have the capacity to reach large numbers of children and may often find themselves in the unique situation of identifying pediatric OSA. Parents are routinely required to complete a health history prior to entering the school system. Including questions about sleep/snoring on an intake questionnaire may identify children who have managed to slip through the cracks. Often children are referred to the nurse's office because of "nodding off" in class, and some children come in voluntarily during a free period to take a nap due to daytime sleepiness. Additionally, school nurses should be cognizant that poor sleep affects a child's school performance and behavior. By the time a child is 5 years of age, more than half of their life will have been spent being asleep and more than one-quarter of their day is spent in school. Daytime symptoms such as mouth breathing, hyperactivity, aggressiveness, learning difficulties, and failure of hearing tests (possibly due to large adenoids) should all alert the school nurse to the possibility of OSA. Parents should be contacted and questioned regarding sleep and snoring, and appropriate referrals should be made.

Adenotonsillectomy is considered first-line therapy and is highly successful in eliminating OSA in children. Although it is considered to be minor surgery, it can be associated with significant complications. While the majority of children tolerate the surgery without difficulties, all children undergoing tonsillectomy or adenoidectomy should be considered to be at increased risk for postoperative complications. These complications may include upper airway edema, pulmonary edema, and respiratory failure, in addition to the usual risks of adenotonsillectomy.

Children with severe OSA have a highly negative intrathoracic pressure due to airway obstruction. Pulmonary edema can occur when airway obstruction is relieved by adenotonsillectomy, causing increased venous return and pulmonary pressure. The challenge for nurses working in the operative and postoperative setting is determining which patients are considered high risk for respiratory complications because polysomnograpy is not a standard preoperative test for children undergoing adenotonsillectomy, even though it is recommended by the American Thoracic Society and the American Academy of Pediatrics.

Studies have demonstrated that children with OSA had a 23% rate of respiratory difficulties after adenotonsillectomy, with the greatest risk seen in children <3 years of age (Statham, Elluru, Buncher, & Kalra, 2006). Children that have been identified as having severe OSA are considered high risk for respiratory compromise. They require overnight inpatient monitoring after surgery in a setting with continuous pulse oximetry so that airway obstruction can be recognized and prompt intervention can occur. Postoperative intensive care unit admission is reserved for very severe OSA, for very young children (<3 years of age), and for those with significant comorbidities (Oron, Marom, Russo, Ezri, & Roth, 2010).

In summary, because of the many complications associated with OSA, it is clear that accurate and timely diagnosis and treatment of the disease can have a positive impact on a child's life. A few simple questions asked during a well child visit or during an emergency room visit or during a trip to the school nurse's office can bring attention to this pervasive problem. Treatment of OSA can turn a cranky, sleepy, hyperactive child into one that is happy, healthy, and growing.

REFERENCES

Amin, R. S., Carroll, J. L., Jeffries, J. L., et al. (2004). Twenty-four-hour ambulatory blood pressure in children with sleep-disordered breathing. *American Journal of Respiratory and Critical Care Medicine, 169*(8), 950–956.

Au, C. T., & Li, A. (2009). Obstructive sleep breathing disorders. *Pediatric Clinics of North America, 56*, 243–259.

Basha, S., Bialowas, C., Ende, K., et al. (2005). Effectiveness of adenotonsillectomy in the resolution of nocturnal enuresis secondary to obstructive sleep apnea. *Laryngoscope, 115*(6), 1101–1103.

Benninger, M., & Walner, D. (2007). Obstructive sleep-disordered breathing in children. *Clinical Cornerstone, 9*(1), 6–12.

Bhattacharjee, R., Kheirandish-Gozal, L., Spruyt, K., et al. (2010). Adenotonsillectomy outcomes in treatment of obstructive sleep apnea in children: A multicenter retrospective study. *American Journal of Respiratory and Critical Care Medicine, 182*, 676–683.

Bonuck, K. A., Freeman, K., & Henderson, J. (2009). Growth and growth biomarker changes after adenotonsillectomy: Systematic review and meta analysis. *Archives of Disease in Childhood, 94*(2), 83–91.

Brouillete, R. T., Manoukian, J. J., Cucharme, F. M., Oudjhane, K., Earle, L. G., Ladan, S., et al. (2001). Efficacy of fluticasone nasal spray for pediatric obstructive sleep apnea. *Journal of Pediatrics, 138*, 838–844.

Capdevila, O. S., Crabtree, V. M., Kheirandish-Gozal, L., et al. (2008). Increased morning brain natriuretic peptide levels in children with nocturnal enuresis and sleep-disordered breathing: A community-based study. *Pediatrics, 121*, e1208–e1214.

Chervin, R. D., Ruzicka, D. L., Bruno, G. J., et al. (2006). Sleep-disordered breathing, behavior, and cognition in children before and after adenotonsillectomy. *Pediatrics, 117*, e769–e778.

Cuhadaroglu, C., et al. (2003). Body position and Obstructive Sleep Apnea Syndrome. *Pediatric Pulmonology, 36*, 335–338.

Goldberg, S., Shatz, A., Picard, I., et al. (2005). Endoscopic findings in children with obstructive sleep apnea: Effects of age and hypotonia. *Pediatric Pulmonology, 40*(3), 205–210.

Gozal, D. (2009). Sleep, sleep disorders and inflammation in children. *Sleep Medicine, 10*, S12–S16.

Gozal, D., Capdevila, O. S., & Kheirandish-Gozal, L. (2008). Metabolic alterations and systemic inflammation in obstructive sleep apnea among non-obese and obese prepubertal children. *American Journal of Respiratory and Critical Care Medicine, 177*(10), 142–149.

Gozal, D., Capdevila, O. S., Kheirandish-Gozal, L., et al. (2007). APOE epsilon 4 allele, cognitive dysfunction, and obstructive sleep apnea in children. *Neurology, 6S*(3), 243–249.

Gozal, D., Crabtree, V. M., Sans Capdevila, O., et al. (2007). C-reactive protein, obstructive sleep apnea, and cognitive dysfunction in school-aged children. *American Journal of Respiratory and Critical Care Medicine, 176*(2), 188–193. 1.

Gozal, D., Daniel, J. M., & Dohanich, G. P. (2001). Behavioral and anatomic correlates of chronic episodic hypoxia during sleep in the rat. *The Journal of Neuroscience, 21*, 2442–2450.

Gozal, D., & Kheirandish, L. (2006). Oxidant stress and inflammation in the snoring child: Confluent pathways to upper airway pathogenesis and end-organ morbidity. *Sleep Medicine Reviews, 10*(2), 83–96.

Gozal, D., & Kheirandish-Gozal, L. (2008). Cardiovascular morbidity in obstructive sleep apnea: Oxidative stress, inflammation, and much more. *American Journal of Respiratory and Critical Care Medicine, 177*(4), 369–375.

Gozal, D., & Kheirandish-Gozal, L. (2009). Obesity and excessive daytime sleepiness in prepubertal children with obstructive sleep apnea. *Pediatrics, 123*(1), 13–18.

Gozal, D., & Kheirandish-Gozal, L. (2010). New approaches to the diagnosis of sleep-disordered breathing in children. *Sleep Medicine, 11*, 708–713.

Gozal, D., Kheirandish-Gozal, L., Serpero, L. D., et al. (2007). Obstructive sleep apnea and endothelial function in school-aged nonobese children: Effect of adenotonsillectomy. *Circulation, 116*(20), 2307–2314.

Gozal, D., Serpero, L. D., Capdevila, O., et al. (2008). Inflammation in non-obese children with obstructive sleep apnea. *Sleep Medicine, S*(3), 254–259.

Guilleminault, C., Pelayo, R., Clerk, A., et al. (1995). Home nasal continuous positive airway pressure in infants with sleep disordered breathing. *The Journal of Pediatrics, 127*, 905–912.

Hoban, T. (2008). Sleep disturbances and attention deficit disorder. *Sleep Med Clin, 3*, 469–478.

Kalra, M., Inge, T., Garcia, V., et al. (2005). Obstructive sleep apnea in extremely overweight adolescents undergoing bariatric surgery. *Obesity Research, 13*, 1175–1179.

Kheirandish, L., & Gozal, D. (2006). Neurocognitive dysfunction in children with sleep disorders. *Developmental Science, 9*(4), 388–399.

Kheirandish-Gozal, L., Capdevila, O. S., Tauman, R., et al. (2006). Plasma C-reactive protein in nonobese children with obstructive sleep apnea before and after adenotonsillectomy. *Journal of Clinical Sleep Medicine, 2*(3), 301–304.

Kiris, M., Muderris, T., Celebi, S., et al. (2010). Changes in serum IGF-1 and IGFBP-3 levels and growth in children following adenoidectomy, tonsillectomy or adenotonsillectomy. *International Journal of Pediatric Otorhinolaryngology, 74*(5), 528–531.

Kohler, M. J. (2009). Differences in the association between obesity and obstructive sleep apnea among children and adolescents. *Journal of Clinical Sleep Medicine, 5*, 506–511.

Kuhle, S., et al. (2009). Interventions for obstructive sleep apnea in children: A systematic review. *Sleep Medicine Reviews, 13*, 123–131.

Lipton, A., & Gozal, D. (2003). Treatment of obstructive sleep apnea in children: Do we really know how? *Sleep Medicine Reviews, 7*(1), 61–80.

Lumeng, J. C., & Chervin, R. D. (2008). Epidemiology of pediatric obstructive sleep apnea. *Proceedings of the American Thoracic Society, 5*, 242–252.

Marcus, C. L., Ward, S. L., Mallory, G. B., et al. (1995). Use of nasal continuous airway positive pressure as treatment of childhood obstructive sleep apnea. *The Journal of Pediatrics, 127*, 88–94.

Marshall, N. S. (2007). Childhood Asthma Prevention Study predictors for snoring in children with rhinitis at age 5. *Pediatric Pulmonology, 42*(7), 584–591.

Meltzer, L., Johnson, C., Crosette, J., et al. (2010). Prevalence of diagnosed sleep disorders in pediatric primary care practices. *Pediatrics, 123*, 1410–1418.

Mindell, J. A., & Owens, J. A. (2003). *A clinical guide to pediatric sleep: Diagnosis and management of sleep problems.* Philadelphia, PA: Lippincott Williams and Williams.

Nakra, N., Bhargava, B., Dzuira, J., et al. (2008). Sleep-disordered breathing with metabolic syndrome: The role of leptin and sympathetic nervous system activity and the effect of continuous positive airway pressure. *Pediatrics, 122*, e634–e642.

Nuckton, T. J., Glidden, D. V., Browner, W. S., et al. (2006). Physical examination: Mallampati score as an independent predictor of OSA. *Sleep, 29*(7), 903–908.

O'Brien, L., & Gozal, D. (2005). Consequences of obstructive sleep apnea syndrome. In S. H. Sheldon, R. Ferber, & M. H. Kryger (Eds.), *Principles and practice of pediatric sleep medicine* (pp. 211–222). Philadelphia: Elsevier Saunders.

O'Brien, L. M., Mervis, C. B., Holbrook, C. R., et al. (2004a). Neurobehavioral implications of habitual snoring in children. *Pediatrics, 114*(1), 44–49.

O'Brien, L. M., Mervis, C. B., Holbrook, C. R., et al. (2004b). Neurobehavioral correlates of sleep-disordered breathing in children. *Journal of Sleep Research, 13*(2), 165–172.

Oron, Y., Marom, T., Russo, E., Ezri, T., & Roth, Y. (2010). Don't overlook the complications of tonsillectomy. *The Journal of Family Practice, 59*(10), 4–9.

Palombini, L., Pelayo, R., & Guilleminault, C. (2004). Efficacy of automated continuous positive airway pressure in children with sleep-related breathing disorders in attended setting. *Pediatrics, 113*, e412–e417.

Perez, I., & Davidson, S. (2008). The snoring child. *Pediatric Annals, 37*(7), 465–469.

Pirelli, P. (2010). Orthodontics and obstructive sleep apnea in children. *The Medical Clinics of North America, 94*, 517.

Ramagopal, M., Mehta, A., Roberts, D. W., et al. (2009). Asthma as a predictor of obstructive sleep apnea in urban African-American children. *The Journal of Asthma, 46*(9), 895–899.

Rich, G. (2003). Efficacy of a therapeutic pillow for snoring and obstructive sleep apnea treatment. *Sleep, 23*(2), 85.

Sheldon, S. H., Ferber, R., & Kryger, M. H. (2005). *Principles and practice of pediatric sleep medicine* (2nd ed.). Philadelphia, PA: Elsevier Saunders.

Spruyt, K., San Capdevila, O., Honaker, S. M., et al. (2008). Obesity, snoring and physical activity in school-aged children. *Sleep, 31*(Suppl.), A76. [Abstract 0230].

Statham, M., Elluru, R., Buncher, R., & Kalra, M. (2006). Adenotonsillectomy for obstructive sleep apnea syndrome in young children: Prevalence of pulmonary complications. *Archives of Otolaryngology—Head & Neck Surgery, 132*(5), 476–480.

Suen, J. S., Arnold, J. E., & Brooks, L. J. (1995). Adenotonsillectomy for treatment of obstructive sleep apnea in children. *Archives of Otolaryngology—Head & Neck Surgery, 121,* 525–530.

Tauman, R., O'Brien, L. M., & Gozal, D. (2007). Hypoxemia and obesity modulate plasma C-reactive protein and interieukin-6 levels in sleep-disordered breathing. *Sleep & Breathing, 11*(2), 77–84.

Wei, J., Barretto, R., & Gerber, M. (2005). Otolarynologic management of sleep-related breathing disorders. In S. H. Sheldon, R. Ferber, & M. H. Kryger (Eds.), *Principles and practice of pediatric sleep medicine* (pp. 249–262). Philadelphia: Elsevier Saunders.

Primary ciliary dyskinesia and bronchiectasis

Rosyln Bravo, BS, MS, APRN, CPNP, AE-C, and
Anita Bhandari, MD

PRIMARY CILIARY DYSKINESIA

Primary ciliary dyskinesia (PCD) is an autosomal recessive disorder that impairs the clearance of mucus from the respiratory system. PCD was initially identified in the 1900s. In the 1970s, this disorder was labeled immotile cilia syndrome. In the 1980s, it was changed to PCD to accurately reflect the reduced or impaired movement of cilia and not the total lack of ciliary movement (Schidlow & Steinfeld, 2005; Greenstone, Rutman, Dewar, Mackay, & Cole, 1988). Due to the impaired movement of the cilia, the majority of clinical manifestations affect the upper and lower airways. However, fertility can also be affected and situs inversus may also occur with Kartagener's syndrome (KS). Although there is no cure for PCD, there are several approaches for management that lessen the disease burden. Progression of the disease can cause serious deterioration of lung function, which usually manifests as a chronic obstructive lung disease. PCD is associated with bronchiectasis due to recurrent inflammation resulting in dilated, scarred airways. Although often observed in PCD, bronchiectasis is a nonspecific finding that is observed in a variety of lung diseases associated with repeated infections such as cystic fibrosis (CF), immunodeficiency, recurrent aspiration, and underlying congenital malformations of the lung (Callahan, 2005; Eastham, Fall, Mitchell, & Spencer, 2004). Nurses

Nursing Care in Pediatric Respiratory Disease, First Edition. Edited by Concettina (Tina) Tolomeo.
© 2012 John Wiley & Sons, Inc. Published 2012 by John Wiley & Sons, Inc.

play an important role in the management of the patient with PCD and bronchiectasis.

Epidemiology

The prevalence of PCD has been found to range from 1:20 to 60,000 live births; however, the reported prevalence varies significantly depending on the population studied (Bi, Bai, & Qiao, 2010; Bush et al., 2007). For instance, in the United Kingdom, Bush et al. (1998) report prevalence ranges from 1:15 to 30,000. In contrast, O'Callaghan, Chetcuti, and Moya (2010) report the prevalence of PCD among an Asian cohort of patients mostly of Pakistani decent as 1:2,265. Of note, 52% of the patients in this cohort were first cousins, suggesting that in a population with high consanguinity, PCD is much more common as expected in an autosomal recessive disorder.

Pathophysiology

PCD is a disorder that results in the impaired function and structure of respiratory cilia, thereby impairing mucociliary clearance (Dell, 2008). A respiratory cilium (Figure 10.1) is made of more than 250 proteins in a "9 + 2" formation consisting of nine peripheral doublets around the central microtubular pair (Bush et al., 2007). Radial spokes connect the doublets to the central microtubular pair (Thai, Gambling, & Carson, 2002). When the doublets slide, a bend in the radial spokes results (Jain et al., 2007). The motion of these cilia resembles a wave with a forward and return stroke; their direction is guided by the central microtubules (Leigh et al., 2009). The cilia are surrounded by a thin fluid that permits their fast action to move the viscous mucus above them, as only the tips of the cilia come in contact with the viscous layer during the forward stroke to move mucus along (Leigh et al., 2009; Sharma, 2008). Cilia beat at a frequency of 1,000–1,500 beats/min; the frequency is slower in the bronchioles than in the larger airway (Sharma, 2008).

Although there are many PCD phenotypes (Bush et al., 2007), only a few are commonly observed. They include the lack of outer dynein arms, a combination of missing inner and outer arms, isolated missing inner arms, or lack of inner arms combined with a radial spoke defect. Rare cases have described a transposition error of the central microtubular pair or a lack of the central microtubular pair. These structural abnormalities are associated with abnormal ciliary movement, which can range from no movement to ineffective movement, such as a windshield wiper or an eggbeater movement (Schidlow & Steinfeld, 2005). Subsequently, the ineffective ciliary movement results in poor airway clearance of mucus, which then leads to recurrent bacterial infections of the airways.

KS is a distinct phenotype of PCD, which comprises situs inversus totalis, recurrent sinusitis, and bronchiectasis (Dell, 2008). KS accounts for half of PCD cases (Schidlow & Steinfeld, 2005). Situs inversus, the complete

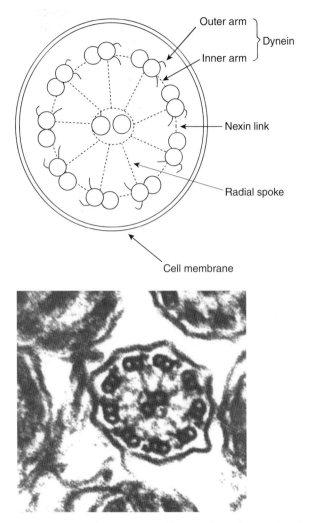

Figure 10.1   Respiratory cilium. Reprinted from Bush et al. (2007) with permission from BMJ Publishing Group, Ltd.

reversal of the abdominal and thoracic organs so that they appear as a mirror image when examined or visualized on a radiograph, is thought to be due to the dysfunction of embryonic node monocilia (Nonaka et al., 1998). More specifically, Nonaka et al. (1998) identified the KIF3B gene, which aids in the creation of motile cilia that participate in the left to right asymmetrical arrangement through nodal flow inside the yolk sac cavity. Nonaka et al. (1998) also observed that in normal mice, nodal cilia are motile in a counterclockwise direction, causing motion of the extra embryonal fluid in a leftward direction. Thus, the rotating movement of the nodal cilia creates asymmetry in the body (Afzelius, 1999), and if these cilia are defective, the normal asymmetry of the internal organs is not established. Furthermore, almost all males with KS are infertile due to the abnormal movement of spermatozoa (Schidlow & Steinfeld, 2005).

Signs and symptoms

Associated findings of PCD differ among age groups. Prenatal presentation is described as the presence of mirror image organ arrangement on ante- natal ultrasound (Bush et al., 2007). Presentation during the newborn period includes rhinorrhea from the first day, respiratory distress or neo- natal pneumonia without any predisposing cause, and positive screening due to positive family history (Bush et al., 2007). Signs and symptoms of PCD that are common in any pediatric age group include rhinitis, cough, and otitis media with effusion (Bush et al., 2007).

Since classical findings (rhinorrhea, recurrent ear infections, cough, and recurrent pneumonia) associated with PCD are common childhood com- plaints, the diagnosis may be delayed unless a thorough review of history is obtained. Coren, Meeks, Morrison, Buchdahl, and Bush (2002) reported that the median age of diagnosis of patients with PCD was 4 years with a range from 0 to 14 years. Twelve out of the 55 children had bronchiectasis, chronic lung damage, at the time of diagnosis, even though 6 of the chil- dren with bronchiectasis had neonatal symptoms and 7 had abnormal situs. In addition, 8 of the 12 had a chronic productive cough. Of the 25 children with abnormal situs and a history of neonatal symptoms, only 13 were diagnosed before 1 year of age and the other 12 received a diagnosis between 4 and 10 years of life. Similarly, in a retrospective review by Jain et al. (2007), only 8 of the 89 patients were diagnosed as neonates, although 43% of them had a history of neonatal respiratory distress.

PCD should be considered in the differential diagnosis for any child with recurrent or persistent pneumonia especially if bronchiectasis is iden- tified on chest X-ray or high-resolution computed tomography (HRCT). Additionally, PCD should be considered in the differential diagnosis of a child with poorly controlled asthma, persistent ear discharge despite myr- ingotomy tubes, or a child with hearing loss (Barbato et al., 2009; Bush et al., 2007).

Although adolescents and adults may have a history of childhood symptoms, they may not be identified as having PCD until they present with fertility issues such as ectopic pregnancy, female subfertility, and male infertility (Bush et al., 2007; Halbert, Patton, Zarutskie, & Soules, 1997). Afzelius and Eliasson (1983) studied fertility among a group of adult males with immotile cilia syndrome and noted that all subjects were infertile. While some had immotile spermatozoa, others had sperms with abnormal appearance, such as coiled sperm tails. In adolescents and adults, addi- tional presenting signs and symptoms include digital clubbing related to chronic pulmonary insufficiency, nasal polyposis, and halitosis from recur- rent sinusitis (Barbato et al., 2009).

Repeated lung infections in undiagnosed cases will cause deterioration of lung function as patients age. In a report by Noone et al. (2004), 47 adults with PCD had a mean forced expiratory volume in 1 second (FEV_1) of 60% predicted compared to 31 children younger than 18 years of age who had a mean FEV_1 of 85%. Additionally, Ellerman and Bisgaard (1997) demonstrated deterioration in lung function over time in a prospective study. In this study, children and adults were followed over a 2- to 16-year time period. The forced vital capacity (FVC) of children ranged from 69 to 117%; for adults, the range was 30–104%. The FEV_1 for children ranged from 53 to 107% compared to 16–99% for adults, suggesting that lung function declines over time with progression of disease (Ellerman and Bisgaard, 1997).

Diagnosis

There are a variety of diagnostic modalities for ciliary dyskinesia; however, electron microscopy remains the gold standard for detecting ultrastructural defects in the cilia (Dell, 2008). Other available diagnostic tests include ciliary beat frequency measurement, ciliary beat pattern analysis, measurement of ciliary disorientation under electron microscopy, and cell culture with regrowth of ciliated epithelium in difficult cases (Bush et al., 2007).

Genetic testing

Genetic testing for the specific mutations of DNAH5 and DNAI1 is also available. However, genetic testing alone is of limited clinical use because testing cannot identify the majority of PCD cases. Mutations in DNAI1, the first gene identified in which mutations were responsible for PCD (Morillas, Zariwala, & Knowles, 2007), accounts for less than 25% of PCD cases (Dell, 2008). More recently, Barbato et al. (2009) listed mutations in DNAHI1, DNA12, KTU, RSPH9, and RSPH4A as being associated with PCD. Other mutations associated with PCD have also been linked to other genetic diseases. The RPGR mutation is also associated with X-linked recessive retinitis pigmentosa and sensory hearing deficits (Barbato et al., 2009). Furthermore, a syndrome of PCD and mental retardation is associated with mutations in OFD1.

Nitric oxide measurement

Identifying a biomarker that could be measured noninvasively and reproducibly has been sought after for the PCD population. Although the measuring fraction of exhaled nitric oxide (FeNO) was initially examined, it is the measurement of nasal nitric oxide (NO) that has been shown to be particularly helpful in this disorder. Nitric oxide in the airways is the result of the enzymatic conversion of amino acids by NO synthase (Moncada & Higgs, 1993). An isoform of this enzyme is inducible NO synthase (iNOS).

It is found mostly in bronchial epithelium in healthy people as well as in asthmatics (Abba, 2010). Nasal NO is extremely low in subjects with PCD (Karadag, James, Gultekin, Wilson, & Bush, 1999; Lundberg et al., 1994). These low levels of NO are mostly related to reduced activity of bronchial iNOS in patients with PCD (Paraskakis, Zihif, & Bush, 2007; Shoemark & Wilson, 2009). Alveolar NO is lower than bronchial NO in PCD (Paraskakis et al., 2007).

Nasal NO is collected from the upper airway via a catheter that is inserted into a nostril. The nasal air is analyzed via a nitric oxide analyzer that uses ozone-based NO_2 chemiluminescence for direct measurement of nitric oxide (Bush et al., 1998). The preferred method to measure NO in children older than 4–5 years of age is by the single-breath online method (American Thoracic Society & European Respiratory Society, 2005). The duration of exhalation must reach at least 4 seconds. As explained by Leigh, Zariwala, and Knowles (2009), the patient must be able to follow directions and proper technique to close the soft palate to limit nasal NO from the lower airway sample. The use of NO measurement may be a good screening tool, but further study is required for test standardization (Leigh et al., 2009).

Saccharin test

The saccharin test, used historically, involves placing a saccharin tablet on the inferior turbinate; the patient then sits forward and the timing of the taste of the saccharin is recorded. The patient is asked to sit while looking downward without sniffing, sneezing, coughing, eating, or drinking for the hour-long test. If the patient detects the taste of saccharin after 60 minutes an abnormality is detected. A positive saccharin test is usually followed by further diagnostics and workup, including a biopsy to confirm diagnosis. Given the difficulty to perform, this test does not lend itself well to the pediatric population.

Complications

Abnormal cilia, abnormal ciliary motion, and poor mucus clearance result in the collection of mucus in the airway, which becomes infected (Weinberger & Abu-Hasan, 2007). Repeated infection with organisms such as *Haemophilus influenzae* and *Pseudomonas aeruginosa* (Schidlow & Steinfeld, 2005) can lead to pneumonia in the majority of patients (Jain et al., 2007). Recurrent pneumonic infections lead to bronchiectasis (Schidlow & Steinfeld, 2005). Bronchiectasis is a chronic condition characterized by dilated bronchi, which have been thickened, inflamed, and provide an excellent milieu for bacterial colonization or overgrowth (Li et al., 2005). Although bronchiectasis can be expected with delayed diagnosis, it has also been reported in young pediatric patients. In a case report by Brown, Pittman, Leigh,

Forman, and Davis (2008), a 6-month-old with PCD and a 33-month-old with PCD both had evidence of bronchiectasis on chest CT.

Mild hemoptysis or blood-streaked mucus may result from coughing through an inflamed airway (Emmons, 2009). A more worrisome but very rare complication is massive hemoptysis, where blood loss exceeds 600 mL in 1 day; although rare, it may be life threatening. Massive hemoptysis usually occurs when there is irritation and infection of collateral vessels that may develop in long-term disease and usually requires emergency embolization (Barker, 2002).

Cilial dysfunction results in chronic infection of both the lower and upper airways. Recurrent infection leading to irreversible lung damage results in loss of lung function over time (Schidlow & Steinfeld, 2005). Children with PCD may also experience sinusitis, rhinorrhea, and hearing difficulty due to fluid buildup in the ear (Barnes, 2009). The lack of normal cilia function often results in chronic sinusitis, chronic rhinitis, rhinopolypsis, frontal sinus abnormalities, and nasosinus aplasia (Barbato et al., 2009; Bi et al., 2010).

Management

Appropriate and timely screening is of great importance with PCD. Aggressive treatment and early institution of airway clearance will prevent progressive loss of lung function and development of bronchiectasis (Barbato et al., 2009). Early diagnosis may also prevent unnecessary ear, nose, and throat procedures and thoracic surgery (Bush et al., 1998). Timely audiology exams are necessary to treat deafness (Bush et al., 1998).

Many PCD therapies have been extrapolated from the clinical guidelines compiled for the management of CF, another genetic disorder that is also associated with chronic obstructive lung disease, bronchiectasis, and low nasal NO. However, the evidence to support their use in patients with PCD is not available. These guidelines recommend that diagnostics at follow-up should include pulmonary function tests (PFTs) and sputum cultures every 3–6 months and yearly, or biannual lung imaging (Barbato et al., 2009; Ellerman and Bisgaard, 1997; Leigh et al., 2009). Patients with PCD should receive all childhood immunizations and a yearly influenza vaccine (Schidlow & Steinfeld, 2005).

Pharmacological treatment

High doses of antibiotics should be used to treat lung infections. Prophylactic antibiotics may be needed if repeated courses of oral antibiotics have been required and the patient is experiencing respiratory or pulmonary function decline (Bush et al., 2007). If *P. aeruginosa* is isolated on sputum cultures, long-term antipseudomonal nebulized antibiotics to prevent exacerbations should be considered (Barbato et al., 2009; Bush et al., 2007). One such agent, Tobi®, a nebulized tobramycin preparation specifically designed for inhalation is available in 300-mg vials and is dosed twice a day. In CF patients, the drug is administered in cycles of 28 days on medication followed by 28 days off (Emmons, 2009). In some instances, respiratory symptoms and pulmonary function may not improve despite frequent oral or inhaled antibiotics; in these cases, a course of intravenous antibiotic therapy is recommended (Bush et al., 2007).

Airway clearance

Although there is no evidence that chest physiotherapy is beneficial in PCD, it is often recommended to promote airway clearance of mucus. There are several options for airway clearance available (Bush et al., 2007). Physical exercise may help with airway clearance (Barbato et al., 2009). In addition, patients may use blowing games (such as blowing bubbles), active cycle breathing (Bush et al., 2007), high-frequency chest wall oscillation (vest therapy), oscillating positive expiratory pressure (PEP) (Acapella®), and huffing to aid in airway clearance.

For huffing, the patient should inhale deeply and hold for a few seconds, followed by two "huff" coughs. As described by Berman, Snyder, Kozier, and Erb (2008), to use huff coughing, the patient should lean forward and exhale forcefully as if with a huff. This allows airways to stay open while clearing mucus out. To prevent mucus from moving back down into the smaller airways, one should follow with short rapid inhalations or "sniffing" (Berman et al., 2008).

A PEP mask or mouthpiece or an oscillating PEP device such as the Acapella (Bush et al., 2007; Volsko, DiFiore & Chatburn, 2003) can be used by itself or in conjunction with nebulized medications to optimize medication delivery to the lower airways. With either device, the goal is to generate 10–25 cm of H_2O of end expiratory pressure, which will stimulate mucus to move out of small airways (Pruitt & Jacobs, 2005). PEP allows for a prolonged expiration period to help open distal airways, thereby increasing available air to cough more effectively and move secretions (Pruitt & Jacobs, 2005).

High-frequency chest wall oscillation therapy is also believed to be beneficial in the treatment of PCD. It is delivered via a nonstretchable vest sized to fit the individual patient's chest. It speeds the clearance of mucus from the peripheral and central airways (Braverman & Stewart, 2007) by delivering oscillating pressures to stimulate the cilia activity (Pruitt & Jacobs, 2005). With rigorous airway clearance, the airways are exposed to irritants for shorter periods of time, thus decreasing inflammation, infections, and bacterial colonization (Braverman & Stewart, 2007).

Although mucolytic agents such as Pulmozyme® (rhDNAase), Mucomyst® (acetylcysteine), and hypertonic saline can be used along with airway clearance techniques, there is little to no evidence to support their efficacy in this patient population. There is a report of hypertonic saline and rhDNAse resulting in symptom relief in PCD patients (Desai, Weller,

& Spencer, 1995; Ten Berge, Brinkhorst, Kroon, & Jongste, 1999). Saline or hypertonic saline in nebulized form has been reported to increase mucus clearance in PCD patients (Barbato et al., 2009; Bush et al., 2007). Hyperosmolar saline is believed to help clear mucus by increasing the movement of water across the lung surface (Amirav, Cohen-Cymberknoh, Shoseyov, & Kerem, 2009) and has been used with an Acapella or a vest to augment airway clearance. Although it has been used in CF patients for decades, Mucomyst (acetylcysteine) was not found to be useful for the treatment of PCD (Stafanger, Garne, Howitz, Morkassel & Koch, 1988). This finding suggests that assuming therapies used in CF should work in PCD may not be a clinically sound approach to therapy.

Imaging

Signs of chronic lung infections on chest radiographs include atelectasis, infiltrates, and hyperinflation (Schidlow & Steinfeld, 2005), all of which can be observed in patients with PCD, as well as bronchiectasis. Other radiographic findings include focal pneumonitis or irregular opacities (Barker, 2002).

In a recent study by Jain et al. (2007), the radiographs of 55 pediatric PCD patients among a cohort of 89 PCD patients were reviewed for abnormalities. Thirty-one patients had dextrocardia; 27 were remarkable for hyperinflation; 54 had bronchial wall thickening and dilatation; 29 had mottled shadows; and 3 had consolidation or collapse, suggesting that there is a wide variety of potential radiographic findings. Additionally, the presence of nodular-cystic lesions or peribronchial thickening on chest X-rays suggests more advanced lung disease and raises suspicion of bronchiectasis, which should be confirmed with HRCT of the chest (Schidlow & Steinfeld, 2005).

Bronchoscopy

Patients may undergo bronchoscopy for direct visualization of the airways to obtain bacterial or fungal cultures and to mechanically clear airways. Bronchoscopy may also document reversed lung anatomy in patients with situs inversus (Sharma, 2008).

Surgical treatment

Persistent sinusitis may require endoscopic sinus surgery or removal of nasal polyps (Sharma, 2008). Nasal sprays and saline rinses may be effective treatment for the sinusitis and rhinorrhea prior to surgery (Barnes, 2009).

Lung transplantation may be considered in cases with severe end-stage lung disease where the FEV_1 is <40%. Other surgical interventions may need to be considered such as lobectomy for focal disease where bronchiectasis has caused the lung tissue to lose function and to become unresponsive to conventional medical treatment (Emmons, 2009; Sharma, 2008).

Otolaryngological treatment

Recently, Campbell, Birman, and Morgan (2009) reviewed the literature on the efficacy of myringotomy tube placement in children with PCD who were experiencing otitis media with effusion. In their review, hearing loss and otitis media with effusion appear to occur in all children with PCD. Moreover, prolonged otorrhea after myringotomy tube placement occurred in 33% of patients with PCD compared to 10–50% occurrence rate in the general population. Lastly, they demonstrated that the largest improvement in hearing after myringotomy tubes were placed occurred in children who had the most significant hearing loss and who had normal hearing on follow-up at 1.5 years.

As otorlaryngolical complications are very common, regular audiology testing and specialty management is necessary. Children with hearing loss may benefit from hearing aids; in some cases, hearing impairment may improve with age (Barnes, 2009).

Nursing care of the child and family

It is important to have a strong relationship with the child with PCD and the family. As with any chronic condition, frequent follow-up is important for improved outcomes in those with PCD.

The nurse's role is multifaceted and includes patient and parent education, patient advocacy, and assessment of adherence issues with daily therapy. In a study by Pifferi et al. (2010), 71.8% of patients found that their quality of life improved after diagnosis. This suggests that making the proper diagnosis, education, and advocacy can have a positive effect on the patient's life. However, the burden of daily treatment regimens can be heavy in children with PCD due to multiple medications and required airway clearance. Assessment and reinforcement of adherence with therapy are the cornerstones of improved quality of life and improved outcomes. With time, patients are less likely to perform daily airway clearance therapy (Pifferi et al., 2010); therefore, strategies to improve knowledge and to elucidate the connection between adherence and improved quality of life need to be emphasized.

As the child grows, he or she needs to become responsible for his or her own health care. Nurses can aid in the transition to adult care. The nurse may also be the one to discuss the need for contraception if the patient does not feel he or she can discuss the topic with his or her long-time health-care provider and parents. Although subfertility is common in females and infertility is common in males, a patient may still be at risk for an unplanned pregnancy and sexually transmitted diseases if birth control is not used (Barnes, 2009).

It is also important to assess the home environment of the child with PCD and to identify a responsible adult to participate in the care of that child. Health-care providers need to know if the child and parent understand the proper method for administering medications and for performing airway clearance. As the child grows, it is important for the family to maintain a healthy home environment. Children with PCD and their families should understand that refraining from and avoiding smoking, exposure to common aeroallergens, and other irritants is helpful (Sharma, 2008).

Children with PCD and their families need to be informed and updated on the name, use, and indications of prescribed medications. Some medications may not be stocked regularly in community pharmacies. Therefore, families need to learn how and where to refill them. The use of airway clearance modalities also need to be reviewed with parents and children. The nurse should also provide children and families with anticipatory guidance to assist them in troubleshooting problems that arise in the daily use of their therapies.

Providing families with adequate support outside the clinical setting is an important role for the nurse. Families must be informed and provided with information for when and how to contact their pulmonary provider for signs of respiratory complications such as increased cough, increased sputum production, changes in color of sputum, or wheezing. In addition, providing professional and accurate sources of information is extremely valuable to patients and families. Helpful Web sites include http://www.pcdfoundation.org and, in the United Kingdom, http://www.pcdsupport.org.uk. Relevant medical information is shared on the sites. Families may find others' experiences with PCD invaluable in helping them navigate and advocate for their child.

Many challenging issues will undoubtedly arise during patient care. PCD is dynamic and requires patient- and family-centered nursing care that addresses issues in a broad and flexible manner.

BRONCHIECTASIS

Epidemiology

The prevalence of bronchiectasis in the United States and in the world is unknown (Barker, 2002; Emmons, 2009). However, between 2001 and 2002, the incidence of non-CF-related bronchiectasis in New Zealand was estimated at 37 per million among children less than 15 years of age (Twiss, Metcalfe, Edwards & Byrnes, 2005). Common childhood illnesses such as pertussis, measles, and tuberculosis place children at risk for developing bronchiectasis (Callahan, 2005). Decreased rates of bronchiectasis in the United States have been attributed to vaccinations for pertussis (Barker, 2002).

Pathophysiology

The lungs are susceptible to infection due to their constant contact with pathogens in the environment (Callahan, 2005) but are usually spared from long-term damage and consequences of this exposure because of robust mucociliary clearance mechanisms and immune responses. However, the airways can fall victim to bacterial and viral infection as well as aspiration events (Callahan, 2005), especially if there is an abnormality in the mucociliary escalator or in host defense. Such exposure and events set the stage for bronchiectasis, which results from repeated infection, inflammation, and destruction of lung tissue (Callahan, 2005). Repeated infections trigger a cycle of inflammation and obstruction causing the muscle layers of the airways to become damaged, leading to destruction of supportive cartilage producing a saccular or dilated airway (Brown & Lemen, 1990).

There are a number of clinical entities that have been associated with bronchectasis including (1) CF (Callahan, 2005); (2) immunodeficiency states including IgG and IgA deficiency, hypogammaglobulinemia, common variable immunodeficiency, and complement pathway defects (Brown & Lemen, 1990); (3) congenital lung malformations, such as congenital lobar emphysema, airway malacia, Williams–Campbell syndrome, and tracheomegaly (Stafler & Carr, 2010); (4) aspiration syndromes, such as recurrent aspiration from abnormal swallow in patients with neurological impairment, foreign body aspiration, and untreated gastroesophageal reflux (Eastham et al., 2004; Stafler & Carr, 2010); and (5) congenital abnormalities, such as tracheoesophageal fistula, or laryngeal cleft (Eastham et al., 2004; Stafler & Carr, 2010).

Signs and symptoms

Children may present with symptoms of a chronic productive cough, shortness of breath, or chest pain (Callahan, 2005; Brown & Lemen, 1990). Occasional presenting symptoms are dyspnea and hemoptysis (Brown & Lemen, 1990). Signs of bronchiectasis may include persistent crackles, wheeze, and digital clubbing (Brown & Lemen, 1990; Callahan, 2005).

Diagnosis

Chest radiographs may show bronchial dilation, volume loss, or bronchial wall thickening (Callahan, 2005). Parallel linear densities associated with bronchiectasis are referred to as the "tram track" sign (Callahan, 2005). After chest X-rays are obtained, a high-resolution chest CT scan (HRCT) should be obtained to confirm diagnosis. On an HRCT, the classical sign of bronchiectasis is the "signet ring," which refers to the bronchial/ pulmonary artery ratio greater than 1, suggesting a dilated airway. Depending on the underlying cause, more diagnostic tests are often needed. For example, if reflux is suspected, a barium swallow may be necessary.

Bronchoscopy may be used to rule out a retained foreign body, broncho-malacia, or other abnormal airway anatomy, to obtain sputum cultures, or to detect fat-laden macrophages associated with aspiration (Stafler & Carr, 2010). Other laboratory tests that might be required include a sweat test to rule out CF, a ciliary biopsy to rule out PCD, and total serum immuno-globulin levels, antibody responses to tetanus, pneumococcal or *H. influenzae* vaccinations, or C3 and C4 complement levels to rule out immunodeficiency, which may predispose patients to recurrent infection and bronchiectasis (Stafler & Carr, 2010).

Complications

Repeated infections in the bronchiectatic areas of the lung are common and may become a focus of recurrent lung infection. Progressive lung damage can lead to chronic respiratory insufficiency, hypercapnia, and pulmonary vascular disease (Chang & Redding, 2006) if bronchiectasis is not treated. Subsequently, it can lead to end-stage pulmonary failure in adults (Stafler & Carr, 2010). The severity and the progression of the disease process have changed with the use of newer and inhaled antibiotics (Chang & Redding, 2006).

Management

The treatment of bronchiectasis depends on the underlying cause. If the cause of the bronchiectasis is due to a noninfectious chronic condition such as CF or PCD, treatment is directed at the underlying problem. A sputum culture should be obtained to guide the decision for appropriate antibiotic therapy (Callahan, 2005). If the patient presents with acute symptoms such as fever, cough, increased sputum production, and a decline in PFTs, the treatment will include aggressive airway clearance and oral or intravenous antibiotics depending on the clinical scenario (Callahan, 2005). Immunoglobulin replacement therapy, along with aggressive antibiotic therapy, may be used for children with immunodeficiency problems (Stafler & Carr, 2010).

Nursing care of the child and family

Nursing care of the child with bronchiectasis includes encouraging adherence to therapies such as antibiotics and airway clearance. Children with bronchiectasis and their families need to be informed and updated on the name, use, and indications of the medications prescribed. For children who use airway clearance regularly, a review of airway clearance techniques should be performed on a regular interval. A portion of this review may be provided directly from a manufacturer but should always be reviewed by the care team. Families should receive anticipatory guidance to help them troubleshoot problems that arise in the daily use of these therapies. Supportive care may include the administration of intravenous antibiotics.

Providing families with adequate support outside the clinical setting is an important role for the nurse. Families must be informed and provided with information for when and how to contact their pulmonary provider for signs of respiratory complications such as increased cough, increased sputum production, changes in the color of sputum, or wheezing. This ensures the institution of early interventions that will help protect the airways from damage over time.

REFERENCES

Abba, A. A. (2010). Exhaled nitric oxide in diagnosis and management of respiratory diseases. *Annals of Thoracic Medicine, 4,* 173–181.

Afzelius, B. A. (1999). Asymmetry of cilia and of mice and men. *International Journal of Developmental Biology, 43,* 283–286.

Afzelius, B. A., & Eliasson, R. (1983). Male and female infertility problems in the immotile-cilia syndrome. *European Journal of Respiratory Diseases, 64,* 144–147.

American Thoracic Society, & European Respiratory Society (2005). Recommendations for the standardized procedures for the online and offline measurement of exhaled lower respiratory nitric oxide and nasal nitric oxide. *American Journal of Respiratory and Critical Care Medicine, 171,* 912–930.

Amirav, I, Cohen-Cymberknoh, M, Shoseyov, D, & Kerem, E (2009). Primary ciliary dyskinesia: Prospects for new therapies, building on the experience in cystic fibrosis. *Pediatric Respiratory Reviews, 10,* 58–62.

Barbato, A., Frisher, T., Kuehni, C., Snijders, I., Azevedo, G., Baktai, L., et al. (2009). Primary ciliary dyskinesia: A consensus statement on diagnostic and treatment approaches in children. *European Respiratory Journal, 34,* 1264–1276.

Barker, A. (2002). Bronchiectasis. *New England Journal of Medicine, 18,* 1383–1393.

Barnes, C. (2009). Diagnosis and management of primary ciliary dyskinesia. *Paediatric Nursing, 21,* 24–27.

Berman, A., Snyder, S., Kozier, B., & Erb, G. (2008). *Kozier & Erb's fundamental of nursing* (8th ed.). Upper Saddle River, NJ: Pearson Prentice Hall.

Bi, J., Bai, C., & Qiao, R. (2010). A 27-year-old Chinese man with recurrent respiratory infections. *Chest, 137,* 990–993.

Braverman, J., & Stewart, B. (2007). The primary ciliary disorders: Underdiagnosed and undertreated. *Respiratory Therapy, 2,* 16–20.

Brown, M. A., & Lemen, R. J. (1990). Bronchiectasis. In V. Chernick & E. L. Kendig (Eds.), *Kendig's disorders of the respiratory tract in children* (pp. 416–429). Philadelphia: W.B Saunders.

Brown, D. E., Pittman, J. E., Leigh, M. W., Forman, L., & Davis, S. D. (2008). Early lung disease in young children with primary ciliary dyskinesia. *Pediatric Pulmonology, 43,* 514–516.

Bush, A., Chodhari, R., Collins, N., Copeland, F., Hall, P., Harcourt, J., et al. (2007). Primary ciliary dyskinesia: Current state of the art. *Archives of Disease in Children*, 92, 1136–1140.

Bush, A., Cole, P., Hariri, M., Mackay, G., Phillips, C., O'Callaghan, C., et al. (1998). Primary ciliary dyskinesia: Diagnosis and standards of care. *European Respiratory Journal*, 12, 982–988.

Callahan, C. (2005). Pneumona and bacterial pulmonary infections. In H. B. Panitch (Ed.), *Pediatric pulmonology the requisites in pediatrics* (pp. 151–171). Philadelphia: Elsevier Mosby.

Campbell, R. G., Birman, C. S., & Morgan, L. (2009). Management of otitis media with effusion in children with primary ciliary dyskinesia: A literature review. *International Journal of Pediatric Otorhinolaryngology*, 73, 1630–1638.

Chang, A. B., & Redding, G. J. (2006). Bronchiectasis. In V. Chernick, T. F. Boat, R. W. Wilmott, & A. Bush (Eds.), *Kendig's disorders of the respiratory tract in children* (pp. 463–477). Philadelphia: W.B Saunders.

Coren, M., Meeks, M., Morrison, I., Buchdahl, R., & Bush, A. (2002). Primary ciliary dyskinesia: Age at diagnosis and symptom history. *Acta Paediatrica*, 91, 667–669.

Dell, S. (2008). Primary ciliary dyskinesia: Myths and realities. *Paediatric Child Health*, 13, 668–670.

Desai, M., Weller, P. H., & Spencer, D. A. (1995). Clinical benefit from nebulized human recombinant DNase in Kartagener's syndrome. *Pediatric Pulmonology*, 20, 307–308.

Eastham, K. M., Fall, A. J., Mitchell, L., & Spencer, D. A. (2004). The need to redefine non-cystic fibrosis bronchiectasis in childhood. *Thorax*, 59, 324–327.

Ellerman, A., & Bisgaard, H. (1997). Longitudinal study of lung function in a cohort of primary ciliary dyskinesia. *European Respiratory Journal*, 10, 2376–2379.

Emmons, E. (2009). Bronchiectasis. Retrieved from http://www.emedicine.medscape.com.

Greenstone, M., Rutman, A., Dewar, A., Mackay, I., & Cole, P. J. (1988). Primary ciliary dyskinesia: Cytological and clinical features. *The Quarterly Journal of Medicine*, 67, 405–423.

Halbert, S., Patton, D., Zarutskie, P., & Soules, M. (1997). Function and structure of cilia in the Fallopin tube of an infertile woman with Kartagener's syndrome. *Human Reproduction*, 12, 55–58.

Jain, K., Padley, S. P. G., Goldstraw, E. J., Kidd, S. J., Hogg, C., Biggart, E., et al. (2007). Primary ciliary dyskinesia in the paediatric population: Range and severity of radiological findings in a cohort of patients receiving tertiary care. *Clinical Radiology*, 62, 986–993.

Karadag, B., James, A. J., Gultekin, E., Wilson, N. M., & Bush, A. (1999). Nasal and lower airway level of nitric oxide in children with primary ciliary dykinesia. *European Respiratory Journal*, 13, 1402–1405.

Leigh, M., Pittman, J., Carson, J., Ferkol, T., Dell, S., Davis, S., et al. (2009). Clinical and genetic aspects of primary ciliary dyskinesia/Kartagener syndrome. *Genetics in Medicine*, 11, 473–487.

Leigh, M. W., Zariwala, M. A., & Knowles, M. R. (2009). Primary ciliary dyskinesia: Improving the diagnostic approach. *Current Opinion in Pediatrics, 21,* 320–325.

Li, A. M., Sonnappa, S., Lex, C., Wong, E., Zacharasiewicz, A., Bush, A., et al. (2005). Non-CF bronchiectasis: Does knowing the aetiology lead to changes in management? *European Respiratory Journal, 26,* 8–14.

Lundberg, J., Weitzberg, E., Nordvall, S., Kuylenstierna, R., Lundberg, J., & Alving, K. (1994). Primarily nasal origin of exhaled nitric oxide and absence in Kargagner's syndrome. *European Respiratory Journal, 7,* 1501–1504.

Moncada, S., & Higgs, A. (1993). The l-arginine-nitric oxide pathway. *New England Journal of Medicine, 329,* 2002–2012.

Morillas, H. N., Zariwala, M., & Knowles, M. (2007). Genetic causes of bronchiectasis: Primary ciliary dyskinesia. *Respiration, 74,* 252–263.

Nonaka, S., Tanaka, Y., Okada, Y., Takeda, S., Harada, A., Kanai, Y., et al. (1998). Randomization of left-right asymmetry due to loss of nodal cilia generating leftward flow of extraembryonic fluid in mice lacking KIF3B motor protein. *Cell, 95,* 829–837.

Noone, P., Leigh, M., Sannuti, A., Minnix, S., Carson, J., Hazucha, M., et al. (2004). Primary ciliary dyskinesia diagnostic and phenotypic features. *American Journal of Respiratory and Critical Care Medicine, 169,* 459–467.

O'Callaghan, C., Chetcuti, P., & Moya, E. (2010). High prevalence of primary ciliary dyskinesia in a British Asian population. *Archives of Disease in Children, 95,* 51–52.

Paraskakis, E., Zihif, N., & Bush, A. (2007). Nitric Oxide production in PCD: Possible evidence for differential nitric oxide synthase function. *Pediatric Pulmonology, 42,* 876–880.

Pifferi, M., Bush, A., Di Cicco, M., Pradal, U., Ragazzo, V., Macchia, P., et al. (2010). Health-related quality of life and unmet needs in patients with primary ciliary dyskinesia. *European Respiratoy Journal, 35,* 787–794.

Pruitt, B., & Jacobs, M. (2005). Clearing away pulmonary secretions. *Nursing, 35,* 37–41.

Schidlow, D. V., & Steinfeld, J. (2005). Primary ciliary dyskinesia (immotile cilia syndrome-Kartagener syndrome). In H. B. Panitch (Ed.), *Pediatric pulmonology the requisites in pediatrics* (pp. 131–139). Philadelphia: Elsevier Mosby.

Sharma, D. (2008). Primary ciliary dyskinesia. Retrieved from http://www.emedicine.medscape.com.

Shoemark, A., & Wilson, R. (2009). Bronchial and peripheral airway nitric oxide in primary ciliary dyskinesia and bronchiectasis. *Respiratory Medicine, 103,* 700–706.

Stafanger, G., Garne, S., Howitz, P., Morkassel, G., & Koch, C. (1988). The clinical effect and the effect on the ciliary motility of oral N-acetylcysteine in patients with cystic fibrosis and primary ciliary dyskinesia. *European Respiratory Journal, 1,* 161–167.

Stafler, P., & Carr, S. B. (2010). Non-cystic fibrosis bronchiectasis: Its diagnosis and management. *Archives of diseases in childhood education and practice edition, 95,* 73–82.

Ten Berge, M., Brinkhorst, G., Kroon, A. A., & de Jongste, J. C. (1999). DNase treatment in primary ciliary dyskinesia—Assessment by nocturnal pulse oximetry. *Pediatric Pulmonology, 27,* 59–61.

Thai, C., Gambling, T., & Carson, J. (2002). Freeze fracture study of airway epithelium from patients with primary ciliary dyskinesia. *Thorax, 57,* 363–365.

Twiss, J., Metcalfe, R., Edwards, E., & Byrnes, C. (2005). New Zealand national incidence of bronchiectasis "too high" for a developed country. *Archives of Disease in Childhood, 90,* 737–740.

Volsko, T., DiFiore, J., & Chatburn, R. (2003). Performance comparison of two oscillating positve expiratory pressure devices: Acpell verus Flutter. *Repiratory Care, 48,* 124–130.

Weinberger, M., & Abu-Hasan, M. (2007). Pseudo-asthma: When cough, wheezing, and dyspnea are not asthma. *Pediatrics, 120,* 855–864.

11

Acute respiratory problems

Marcia Winston, MSN, CPNP, AE-C, and Catherine Kier, MD

INTRODUCTION

Acute respiratory conditions can result in poor outcomes for the child if they are not quickly diagnosed and treated. This chapter provides information regarding the diagnosis and management of foreign body aspiration (FBA), pneumothorax, and respiratory failure.

FBA

FBA of the airway could be life threatening with obvious clinical symptoms such as choking and sudden respiratory distress. However, unwitnessed FBA may present with subtle symptoms. Therefore, any suspicion of FBA warrants a careful clinical evaluation to avoid long-term complications.

Epidemiology

FBA is common in the younger age group. Children younger than 3 years of age account for approximately 80% of cases (Holinger, 2007). Round hard objects are the most common choking hazard for children. Approximately 17,537 children aged 14 years old and younger were seen in the emergency departments for choking-related episodes in 2001; many episodes were associated with candy/gum (19.0%) and coins (12.7%).

Nursing Care in Pediatric Respiratory Disease, First Edition. Edited by Concettina (Tina) Tolomeo.
© 2012 John Wiley & Sons, Inc. Published 2012 by John Wiley & Sons, Inc.

There is no readily available data about FBA in adolescents. However, as piercings in adolescents are popular, including those of the tongue, nose, and lip, they should be considered as potential sources of aspiration. Intoxication and use of sedatives are also risk factors.

National mortality data in 2000 reported 160 children aged 14 years old and younger died from obstruction of the respiratory tract associated with inhaled or ingested foreign bodies (FBs) (Gotsch, Annest, & Holmgreen, 2002). Food and nonfood substances were associated with 41 and 59% of these deaths, respectively. Death caused by suffocation following FBA is the fifth most common cause of mortality due to unintentional injury in the United States and is the leading cause of mortality due to unintentional injury in children younger than 1 year (National Center for Injury Prevention and Control, 2010).

Pathophysiology

FBA is common in children younger than 3 years, with the peak incidence between 1 and 2 years of age. Most children at this age are able to stand and like to explore their environment via the oral route. They have the fine motor skills to put a small object into their mouths, but they do not have molars to chew food adequately (Chernick, Boat, Wilmott, & Bush, 2006), placing them at risk for FBA. Access to foods and small objects not appropriate for their age and older siblings (who may give them food or small objects) are additional risk factors. In older children, loss of consciousness, alcohol intoxication, and neurological disorders predispose to FBA.

Laryngeal (3%) and tracheal FBs (13%) are less common. The most common location of aspirated FBs in children is in the bronchi (Black, Johnson, & Matlak, 1994; Eren, Balci, Dikici, Doblan, & Eren, 2003; Tan et al., 2000). Since the right mainstem bronchus forms a less acute angle with the trachea compared to the left mainstem bronchus, most aspirated FBs are lodged in the right lung (59%) as follows: right mainstem bronchi (52%), right lower lobe bronchus (6%), and right middle lobe bronchus (<1%). FBs may become lodged in the left lung (23%) as follows: left mainstem bronchus (18%) and left lower bronchus (5%). Bilateral FBA has occurred in about 2% of cases (Eren, Balci, Dikici, Doblan, & Eren, 2003).

Large, bulky FBs (such as food) and FBs with irregular edges usually become lodged in the laryngotracheal area. This is particularly common in ages less than 1 year. Their weak respiratory effort and narrow trachea caliber place them at risk for laryngotracheal FBA. Laryngotracheal FBs are associated with increased morbidity and mortality because of the increased chance of suffocation (Lima, 1989).

Signs and symptoms

The clinical presentation of FBA is dependent on a number of associated factors such as (1) whether the event was witnessed, (2) time of suspicion or diagnosis since the event, (3) age of the child, (4) type of object aspirated, and (5) location of the object.

History

Medical history is important for the diagnosis of FBA. In a recent review of approximately 100 cases, main symptoms in children with FBA were choking (77%), prolonged cough (15%), dyspnea (4%), and nonresolving pneumonia (2%) (Even et al., 2005). Although most cases of FBA are diagnosed within 24 hours of presentation (about 50–75% of cases), diagnosis may be delayed (20% of cases in one series) greater than 4 weeks after aspiration (Blazer, Naveh, & Friedman, 1980).

Children who aspirate an FB may present with obvious clinical symptoms such as severe respiratory distress, cyanosis, inability to communicate, altered mental status, and even loss of consciousness. Such presentations are medical emergencies and require the institution of immediate life support, including attempts to dislodge the FB, establishment of an airway, and immediate transfer to a medical facility for bronchoscopic removal of the FB.

More commonly, the clinical presentation is less emergent. A choking episode, if witnessed, is usually characterized by a sudden onset of cough and may be accompanied by difficulty breathing and, at times, cyanosis. Choking is a sign of mechanical obstruction of the airway and prevents breathing. The associated cough is the body's protective reflex in an attempt to clear the airway. Choking is usually self-limited. The aspirated FB may be cleared and coughed up to the upper airway, out through the mouth, or eventually swallowed. However, there are instances when the FB stays lodged in the airway, and it is important to continue to monitor for symptoms.

Persistent coughing and wheezing in a previously healthy child should warrant further investigation for FBA. Delay in diagnosis is common with lower airway involvement because nonspecific respiratory symptoms are dismissed as new onset asthma. Subtle symptoms of chronic cough and intermittent fevers are attributed to recurrent upper respiratory viral infections, especially if the episode occurred during the winter months.

The aspiration event may not have been witnessed or may not be readily recalled by the parent. In such cases, it is important to elicit the history carefully and to guide the parent in recalling the events prior to the presentation of the persistent cough and/or wheeze. There should be a high suspicion of FBA especially if the child had no prior respiratory symptoms before the event.

Physical examination

The physical examination may be normal, but this should not stop the health-care provider from further evaluating for FBA especially if there is high suspicion based on history. Findings in physical examination that are suspicious for FBA include coughing and wheezing. Wheezing may be generalized or focal.

Homophonous or monophonic wheezing, a constant audible sound throughout the lung (though this may vary in loudness depending on the distance from the site of obstruction), is more characteristic of FBA, as opposed to heterogeneous or polyphonic wheezing, wherein the degree of narrowing varies from place to place within the lung. Homophonous wheezing is associated with central airway involvement, whereas hetero-phonous wheezing is associated with small airway obstruction, often heard in acute inflammatory conditions such as asthma exacerbation or bronchi-olitis. The clinician should perform a careful, thorough physical exam focusing on the characteristic and regional variation of the breath sounds, preferably when the child is quiet, with minimal ambient noise.

Location of the object

FBA signs and symptoms vary according to the location of the FB. Sudden significant acute respiratory distress with increased respiratory effort, upper airway sounds of stridor, and hoarseness usually signify laryngo-tracheal FBA. Complete airway obstruction is possible and is a true medical emergency, requiring immediate intervention.

In contrast, children with lower airway FBA have symptoms that include cough, wheeze, decreased breath sounds, and fever. A history of choking and respiratory distress may precede the above-mentioned symptoms.

Type of object aspirated

Large round objects tend to get lodged in the upper airway. Smaller objects usually end up aspirated in the lower airway.

The risks of complications with FBA depend on the size, shape, or make of the FB. Pointed or sharp-edged objects such as pins or tacks may pen-etrate the airway mucosa, causing intense inflammation or bleeding. Larger, sharp objects may even penetrate through the airway into the esophagus posteriorly. Objects with corrosive chemicals such as watch batteries are caustic to the mucosa and cause burns and eventual scarring. Food material such as salted peanut can cause irritation and pneumonitis in the lower airway mucosa. Vegetable and organic materials could be a nidus for infection and pneumonia.

Diagnosis

Medical history is very helpful in the diagnosis of FBA. Physical exam may be helpful if there are positive findings, but a negative physical exam does not rule out the diagnosis.

Radiopaque objects are visible on chest X-ray (see Figure 11.1). Unfortunately, most aspirated objects are radiolucent. If the aspirated object is not visible, there are some clues to indicate the presence of airway obstruction. When the airway is obstructed at the laryngotracheal level, a

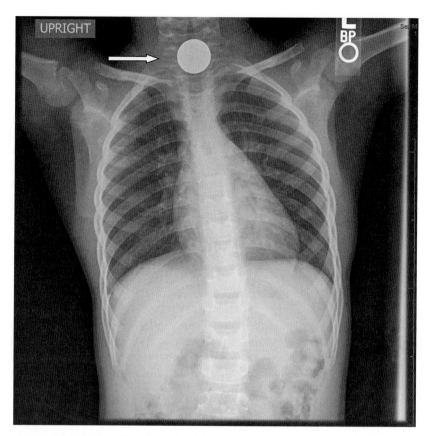

Figure 11.1   Chest X-ray film of a child (PA view) showing a coin—a radiopaque object. The child appeared in no respiratory distress. The coin was swallowed. Courtesy of Dr. Jeffrey Hellinger.

properly performed lateral neck film, or a posteroanterior chest X-ray, will reveal evidence of subglottic involvement. Normally, the airway is seen as an outline of air column (black) with its surrounding soft tissue structures like the epiglottis and the adenoids (lighter density). On careful review of a lateral neck film or a posteroanterior chest X-ray film, a subtle density in the air column may represent an aspirated object, or a narrowed area of the air column may represent airway obstruction at that level with associated swelling of the surrounding structures.

When the level of airway obstruction is at the lower airway, chest X-ray findings may include hyperinflation, atelectasis, pneumonia, and mediastinal shift. Hyperinflation occurs when there is a "ball-valve" mechanism secondary to partial airway obstruction, allowing air to flow in during inspiration but not out during expiration, resulting in air trapping. Hyperinflation of the unaffected airway may also occur in some instances because of preferential ventilation of the unobstructed airway (least resistance of airflow). Atelectasis eventually develops as a result of complete obstruction of the affected airway. Mediastinal shift may be prominent or may be subtle. Pneumonia may eventually develop, with the FB as a nidus of infection. This usually manifests as a persistent infiltrate. Lung abscess or bronchiectasis could be a late finding for an undiagnosed and retained FB.

Additional radiographic procedures may be helpful if the standard chest X-ray does not reveal abnormal findings. For older cooperative children, an expiratory chest X-ray may reveal hyperinflation of the affected area because of air trapping distal to the FB. In addition, mediastinal shift away from the affected side (where the FB is) may manifest in an expiratory film. For younger children and infants, a lateral decubitus film could be obtained. Normally, the side that is down (the side the child or infant is lying) will be of smaller volume because of the effect of gravity. Persistent hyperinflation of the side that is down suggests the presence of an FB on that side. It is important to remember that the absence of any of these findings on chest X-ray does not rule out the diagnosis of FBA.

Computed tomography (CT) scan or magnetic resonance imaging (MRI) of the chest is used only when the chest X-ray is nonconclusive but the presentation is very suspicious for FBA. These procedures tend to take longer to perform compared to the chest radiographs, may require sedation, and expose the patient to an increased amount of radiation.

Complications

The most serious complication of FBA is complete airway obstruction, which may lead to death. This is almost always at the laryngeal level. Death tends to occur in infants and younger children because of their small airway size. Delayed removal of the FB may also lead to severe hypoxia and neurological injury.

Retained FB, when it remains undiagnosed, may lead to infection, such as persistent pneumonia. Unresolved pneumonia with persistent infiltrate on chest X-ray series warrants visualization of the airway to rule out FBA. Late manifestations may include lung abscesses and bronchiectasis, leading to chronic lung disease.

Management

Complete airway obstruction with life-threatening symptoms (i.e., severe respiratory distress, no cough, inability to communicate, cyanosis, altered mental status) is a medical emergency. Dislodgement of the FB to relieve the airway obstruction should be attempted immediately. Knowledge of basic life support maneuvers is very important. Heimlich maneuver for older children, back blows, and chest compressions for infants and younger children are recommended. Children who can cough and speak should be allowed to relieve the obstruction themselves because Heimlich or back blows may convert a partial to a complete airway obstruction.

Establishment of an airway is of primary importance. If the obstruction is deemed to be at the laryngeal level, cricothyrotomy may be performed to bypass the obstruction. For lower obstruction, intubate the trachea, force the FB down into one of the mainstem bronchi, and ventilate the patient through the unobstructed lung while awaiting endoscopic removal of the FB.

FB removal in children is performed using rigid bronchoscopy under general anesthesia (Ciftci, Bingol-Kologlu, Senocak, Tanyel, & Buyukpakcu 2003). Rigid bronchoscopy provides the ability to ventilate the patient during the procedure, a wider angle visualization of the airway, and the ability to pass instruments such as forceps for extraction of the FB.

Flexible bronchoscopy may be initially performed to scout for possible FB. It is a relatively safe procedure that can be performed under conscious sedation. When an FB is visualized, a rigid bronchoscopy is then performed.

Nursing care of the child and family

FBA is completely preventable. Education is the key to its prevention. It is the responsibility of nurses to provide education to parents about the risk factors for FBA. The risk of aspiration should be discussed in the context of a growing and developing child that is exploring the world. Caregivers should be educated about the following:

- Safe and developmentally appropriate foods (in young children, encourage the avoidance of foods in shapes, sizes, and textures that the children are not ready to handle, such as hotdogs, grapes, popcorn, nuts, candy, and gum).
- Developmentally appropriate toys (emphasize the dangers associated with batteries and magnets).
- Childproofing their home (remind parents about risks associated with small, attractive parts when decorating for holidays or outside).

All parents should also be educated on early detection and initial management of FBA.

PNEUMOTHORAX

Pneumothorax is the accumulation of air in the pleural space. Air enters into the pleural space either from the alveoli or from the atmosphere. Pneumothorax can be traumatic or spontaneous when it occurs in the absence of trauma. The spontaneous form will be discussed in this chapter.

Spontaneous pneumothorax can be primary (i.e., with no underlying lung pathology) or secondary (i.e., when there is identified lung pathology). Risk factors for the development of pneumothorax include asthma, cystic fibrosis, chronic lung disease, certain congenital anomalies, and presence of apical blebs. Pneumothorax is more common in tall, thin individuals. The upper lobes of the lungs are normally more expanded compared with the dependent lower regions due to the more negative transalveolar pressures in the apices. The difference in transpulmonary pressures is exaggerated in thin, tall individuals, which predisposes them to the formation of apical blebs and, eventually, pneumothorax.

Pneumothorax could be life threatening but can result in a good prognosis with careful and immediate attention. Recurrence is common in patients diagnosed with pneumothorax particularly if the pneumothorax is spontaneous.

Epidemiology

Pneumothorax is less common in the general pediatric population compared to adults (Davis, Wensley, & Phelan, 1993; Poenaru, Yazbeck, & Murphy, 1994; Wilcox, Glick, Karamanoukian, Allen, & Azizkhan, 1995). The reported incidence of pneumothorax in adults is about 5–10 per 100,000 populations/year. The exact incidence of pneumothorax in children in the general population is not reported in the literature. There are few published reports of cohorts of pneumothorax in children, most of which are observed cases over a period of time from large institutions like children's hospitals (Davis, Wensley, & Phelan, 1993; Poenaru, Yazbeck, & Murphy, 1994; Wilcox, Glick, Karamanoukian, Allen, & Azizkhan, 1995). Demographics, clinical course and response to treatment have been described, and differences were compared to pneumothorax in adults. Underlying pathology is more frequently observed in children and recurrence is less common. Pneumothorax is more common in males (Kirby & Ginsberg, 1992; Paape & Fry, 1994; Sahn & Heffner, 2000; Weissberg & Refaely, 2000). Studies in young children also report a male preponderance (Davis 1993; Wilcox, Glick, Karamanoukian, Allen, & Azizkhan, 1995).

The rate of pneumothorax is relatively high in newborns. A report of spontaneous pneumothorax in term newborns was 0.17 per 1,000 live births (Al Tawil et al., 2004). The incidence rate of spontaneous pneumothorax in preterm newborns with birth weights of 500–1,500 g is even higher at 6.3% of 26,007 infants (Horbar et al., 2002). Reasons may include the fact that the majority of preterm neonates develop lung disease, such as respiratory distress syndrome, and are placed on positive pressure ventilation. Chronic lung disease of infancy and bronchopulmonary dysplasia (BPD) are also associated with a higher risk for pneumothorax. Other risk factors for developing pneumothorax during the newborn period and infancy include meconium aspiration syndrome (Wiswell & Henley, 1992; Wiswell, Tuggle, & Turner, 1990), transient tachypnea of the newborn, pulmonary hypoplasia and other congenital anomalies, pneumonia, and infection.

Risk factors associated with spontaneous pneumothorax apart from body habitus are smoking, marijuana smoking, and cocaine inhalation (Feldman, Sullivan, Passero, & Lewis, 1993; Luque, Cavallaro, Torres, Emmanual, & Hillman, 1987). There were familial cases of spontaneous pneumothorax, namely, autosomal dominant and X-linked recessive inheritance described in the literature (Abolnik, Lossos, Zlotogora, & Brauer, 1991; Morrison, Lowry, & Nevin, 1998). A rare genetic disorder, Birt–Hogg–Dubé syndrome, may cause spontaneous pneumothorax in families as a result of lung cyst formation (Menko et al., 2009).

The underlying pulmonary conditions associated with secondary spontaneous pneumothorax found in children and adolescents are cystic fibrosis, asthma, acute respiratory infections especially necrotizing pneumonia and lung abscess, FBA, congenital malformations such as congenital cystic adenomatoid malformation and congenital lobar emphysema, lung diseases including interstitial lung disease, sarcoidosis, and Langerhans cell granulomatosis; and connective tissue disorders including Marfan's syndrome and Ehlers–Danlos syndrome (Robinson, Cooper, & Ranganathan, 2009). Catamenial pneumothorax (occurring in relation to the menstrual cycle) with endometriosis in the chest may be found in adolescent females (Johnson, 2004; Joseph & Sahn, 1996).

Pathophysiology

Air leak through the visceral and/or parietal pleura results in pneumothorax. Significant transalveolar pressures (i.e., the difference between the alveolar pressure and the intrapleural pressure) cause the alveoli to distend and eventually to rupture. These pressure differences typically occur with increases in alveolar pressure such as during positive pressure ventilation or Valsalva maneuver, or with more negative intrapleural pressure such as with severe asthma exacerbation.

Subpleural blebs, when present, are usually found in the apices of the lungs due to the difference in transalveolar pressure between the apices and the bases of the lungs (West, 2007; Jenkinson, 1985). The blebs can rupture directly into the pleural space leading to a pneumothorax. Occasionally, blebs can rupture into other anatomical spaces such as the mediastinum, soft tissues, and peribronchial tissues leading to pneumomediastinum, subcutaneous emphysema, and pulmonary interstitial emphysema, respectively.

Pneumothorax could also occur as a result of direct injury to the visceral pleura. This commonly occurs secondary to an underlying lung disease such as infections (e.g., lung abscess, necrotizing pneumonia, tuberculosis, and exacerbation/infection in cystic fibrosis) or malignancies. Bronchopleural fistula may occur as a result of a persistent connection between the airways and pleural space.

Physiological disturbances depend on the size of the pneumothorax. A small amount of air leak is usually tolerated with minimal symptoms. The air leak is eventually resorbed without any interventions. When the pneumothorax is large, the buildup of pressure in the intrapleural space leads to lung collapse. This is called tension pneumothorax. The significantly increased intrapleural pressure shifts the mediastinum away from the affected side, leading to compromised venous return, decreased ventricular size during diastole, decreased cardiac output, and cardiovascular collapse (Leigh-Smith & Harris, 2005; Montgomery, 2006).

The signs and symptoms of a pneumothorax may be attenuated by preexisting adhesions in the pleural space. Despite its size, lung collapse and the accompanying effects of a tension pneumothorax may not occur when the visceral pleura is tethered to the parietal pleura due to the adhesions.

Signs and symptoms

The signs and symptoms of a pneumothorax may be subtle with nonspecific chest pain or vague symptoms of feeling uncomfortable, or may present with acute respiratory distress with cardiopulmonary compromise. The clinical presentation depends on a number of factors including the size of the pneumothorax (amount of air leak in the pleural space), the degree of lung collapse, the speed of equilibration (rapid vs. slow), the presence of tension within the pleural space (increased intrathoracic pressure), and the patient's underlying condition (including age and severity of illness).

History

Sudden onset of chest pain and dyspnea is the usual complaint of a patient with a large pneumothorax. The pain is described as sharp or stabbing, and can even be preceded by a sensation of "popping" on the affected side. The pain typically is diffuse on the affected side with radiation to the ipsilateral shoulder. A small pneumothorax may present with minimal to no symptoms and may be an incidental finding on a chest imaging for another indication. Patients presenting with spontaneous pneumothorax should always be investigated for potential underlying conditions that may predispose them to develop the pneumothorax.

Physical examination

Physical findings associated with a large pneumothorax may include decreased breath sounds, decreased chest rise during inspiration, and hyperresonance on percussion on the affected side. Respiratory compromise may include tachypnea, increased work of breathing, and cyanosis. Patients should be examined for signs of tension pneumothorax, such as tracheal shift to the opposite side, decreased heart sounds, and apical impulse shifted to the opposite side. Crepitations usually imply the presence of subcutaneous emphysema and can be palpitated on the chest wall and the neck.

Diagnosis

Chest X-ray confirms the diagnosis of pneumothorax. Both anteroposterior and lateral views will be helpful in delineating the pleural air especially for the small pneumothorax. Intrapleural air presents on a chest X-ray with a pleural line that outlines the visceral pleura (see Figure 11.2) together with a hyperlucent area devoid of lung and vascular markings. A large pneumothorax presents with more obvious findings including a hyperlucent area surrounding the collapsed lung on the affected side, flattening of the diaphragm on the affected side, and tracheal and/or mediastinal shift to the opposite side of the pneumothorax. A lateral decubitus film with the affected side up may also be helpful, especially in an infant.

A CT of the chest is not usually needed to diagnose a pneumothorax. However, CT is most helpful in determining the underlying lung pathology (Choudhary, Sellar, Wallis, Cohen, & McHugh, 2005). In newborns, transillumination of the chest in a darkened room may help make the diagnosis of pneumothorax immediately, especially in an emergency. A high-intensity fiber-optic probe is placed against the chest wall of the neonate. Positive transillumination is highly suggestive of a pneumothorax (Kuhns, Bednarek, Wyman, Roloff, & Borer, 1975).

Complications

Tension pneumothorax is a life-threatening medical emergency. The prognosis significantly improves with immediate diagnosis and intervention.

The recurrence of spontaneous pneumothorax is common. In adults, recurrence of spontaneous pneumothorax is about 30% (Kirby & Ginsberg, 1992; Paape & Fry, 1994). Reports in children are limited (Davis, Wensley, & Phelan, 1993; Wilcox, Glick, Karamanoukian, Allen, & Azizkhan, 1995). In a report of 58 children with spontaneous pneumothorax, the risk of recurrence was 50%, with each recurrence increasing the risk of further recurrences (Poenaru, Yazbeck, & Murphy, 1994).

Activities associated with drastic changes in pressure like scuba diving and flying in unpressurized aircrafts should be avoided to decrease recurrence. In addition, patients are advised to avoid contact sports, playing wind musical instruments, or air travel at least 4 weeks after an episode of pneumothorax (Montgomery, 2006).

Management

Management depends on the severity of symptoms, size of the pneumothorax, and the underlying lung problem. Ideally, children with pneumothorax should be observed in the hospital initially.

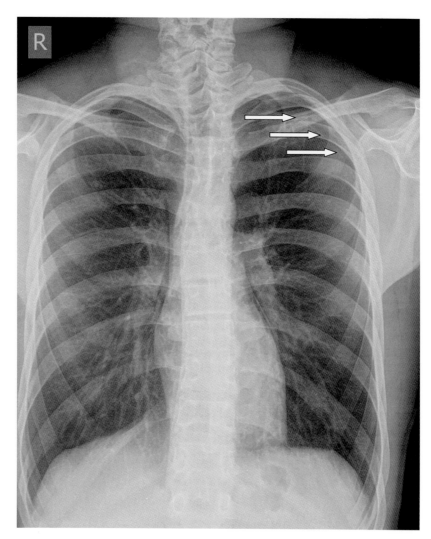

Figure 11.2 Chest X-ray (PA view) showing a small pneumothorax (<25% of the left hemithorax). Note the pleural line (white line) outlining the visceral pleura on the left apex with a small area of hyperlucency with no lung and vascular markings (as compared to the rest of the lung fields). There is also the presence of pneumomediastinum, with note of air (black line) outlining the mediastinal area. Courtesy of Dr. Jeffrey Hellinger.

Conservative management

For a small pneumothorax (i.e., less than 25% of the affected hemithorax) with minimal symptoms, treatment is conservative, mainly with supplemental oxygen and close observation. Treatment of the underlying lung disease, if any is identified, should be addressed.

Supplemental oxygen is usually used to enhance the resorption of the intrapleural air. Unless the patient is inhaling supplemental oxygen when the pneumothorax occurred, air in the intrapleural space is room air with 21% oxygen and 79% nitrogen. Inhalation of 100% oxygen creates a steep gradient for nitrogen absorption from the intrapleural space into the alveolar space. Eventually, the air in the intrapleural space gets converted into 100% oxygen, which is more easily resorbed by the body compared with nitrogen. Oxygen at 100% can only be delivered to a nonventilated patient via a non-rebreather mask. Pain control with analgesics and supportive care should be provided.

Evacuation of the pleural air

For children with a large pneumothorax (i.e., more than 25% of the affected hemithorax) who typically present with more significant symptoms such as dyspnea, hypoxemia, and pain, evacuation of the pleural air is needed. Needle aspiration and chest tube placement are options for evacuation of the pleural air (Camuset et al., 2006). In an emergency, air can be evacuated from the intrapleural space with a large-bore intravenous catheter placed anteriorly in the second intercostal space of the affected site. The catheter can be connected to a large syringe via a three-way stopcock or to a tubing with the opposite end submerged in water. Air can be easily withdrawn with the syringe until resistance is felt. In this case, the pneumothorax has been evacuated. This method provides an estimate of the size of the pneumothorax. If the latter method is used, where the tubing is submerged in water, bubbles should form until the pneumothorax is completely evacuated. The temporary catheter is typically converted into a chest tube (pigtail catheter or thoracostomy tube) until the source of the air leak is identified and addressed or no more air leak is present.

The chest tube uses a one-way Heimlich valve or water seal device to prevent reaccumulation of air. Suction is applied to a water seal device if the lung does not fully expand after the drainage. The chest tube is usually clamped when no bubbles are seen on the water seal from the patent tube after approximately 12 hours. The chest tube is then removed after 24 hours if there is no radiographic or clinical evidence of recurrence of the pneumothorax.

Pleurodesis

Pleurodesis is the injection of sclerosing agents at the time of thoracostomy tube placement to decrease the risk of recurrence. Agents used are talc, tetracycline, and fibrin glue (Cardillo et al., 2006; Chen et al., 2006). Pleural abrasion with dry gauze has also been used (Casadio et al., 2002). In a report of about 200 spontaneous pneumothorax cases, the recurrence rate in the intrapleural tetracycline group (25%) was significantly less than that in the control group (41%)(Light et al., 1990).

Surgical intervention

Surgery is indicated for persistent air leaks and is needed more often in secondary rather than in primary pneumothorax. Surgical approaches include video-assisted thoracoscopic surgery (VATS), minithoracotomy, and conventional thoracotomy (Chan, Clarke, Daniel, Knight, & Seevanayagam, 2001; Hatz et al., 2000; Lang-Lazdunski, Kerangal, Pons, & Jancovici, 2000; Nazari, Buniva, Aluffi, & Salvi, 2000; Yamamoto et al., 2000). Thoracoscopic treatment of spontaneous pneumothorax is safe and effective in children. Recently, VATS has been used often, especially in children, because it provides adequate exposure for resection or stapling (Ozcan, McGahren, & Rodgers, 2003). Surgical intervention includes stapling or oversewing of ruptured blebs or tears, and resection of abnormal lung tissue, if found.

Nursing care of the child and family

Nursing care of the child with a pneumothorax requires a comprehensive understanding of normal respiratory anatomy and physiology in order to understand the process that led to the accumulation of air in the pleural space and the rationale for the treatment in an individual patient. Needle aspiration or chest tube placement may be needed to remove the air, restore negative pressure, and re-expand the lung.

Chest tube insertion requires pain management. Once a chest tube is placed, the nurse should consult with the medical team to confirm that a chest X-ray was performed and should document proper placement of the tube. The nurse must also ensure the tube is secure to prevent displacement. In the event of tube displacement, the site should be covered with a sterile petroleum dressing to prevent ambient air from entering the pleural space and from enlarging the pneumothorax. If displacement occurs, the physician should be contacted immediately. Furthermore, if the tube becomes disconnected, place the end of the tube in a bottle of sterile water until a new unit is established (Verger & Lebet, 2008).

When treating a small pneumothorax with 100% supplemental oxygen, the nurse must ensure that the non-rebreather mask is maintained in place and that it has adequate flow from the oxygen flow meter. Nursing care of the patient with a chest tube includes managing and monitoring the chest tube system function. A chest tube is connected to a drainage system and the specific system used varies according to the institution. Nurses should consult their institution's policy and procedure manual for operational information about the chest tube system.

Wall suction may or may not be ordered. The amount of sterile water in the water seal chamber and negative pressure are dictated by the manufacturer. Constant bubbling in the water seal chamber indicates an air leak. The tubing should be kept in a dependent position free of loops that could impede the evacuation of air. Milking or stripping chest tubes causes large fluctuations in intrapleural pressure and may cause air leak, bleeding from entrapment of pleural tissue in the drainage system, or worsening of the pneumothorax (Halm, 2007).

The integrity of the suture made at the time of tube placement should be assessed. Care must be taken to limit the risk of displacing the tube. The chest tube insertion site should also be evaluated on a regular basis. Assessment includes observing the insertion site for signs of infection such as redness, swelling, warmth, and drainage (color and amount). An occlusive petroleum dressing is applied to the insertion site to prevent air leaks. The frequency of dressing changes depends on institutional policy.

All patients with pneumothorax require continuous cardiopulmonary and pulse oximetry monitoring. The nurse must monitor vital signs and respiratory status including auscultation of breath sounds in all lung fields. Auscultation helps to determine progress or signs of deterioration.

A tension pneumothorax is a medical emergency, and the nurse must communicate signs of a tension pneumothorax to the child's physician immediately. Signs of a tension pneumothorax include tachycardia, hypotension, dyspnea, chest pain, decreased oxygen saturation, and tracheal deviation (a relatively late finding).

Nursing care of patients with a pneumothorax also includes regular encouragement of deep breathing and position changes. Pain management should be ongoing to prevent the child from splinting (especially during coughing or deep breathing), which could prevent optimal lung re-expansion.

As children are recovering from a pneumothorax, education should be provided cautioning patients against certain activities. Children should avoid flying, contact sports, scuba diving, and playing musical wind instruments.

RESPIRATORY FAILURE

Respiratory distress occurs often in children and is one of the most common complaints in an emergency room (Krauss, Harakal, & Fleisher, 1991). Infants and younger children with respiratory problems can deteriorate quickly. Therefore, it is very important to be able to recognize early signs immediately and to intervene appropriately.

There are several anatomical and physiological differences in the respiratory system in infants and younger children as they develop. These differences may explain the higher incidence of respiratory failure in the younger age group. The upper airway is funnel shaped, with its narrowest portion at the subglottic area. This is a likely site for obstruction as in the case of croup. The infant's thoracic cage is soft, with the ribs more horizontally positioned, resulting in a disadvantage for chest expansion. Another disadvantage is the infant's diaphragm, which is more flattened. In addition, the younger child's diaphragm has a higher percentage of type

II respiratory muscle fibers (responsible for bursts of motor activity) than type I fibers (responsible for sustained muscle activity), making the diaphragm easier to fatigue. The nervous system of the infant is immature and, thus, more prone to apnea. Finally, the infant's lower airways are smaller and more prone to significant airway obstruction during illness as in the case of bronchiolitis.

Respiratory failure occurs when the respiratory system cannot sustain adequate gas exchange, particularly oxygen and carbon dioxide. A partial pressure of oxygen (paO_2) is decreased below 60 mmHg (hypoxemia), or a partial pressure of carbon dioxide ($paCO_2$) above 50 mmHg (hypercarbia) with blood pH below 7.35 is frequently used to define respiratory failure (Pope & McBride, 2004). Even with significant impairment in gas exchange, children may be clinically stable until rapid deterioration happens.

Respiratory failure can be "acute" or "chronic." Acute respiratory failure presents with rapid onset (i.e., minutes to hours), such as in toxic inhalation, whereas chronic respiratory failure presents with an insidious onset (i.e., weeks to months), such as in muscular dystrophy. Some patients may have an acute-on-chronic respiratory failure. High-risk children with chronic respiratory insufficiency (as seen in neuromuscular disease) may have acute deterioration during an intercurrent respiratory infection.

Epidemiology

Respiratory failure can be caused by abnormalities of one or any combination of the following three main categories:

(1)   Central nervous system (respiratory drive)
(2)   Chest wall and respiratory muscles (respiratory pump)
(3)   Lungs (gas exchange)

The representative causes of respiratory failure in children categorized into the three main areas are shown in Table 11.1.

The incidence of respiratory failure is higher in younger children. Two-thirds of the cases in children occur in the first postnatal year, and one-half is seen in the neonatal period (Nitu & Eigen, 2009).

Pathophysiology

Respiratory failure occurs when there is derangement in oxygenation and/or ventilation. In respiratory failure, the paO_2 is decreased (hypoxemia) and/or the $paCO_2$ is increased (hypercarbia).

For oxygen to be used by the tissues, it needs to enter the alveoli from the atmosphere. Oxygen binds to hemoglobin and is transported to the tissues for use by the cells. When the overall process of oxygen delivery is impaired, hypoxia occurs. It may involve the whole body (generalized

Table 11.1   Representative causes of respiratory failure in children categorized in three main areas.

Disorders of the central nervous system (respiratory drive)
   Head trauma
   Toxic ingestion
   Congenital hypoventilation syndrome
   Apnea of prematurity
Disorders of the chest wall and respiratory muscles (respiratory pump)
   Neuromuscular disease (myopathies/muscular dystrophies)
   Spinal cord injury
   Respiratory muscle fatigue during an acute respiratory infection in a previously healthy infant
Disorders of the lungs (gas exchange)
   Asthma
   Bronchiolitis
   Pneumonia

hypoxia) or a region of the body (tissue hypoxia). Hypoxia differs from hypoxemia. Hypoxemia refers to a low paO_2 within the arterial blood. It is possible to experience hypoxia (e.g., due to anemia) yet maintain high paO_2 in the blood.

The most frequent cause of hypoxemia is an imbalance of ventilation (V) and perfusion (Q) or V/Q mismatch. Ventilation refers to the air that reaches the lungs, while perfusion refers to the blood that reaches the lungs. The V/Q ratio is a measure of the efficiency and adequacy of the matching between these two variables. The ideal ratio is approximately 1.0. Shunt and dead space ventilation are the extreme forms of V/Q mismatch. If there is no ventilation but blood continues to perfuse the lungs, a shunt exists. If there is no blood flow but air continues to ventilate the lungs, dead space ventilation exists. A shunt leads to hypoxemia, while dead space ventilation leads to hypercarbia in the absence of compensation. Shunts may be intrapulmonary such as in areas of atelectasis where blood continues to perfuse the collapsed lung areas. Shunts may also be intracardiac as in tetralogy of Fallot, where blood from the right ventricle bypasses the lungs through the ventricular septal defect. An example of dead space ventilation is in areas of pulmonary embolus. Blood does not flow in the obstructed segments of the pulmonary artery, while air continues to ventilate the lung units.

Hypoxia can be classified as anoxic, anemic, stagnant, and cytochemical based on the oxygen delivery process. Anoxic hypoxia occurs when the inhaled air has a low oxygen content, as in ascending to high altitude or diving underwater while breathing into a closed-circuit rebreather system. Anoxic hypoxia can also occur when the absolute amount of oxygen in the blood is decreased despite adequate oxygen from the air. This happens in shunts.

Anemic hypoxia occurs when there is a problem with the hemoglobin that is used to transport oxygen from the lungs to the peripheral tissues. Examples include anemia (low hemoglobin) and hemoglobinopathies (e.g., sickle cell disease). The amount of oxygen in the blood may be sufficient and the hemoglobin carrying the oxygen is appropriate; however, if blood is not flowing, oxygen cannot be transported to the peripheral tissues. This occurs with stagnant hypoxia, such as with heart failure or septic shock. Lastly, if the cells cannot utilize oxygen, cytochemical hypoxia occurs. Cyanide poisoning is an important example of cytochemical hypoxia.

Ventilation, which mainly affects carbon dioxide removal, is determined by the alveolar minute ventilation. Minute ventilation is the product of respiratory rate and tidal volume, while tidal volume is divided between the air that goes through the conducting airways and air that reaches the alveoli. Since no gas exchange occurs in the conducting airways, only alveolar tidal volume affects carbon dioxide elimination. Ventilatory failure occurs in conditions that decrease respiratory rate (bradypnea) or alveolar tidal volume (shallow breathing). Increases in dead space ventilation by limiting effective alveolar minute ventilation also lead to hypercarbia.

Signs and symptoms

Early identification of impending respiratory failure is crucial in achieving good outcomes. Signs of increased work of breathing or respiratory distress include stridor, wheeze, tachypnea, or hyperpnea, use of accessory muscles, and/or retractions. Children with neuromuscular disease or breathing impairment from a central neurological cause may not manifest increased work of breathing and yet be in respiratory failure. A change in respiratory pattern from the child's baseline is an indication for assessment and intervention as appropriate.

History

A detailed history should only be obtained once the child's respiratory status is stabilized. Helpful historical information includes history of trauma; onset and duration of symptoms such as gagging or choking; change in voice, which usually signifies upper airway involvement; associated symptoms such as fever, which may suggest an infectious etiology; exposures to possible toxins, medications, or allergens; prior episodes such as asthma; and underlying medical condition or chronic illness.

Physical exam

Physical examination of the respiratory system starts with an assessment of the child's sensorium. Prolonged, undetected respiratory failure presents with decreased sensorium due to carbon dioxide narcosis and/or cerebral hypoxia. A child who was previously working hard to breathe but is now quiet and minimally responsive is at high risk for cardiopulmonary arrest. This should be recognized on initial contact with the child.

An orderly examination of the respiratory system may follow once the child is deemed stable. Assess the child's work of breathing. Increased work of breathing includes nasal flaring, intercostal and substernal retractions, and head bobbing. Inspection of the chest wall includes the shape of the thoracic cage and movement (asymmetric chest rise may indicate a unilateral process such as pneumothorax). Auscultate the chest for breath sounds including quality and symmetry of air entry and adventitious breath sounds such as stridor, wheezes, or crackles. Asymmetric breath sounds should raise the suspicion of an FBA or airway obstruction as with mucus plugging or mass. Stridor is usually an inspiratory sound suggesting narrowing of the upper airway as with croup. Wheezing is typically an expiratory sound suggesting intrathoracic airway obstruction as with asthma and bronchiolitis. Crackles indicate an alveolar process such as pneumonia or pulmonary edema.

Heart examination for abnormal heart sounds, abnormal rhythm, or presence of murmurs may indicate a possible heart disease as the cause of the respiratory problem. Also, assess the child's perfusion as a measure of cardiac function. Monitor the caliber of the pulse and the capillary refill time (Baraff, 1993).

In addition to the sensorium, neurological examination may reveal conditions that may lead to chronic respiratory failure. Muscle strength is decreased in myopathies such as in Duchenne muscular dystrophy. Delayed or loss of motor milestones may be the first clue to a hereditary myopathy.

Diagnosis

Pulse oximeter

Pulse oximetry is a convenient tool used for respiratory monitoring. It is a noninvasive method that indirectly measures oxygen saturation. Direct measurement is done through arterial blood gas. Pulse oximetry allows for continuous monitoring through light absorption of oxyhemoglobin to estimate oxygen saturation of hemoglobin. An oxygen saturation of 90% is approximately a paO_2 of 60 mmHg based on the sigmoid shape of the oxyhemoglobin dissociation curve.

Pulse oximetry is helpful, but one should be careful not to rely solely on the pulse oximeter readings. Pulse oximetry has several limitations. Oxygen saturation does not necessarily reflect oxygen content or oxygen delivery. A child with anemia may have normal saturation by pulse oximetry, but O_2 delivery is impaired and could lead to tissue hypoxia. Oxygen saturation may also be artificially increased when carboxyhemoglobin concentrations are high, as with smoke inhalation and carbon monoxide poisoning. Conversely, it may be decreased artificially in the presence of intravenous dyes. Presence of methemoglobin in the blood will also alter (may decrease or increase) the measured oxygen saturation. As pulse oximetry relies on light absorption, signal detection is poor for children with decreased peripheral perfusion, as with hypovolemia or hypothermia. A reliable pulse oximetry reading does not fluctuate, and the recorded pulse rate on the oximeter should match the child's heart rate.

Oxygen saturation should never be used as a sole measure of respiratory status. The child may be maintaining a high oxygen saturation at the expense of tachypnea and hyperventilation or the oxygen saturation may be maintained because of supplemental oxygen. Respiratory failure may still ensue because of carbon dioxide retention. End tidal monitors are available for the spontaneously breathing child. They provide an estimate of the child's pCO_2. Transcutaneous CO_2 monitors are also being developed to provide a noninvasive method of measuring CO_2 in the blood.

Cyanosis is an ominous sign, as this occurs late in the course of respiratory failure. Cyanosis may not be evident in children with anemia until much lower levels of paO_2 because cyanosis is related to the absolute amount of reduced hemoglobin.

Heart rate monitoring is also helpful in assessing the respiratory status as this reflects the work of breathing. Tachycardia, like tachypnea, is a compensatory mechanism for maintaining adequate oxygen delivery. Eventually, bradycardia ensues because of severe hypoxemia. Similar to bradypnea, bradycardia is a sign of impending cardiopulmonary arrest.

Blood pressure usually is high in an agitated child. Low blood pressure is an ominous sign suggesting poor perfusion, and is an indication for prompt hemodynamic and respiratory intervention.

Laboratory and radiological evaluation

Laboratory and radiographic evaluations are important tools for monitoring respiratory status and for assessing the child's response to intervention. However, aggressive intervention should not be delayed pending laboratory and radiological evaluation. A rapid clinical assessment should be enough to make immediate clinical decisions regarding respiratory management.

Arterial blood gas assesses the current oxygen and carbon dioxide tensions and acid–base status. Blood gas results require careful interpretation and should always be correlated with the child's clinical status. Normal paO_2 or normal $paCO_2$ per se is not reassuring. Normal or even high paO_2 may be due to a high FiO_2 requirement in a patient in impending respiratory failure. Normal or even low $paCO_2$ may be due to severe tachypnea (thereby "blowing off" carbon dioxide), in a patient with impending respiratory failure.

In acute respiratory failure, the arterial pH falls because the serum bicarbonate concentration only rises slightly, as there is not enough time for metabolic (renal) compensation. As the paCO$_2$ continues to remain elevated, the kidneys eventually conserve bicarbonate. The serum bicarbonate concentration increases, and the arterial pH returns toward normal. Metabolic (renal) compensation usually begins within 24 hours of respiratory failure onset.

In children with suspected chronic respiratory failure, a complete blood count may show polycythemia. Hemoglobin increases as the body attempts to improve oxygen content. Serum bicarbonate levels are also elevated in children with chronic respiratory failure.

Complications

Children with acute respiratory distress can develop severe hypoxemia and hypercarbia, leading to respiratory arrest. Respiratory failure is the most common cause of cardiopulmonary arrest in children. Early recognition and aggressive intervention is necessary to prevent this outcome (Donoghue et al., 2005; Nadkarni et al., 2006).

Management

It cannot be overemphasized that respiratory failure should be identified as soon as possible. Inability to recognize and to intervene promptly can lead to devastating cardiopulmonary arrest.

Initial management for respiratory failure revolves around basic life support guidelines. The management should proceed in an orderly manner beginning with the airway, breathing, and then circulation.

In children who are relatively stable, the pathophysiological cause of the respiratory failure should be identified as much as possible. For example, children who are hypoxemic due to hypoventilation should be treated for hypoventilation and should not be simply placed on supplemental oxygen. If supplemental oxygen is needed, it can be delivered in different ways depending on the child's requirement. Oxygen can be delivered by nasal cannula, high flow nasal cannula, face mask, or non-rebreather mask. Only low-flow oxygen can be delivered by nasal cannula. Prolonged use of nasal cannula can cause nasal mucosa dryness and irritation.

Some patients could benefit from noninvasive ventilation such as continuous positive airway pressure (CPAP) or bilevel positive airway pressure (BiPAP). In these modes, positive pressure is delivered through a tight-fitting face mask or nasal prongs. Children should have a good respiratory drive when on noninvasive ventilation. The goal is to decrease the child's work of breathing by assisting their ventilation and to support the child's respiratory muscles. Children should be closely monitored as they may continue to worsen and require invasive ventilation.

CPAP provides a single level of airway pressure, whereas BiPAP provides two levels of pressure: an inspiratory positive airway pressure and an expiratory positive airway pressure. The choice between CPAP and BiPAP is determined by the amount of respiratory support the child requires. BiPAP provides a higher level of support than CPAP. BiPAP is often utilized for chronic respiratory failure in an attempt to avoid tracheostomy and mechanical ventilation. The use of CPAP and BiPAP may be limited due to the development of pressure ulcers.

In children who progress to respiratory failure, tracheal intubation and mechanical ventilation may be necessary. A quality team with an identified leader and good communication is the key to a successful intubation. Proper positioning of the airway, with the neck slightly hyperextended, will ensure a patent airway. Bag–mask ventilation with 100% oxygen should be initiated while preparing to intubate the trachea. The appropriate size of the endotracheal tube can be estimated based on the child's age. Endotracheal tubes bigger and smaller than the predicted size should also be readily available. Sedation and neuromuscular blockade are oftentimes used for intubation.

Difficult intubation should be anticipated so that an alternative device or procedure could be considered to support the airway. Laryngeal mask airway (LMA) is an alternative device. It is essentially an endotracheal tube with an inflatable mask at the end. It is inserted blindly into the upper airway through the patient's mouth. The mask forms a seal around the laryngeal area, and positive pressure ventilation can be initiated until definitive intubation can be arranged. There is a risk of aspiration of stomach contents with LMA use. Intubation using fiber-optic scopes is also helpful for accessing anatomically difficult airways.

There are different types and brands of mechanical ventilators. Newer generations of mechanical ventilators are more compact, lighter, and convenient for transport and mobility. There are also numerous modes of conventional ventilation, some of which are discussed next. In cases of severe respiratory failure, other modalities may be used.

The assist control (AC) mode provides a full mechanical breath (preset tidal volume or peak pressure) with each spontaneous breath. The synchronized intermittent mechanical ventilation (SIMV) mode provides a mechanical breath every set number of seconds. The breath is provided in synchrony with the child's own spontaneous breath. If the child does not take a breath within a certain amount of time, the ventilator provides a mandatory breath. The SIMV mode can be used with pressure support (PS). SIMV-PS gives a combination of full mechanical breaths every set number of seconds plus partially supported patient-initiated spontaneous breaths; thus, some work is done by the ventilator and some by the child.

High-frequency ventilation (HFV) is the delivery of smaller tidal volumes with a rate greater than 150 breaths/min to minimize the complications of barotrauma (high pressure changes) and volutrauma (high tidal volume ventilation). HFV should be considered in children who require high supplemental oxygen and high airway pressure (>35 mmHg) (Arnold, 2000).

The instillation of a surfactant can improve the outcome of respiratory distress syndrome especially in preterm infants (Lotze et al., 1998). A surfactant for the treatment of acute respiratory distress syndrome (ARDS) in the older pediatric age group has also been used and is now being studied systematically. In addition, inhaled nitric oxide has been administered to patients with pulmonary hypertension (Neonatal Inhaled Nitric Oxide Study Group, 1997). Nitric oxide may improve oxygenation by relaxing the pulmonary vasculature.

The general indication for extracorporeal membrane oxygenation (ECMO) is a reversible underlying illness for children with respiratory failure who have failed conventional ventilator strategies. ECMO allows the lungs to "rest" and not be subjected to the additional lung injury caused by high-pressure ventilation. It provides gas exchange through an extracorporeal system. Survival is determined primarily by the underlying illness. Meconium aspiration syndrome requiring ECMO carries the best prognosis, with a survival rate of 94% compared to older children undergoing ECMO for viral pneumonia with a survival rate of 64% (Radhakrishnan, Lally, Lally, & Cox, 2007).

Nursing care of the child and family

Nursing care of the child with impaired gas exchange whereby the respiratory system cannot meet the body's metabolic demands is a medical emergency (Burg, 2006). The nurse must identify the signs and symptoms of impending acute respiratory failure quickly and must communicate this assessment to the medical team in order for it to be managed effectively. Early identification and management of impending respiratory failure, acute respiratory failure, or acute-on-chronic respiratory failure promotes the safety and well-being of the child.

Early signs and symptoms of respiratory failure include rapid, shallow breathing, nasal flaring, grunting, retractions, increased work of breathing, use of accessory muscles, and chest pain. The increased work of breathing may lead to muscle fatigue and acute respiratory failure. Other less specific signs of respiratory failure are mood changes, headache, anxiety, mental confusion, restlessness, irritability, and depressed level of consciousness (Wilson & Thompson, 1990). An ominous sign is when a child does not recognize or respond to his parents or to a noxious stimulus such as pain.

Continuous cardiorespiratory and pulse oximetry monitoring must be instituted if the child is experiencing increased work of breathing or impending respiratory failure. End tidal CO_2 should also be employed if available. The nurse must maintain the airway, breathing, and circulation (ABC) of basic life support at all times. Supplemental oxygen, suction, airway equipment, and a means of ventilating the child with an Ambu bag–mask assembly should be readily available at the bedside.

The bedside nurse should also be constantly monitoring the child's vital signs and clinical symptoms while awaiting transfer to an intensive care unit or immediate medical intervention.

If the child has an endotracheal tube in place, the nurse must ensure that the tube remain patent. The child should be suctioned via the endotracheal tube as needed. Some institutions use in-line suction catheters. The nurse must also ensure that the tube remain secure. Each institution has its own policy for how the endotracheal tube should be secured and how often the tapes should be changed.

The child with impaired gas exchange and his/her family are often frightened. The family and child require a clear, concise, and developmentally appropriate explanation of the situation including the urgency of medical interventions. Parents should be allowed to stay with their child even in the most serious situations such as intubation. Allowing the child the comfort of their parents' presence may decrease the child's anxiety and work of breathing.

Care for the child with respiratory failure requires a team approach. Working together, the physician or advanced practice nurse, the bedside nurse, the respiratory therapist, and the social worker can ensure the best outcome for the child who needs intubation to manage respiratory failure.

ACKNOWLEDGMENTS

The authors would like to thank Dr. Jeffrey Hellinger, Children's Hospital of Philadelphia, for the images he provided, and Natalie DiFeo, RRT, CRNP, and Laura Miske, MSN, CNS, for sharing their expertise in the nursing care of children with acute respiratory problems.

REFERENCES

Abolnik, I., Lossos, I., Zlotogora, J., & Brauer, R. (1991). On the inheritance of primary spontaneous pneumothorax. *American Journal of Medical Genetics, 40*(2), 155–158.

Al Tawil, K., Abu-Ekteish, F. M., Tamimi, O., Al Hathal, M. M., Al Hathlol, K., & Laimun, B. A. (2004). Symptomatic spontaneous pneumothorax in term newborn infants. *Pediatric Pulmonology, 37*(5), 443–446.

Arnold, J. H. (2000). High frequency ventilation in the pediatric intensive care unit. *Pediatric Critical Care Medicine, 1*, 93–99.

Baraff, L. J. (1993). Capillary refill: Is it a useful clinical sign? *Pediatrics, 92*(5), 723–724.

Black, R. E., Johnson, D. G., & Matlak, M. E. (1994). Bronchoscopic removal of aspirated foreign bodies in children. *Journal of Pediatric Surgery, 29*(5), 682–684.

Blazer, S., Naveh, Y., & Friedman, A. (1980). Foreign body in the airway. A review of 200 cases. *American Journal of Diseases of Children, 134*(1), 68–71.

Burg, F., Inglefinger, J., Polin, R., & Gerson, A. (2006). *Current pediatric therapy* (18th ed.). Ames, IA; Philadelphia: Saunders Elsevier.

Camuset, J., Laganier, J., Brugière, O., Dauriat, G., Jebrak, G., Thabut, G., Mal, H. (2006). Needle aspiration as first-line management of primary spontaneous pneumothorax. *Presse Médicale, 35*(5, Pt 1), 765–768.

Cardillo, G., Carleo, F., Giunti, R., Carbone, L., Mariotta, S., Salvadori, L., Martelli, M. (2006). Videothoracoscopic talc poudrage in primary spontaneous pneumothorax: A single-institution experience in 861 cases. *The Journal of Thoracic and Cardiovascular Surgery, 131*(2), 322–328.

Casadio, C., Rena, O., Giobbe, R., Rigoni, R., Maggi, G., & Oliaro, A. (2002). Stapler blebectomy and pleural abrasion by video-assisted thoracoscopy for spontaneous pneumothorax. *The Journal of Cardiovascular Surgery, 43*(2), 259–262.

Chan, P., Clarke, P., Daniel, F. J., Knight, S. R., & Seevanayagam, S. (2001). Efficacy study of video-assisted thoracoscopic surgery pleurodesis for spontaneous pneumothorax. *The Annals of Thoracic Surgery, 71*(2), 452–454.

Chen, J., Hsu, H., Chen, R., Kuo, S., Huang, P., Tsai, P., Lee, Y. (2006). Additional minocycline pleurodesis after thoracoscopic surgery for primary spontaneous pneumothorax. *American Journal of Respiratory and Critical Care Medicine, 173*(5), 548–554.

Chernick, V., Boat, T., Wilmott, R., & Bush, A. (2006). *Kendig's disorders of the respiratory tract in children* (7th ed.). Ames, IA; Philadelphia: Saunders Elsevier.

Choudhary, A. K., Sellar, M. E., Wallis, C., Cohen, G., & McHugh, K. (2005). Primary spontaneous pneumothorax in children: The role of CT in guiding management. *Clinical Radiology, 60*(4), 508–511.

Ciftci, A. O., Bingol-Kologlu, M., Senocak, M. E., Tanyel, F. C., & Buyukpakcu, N. (2003). Bronchoscopy for evaluation of foreign body aspiration in children. *Journal of Pediatric Surgery, 38*(8), 1170–1176.

Davis, A. M., Wensley, D. F., & Phelan, P. D. (1993). Spontaneous pneumothorax in paediatric patients. *Respiratory Medicine, 87*(7), 531–534.

Donoghue, A. J., Nadkarni, V., Berg, R. A., et al. (2005). Out-of-hospital pediatric cardiac arrest: An epidemiologic review and assessment of current knowledge. *Annals of Emergency Medicine, 46*(6), 512–522.

Eren, S., Balci, A. E., Dikici, B., Doblan, M., & Eren, M. N. (2003). Foreign body aspiration in children: Experience of 1160 cases. *Annals of Tropical Paediatrics, 23*(1), 31–37.

Even, L., Heno, N., Talmon, Y., Samet, E., Zonis, Z., & Kugelman, A. (2005). Diagnostic evaluation of foreign body aspiration in children: A prospective study. *Journal Pediatric Surgery, 40*(7), 1122–1127.

Feldman, A., Sullivan, J., Passero, M., & Lewis, D. (1993). Pneumothorax in polysubstance abusing marijuana and tobacco smokers: Three cases. *Journal of Substance Abuse, 5*(2), 183–186.

Gotsch, K., Annest, J. L., & Holmgreen, P. (2002). Nonfatal choking-related episodes among children—United States, 2001. *MMWR. Morbidity and Mortality Weekly Report, 51*, 945.

Halm, M. A. (2007). To strip or not to strip? Physiological effects of chest tube manipulation. *American Journal of Critical Care, 16*(6), 609–612.

Hatz, R. A., Kaps, M. F., Meimarakis, G., Loehe, F., Müller, C., & Fürst, H. (2000). Long-term results after video-assisted thoracoscopic surgery for first-time and recurrent spontaneous pneumothorax. *The Annals of Thoracic Surgery, 70*(1), 253–257.

Holinger, L. (2007). Foreign bodies of the airway. In R. Kliegman (Ed.), *Nelson textbook of pediatrics* (18th ed., pp. 1769–1770). Chap 384. Ames, IA; Philadelphia: Saunders Elsevier.

Horbar, J. D., Badger, G. J., Carpenter, J. H., Fanaroff, A. A., Kilpatrick, S., LaCorte, M., . . . Soll, R. F. (2002). Trends in mortality and morbidity for very low birth weight infants, 1991–1999. *Pediatrics, 110*(1), 143–151.

Jenkinson, S. (1985). Pneumothorax. *Clinics in Chest Medicine, 6,* 153.

Johnson, M. (2004). Catamenial pneumothorax and other thoracic manifestations of endometriosis. *Clinics in Chest Medicine, 25*(2), 311–319.

Joseph, J., & Sahn, S. A. (1996). Thoracic endometriosis syndrome: New observations from an analysis of 110 cases. *The American Journal of Medicine, 100*(2), 164–170.

Kirby, T., & Ginsberg, R. (1992). Management of the pneumothorax and barotrauma. *Clinics in Chest Medicine, 13*(1), 97–112.

Krauss, B. S., Harakal, T., & Fleisher, G. R. (1991). The spectrum and frequency of illness presenting to a pediatric emergency department. *Pediatric Emergency Care, 7*(2), 67–71.

Kuhns, L., Bednarek, F., Wyman, M., Roloff, D., & Borer, R. (1975). Diagnosis of pneumothorax or pneumomediastinum in the neonate by transillumination. *Pediatrics, 56*(3), 355–360.

Lang-Lazdunski, L., de Kerangal, X., Pons, F., & Jancovici, R. (2000). Primary spontaneous pneumothorax: One-stage treatment by bilateral videothoracoscopy. *The Annals of Thoracic Surgery, 70*(2), 412–417.

Leigh-Smith, S., & Harris, T. (2005). Tension pneumothorax—Time for a rethink? *Emergency Medicine Journal, 22*(1), 8–16.

Light, R., O'Hara, V. S., Moritz, T. E., McElhinney, A., Butz, R., Haakenson, C., Berger, R. (1990). Intrapleural tetracycline for the prevention of recurrent spontaneous pneumothorax. *The Journal of the American Medical Association, 264*(17), 2224–2230.

Lima, J. (1989). Laryngeal foreign bodies in children: A persistent, life-threatening problem. *The Laryngoscope, 99*(4), 415–420.

Lotze, A., Mitchell, B. R., Bulas, D. I., et al. (1998). Multicenter study of surfactant (beractant) use in the treatment of term infants with severe respiratory failure. *Journal of Pediatrics, 132,* 40–47.

Luque, M., III, Cavallaro, D., Torres, M., Emmanual, P., & Hillman, J. (1987). Pneumomediastinum, pneumothorax, and subcutaneous emphysema after alternate cocaine inhalation and marijuana smoking. *Pediatric Emergency Care, 3*(2), 107–109.

Menko, F. H., van Steensel, M. A. M., Giraud, S., Friis-Hansen, L., Richard, S., Ungari, S., et al. (2009). Birt-Hogg-Dubé syndrome: Diagnosis and management. *The Lancet Oncology, 10*(12), 1199–1206.

Montgomery, M., & Sigalet, D. (2006). Air and liquid in the pleural space. In V. Chernick, T. Boat, R. Wilmott, & A. Bush et al. (Eds.), *Kendig's disorders of the respiratory tract in children* (7th ed., pp. 368–387). Philadelphia: Saunders.

Morrison, P., Lowry, R., & Nevin, N. (1998). Familial primary spontaneous pneumothoraxconsistent with true autosomal dominant inheritance. *Thorax, 53*(2), 151–152.

Nadkarni, V. M., Larkin, G. L., Peberdy, M. A., Carey, S. M., Kaye, W., Mancini, M. E., for the National Registry of Cardiopulmonary Resuscitation Investigators (2006). First documented rhythm and clinical outcome from in-hospital cardiac arrest among children and adults. *Journal of the American Medical Association, 295*(1), 50–57.

National Center for Injury Prevention and Control (2010). WISQARS leading causes of death reports. CDC. Retrieved from http://www.cdc.gov/injury/wisqars/fatal.html (accessed July 3, 2010).

Nazari, S, Buniva, P, Aluffi, A, & Salvi, S (2000). Bilateral open treatment of spontaneous pneumothorax: A new access. *European Journal of Cardio-Thoracic Surgery: Official Journal Of The European Association For Cardio-Thoracic Surgery, 18*(5), 608–610.

Neonatal Inhaled Nitric Oxide Study Group (1997). Inhaled nitric oxide in full-term and nearly full-term infants with hypoxic respiratory failure. *New England Journal of Medicine, 336*(9), 597–604.

Nitu, ME, & Eigen, H (2009). Respiratory failure. *Pediatrics in Review, 30,* 470–478.

Ozcan, C., McGahren, E. D., & Rodgers, B. (2003). Thoracoscopic treatment of spontaneous pneumothorax in children. *Journal of Pediatric Surgery, 38*(10), 1459–1464.

Paape, K., & Fry, W. (1994). Spontaneous pneumothorax. *Chest Surgery Clinics of North America, 4*(3), 517–538.

Poenaru, D., Yazbeck, S., & Murphy, S. (1994). Primary spontaneous pneumothorax in children. *Journal of Pediatric Surgery, 29*(9), 1183–1185.

Pope, J., & McBride, J. (2004). Consultation with the specialist: Respiratory failure in children. *Pediatrics in Review, 25,* 160–167.

Radhakrishnan, R. S., Lally, P. A., Lally, K. P., & Cox, C. S., Jr. (2007). ECMO for meconium aspiration syndrome: Support for relaxed entry criteria. *American Society of Artificial Internal Organs Journal, 53,* 489–491.

Robinson, P., Cooper, P., & Ranganathan, S. (2009). Evidence-based management of paediatric primary spontaneous pneumothorax. *Paediatric Respiratory Reviews, 10*(3), 110–117.

Sahn, S., & Heffner, J. (2000). Spontaneous pneumothorax. *The New England Journal of Medicine, 342*(12), 868–874.

Tan, H. K., Brown, K., McGill, T., Kenna, M. A., Lund, D. P., & Healy, G. B. (2000). Airway foreign bodies (FB): A 10-year review. *International Journal of Pediatric Otorhinolaryngology, 56*(2), 91–99.

Verger, J., & Lebet, R. (2008). *American association of critical care nurses procedure manual for pediatric acute and critical care.* Ames, IA; St. Louis, MO: Saunders Elsevier.

Weissberg, D., & Refaely, Y. (2000). Pneumothorax: Experience with 1,199 patients. *Chest, 117*(5), 1279–1285.

West, J. (2007). *Pulmonary pathophysiology: The essentials* (7th ed.). Ames, IA: Lippincott Williams and Wilkins.

Wilcox, D., Glick, P., Karamanoukian, H., Allen, J., & Azizkhan, R. (1995). Spontaneous pneumothorax: A single-institution, 12-year experience in patients under16 years of age. *Journal of Pediatric Surgery, 30*(10), 1452–1454.

Wilson, S., & Thompson, J. (1990). *Mosby's clinical nursing series respiratory disorders* (2nd ed.). Ames, IA: Mosby Year Book.

Wiswell, T., & Henley, M. (1992). Intratracheal suctioning, systemic infection, and the meconium aspiration syndrome. *Pediatrics, 89*(2), 203–206.

Wiswell, T., Tuggle, J., & Turner, B. (1990). Meconium aspiration syndrome: Have we made a difference? *Pediatrics, 85*(5), 715–721.

Yamamoto, H., Okada, M., Kanehira, A., Tachibana, S., Saito, H., Maniwa, Y., et al. (2000). Video-assisted blebectomy using a flexible scope and a bleb implement. *Surgery Today, 30*(3), 241–243.

Index

Page numbers in *italics* denote figures; those in **bold**, tables.

Nursing Care in Pediatric Respiratory Disease, First Edition. Edited by Concettina (Tina) Tolomeo.
© 2012 John Wiley & Sons, Inc. Published 2012 by John Wiley & Sons, Inc.